AF556702

Molecular Approaches to Immunology

MIAMI WINTER SYMPOSIA

---

1. *W. J. Whelan and J. Schultz, editors:* HOMOLOGIES in ENZYMES AND METABOLIC PATHWAYS *and* METABOLIC ALTERATIONS IN CANCER,* 1970

2. *D. W. Ribbons, J. F. Woessner, Jr., and J. Schultz, editors:* NUCLEIC ACID-PROTEIN INTERACTIONS *and* NUCLEIC ACID SYNTHESIS IN VIRAL INFECTION,* 1971

3. *J. F. Woessner, Jr. and F. Huijing, editors:* THE MOLECULAR BASIS OF BIOLOGICAL TRANSPORT, 1972

4. *J. Schultz and B. F. Cameron, editors:* THE MOLECULAR BASIS OF ELECTRON TRANSPORT, 1972

5. *F. Huijing and E. Y. C. Lee, editors:* PROTEIN PHOSPHORYLATION IN CONTROL MECHANISMS, 1973

6. *J. Schultz and H. G. Gratzner, editors:* THE ROLE OF CYCLIC NUCLEOTIDES IN CARCINOGENESIS, 1973

7. *E. Y. C. Lee and E. E. Smith, editors:* BIOLOGY AND CHEMISTRY OF EUCARYOTIC CELL SURFACES, 1974

8. *J. Schultz and R. Block, editors:* MEMBRANE TRANSFORMATION IN NEOPLASIA, 1974

9. *E. E. Smith and D. W. Ribbons, editors:* MOLECULAR APPROACHES TO IMMUNOLOGY, 1975

10. *J. Schultz and R. C. Leif, editors:* CRITICAL FACTORS IN CANCER IMMUNOLOGY, 1975

MIAMI WINTER SYMPOSIA - VOLUME 9

Molecular Approaches to Immunology

edited by

E. E. Smith

D. W. Ribbons

DEPARTMENT OF BIOCHEMISTRY
UNIVERSITY OF MIAMI
MIAMI, FLORIDA

Proceedings of the Miami Winter Symposia, January 13 - 17, 1975 sponsored by the Department of Biochemistry, University of Miami Miami, Florida

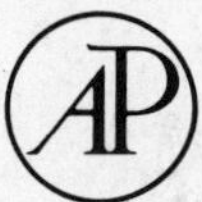

ACADEMIC PRESS, INC. New York San Francisco London 1975
A Subsidiary of Harcourt Brace Jovanovich, Publishers

ACADEMIC PRESS, INC.
111 Fifth Avenue, New York, New York 10003

United Kingdom Edition published by
ACADEMIC PRESS, INC. (LONDON) LTD.
24/28 Oval Road, London NW1

Library of Congress Cataloging in Publication Data
Main entry under title:

Molecular approaches to immunology.

(Miami winter symposia; 9)
Bibliography: p:
1. Immunology–Congresses. I. Smith, Eric Ernest, (date) II. Ribbons, Douglas W. III. Miami, University of, Coral Gables, Fla. Dept. of Biochemistry. IV. Series.
QR180.3.M64 574.2'9 74-27794
ISBN 0-12-651050-4

PRINTED IN THE UNITED STATES OF AMERICA

CONTENTS

CONTENTS

SPEAKERS, CHAIRMEN, AND DISCUSSANTS

Bell, C., University of Illinois Medical Center, Chicago, Illinois

Briles, E., Washington University School of Medicine, St. Louis, Missouri

Chang, C. H., Tufts Cancer Research Center, Boston, Massachusetts

Citronbaum, R., University of Southern California, Los Angeles, California

Claman, H. N., University of Colorado Medical Center, Denver, Colorado

Cohen, G., University of Texas Medical Branch, Galveston, Texas

Cohn, M., The Salk Institute for Biological Studies, San Diego, California

Cunningham, B. A., Rockefeller University, New York, New York

Edelman, G. M., (Session Chairman) The Rockefeller University, New York, New York

Fudenberg, H. H., University of California, School of Medicine, San Francisco, California

Gershon, R. K., Yale University of Texas Medical Branch, Galveston, Texas

Grant, N., Wyeth Laboratories, Philadelphia, Pennsylvania

Greer, S. B., University of Miami School of Medicine, Miami, Florida

Haber, E., Harvard Medical School, Boston, Massachusetts

Haurowitz, F., Indiana University, Bloomington, Indiana

Heiniger, H., Jackson Laboratory, Bar Harbor, Maine

Herzenberg, L. A., Stanford University, Stanford, California

Holley, R. W., The Salk Institute for Biological Studies, San Diego, California

Kabat, E. A., (Session Chairman) Columbia University College of Physicians and Surgeons, New York, New York

Katz, D. H., Harvard Medical School, Boston, Massachusetts

Koch, G., Roche Institute of Molecular Biology, Nutley, New Jersey

Kondracki, E., Department of Microbiology, Buffalo, New York

Kramer, G., University of Texas, Austin, Texas

Lamon, E. W., University of Alabama, Dept. of Surgery, Birmingham, Alabama

Leder, P., National Institute of Health, Bethesda, Maryland

Leif, R. C., Papanicolaou Cancer Research Institute, Miami, Florida

Levine, B. B., New York University School of Medicine, New York, New York

Longton, R. W., Naval Medical Research Institute, National Naval Medical Center, Bethesda, Maryland

Milstein, C., MRC Laboratory of Molecular Biology, Cambridge, England

Poulik, M. D., William Beamont Hospital, Royal Oak, Michigan

Putnam, F. W., (Session Chairman) Indiana University, Bloomington, Indiana

Quintans, J., Basel Institute for Immunology, Basel, Switzerland

Raam, S., Tufts Cancer Research Center, Boston, Massachusetts

Roelants, G. E., Basel Institute for Immunology, Basel, Switzerland

Scharff, M. D., (Session Chairman) Albert Einstein College of Medicine, New York, New York

Schienkeim, I., New York University School of Medicine, New York, New York

Schulman, R., Bell Laboratories, New Jersey

Sigel, M. M., (Session Chairman) University of Miami, Miami, Florida

Stanford, H. K., (Session Chairman) President, University of Miami, Coral Gables, Florida

Taylor, S., Northwestern University, Evanston, Illinois

Teodorescu, M., University of Illinois, Urbana, Illinois

Thilly, W., Massachusetts Institute of Technology, Cambridge, Massachusetts

White, A., Syntex Research, Palo Alto, and Stanford University, Stanford, California

Whitten, H., University of Alabama, Birmingham, Alabama

Williamson, A. R., University of Glasgow, Glasgow, Scotland

Wu, T., Northwestern University, Evanston, Illinois

PREFACE

This volume is the ninth of a continuing series published under the title: "Miami Winter Symposia." In January 1969, the Department of Biochemistry of the University of Miami and the University-affiliated Papanicolaou Cancer Research Institute joined in sponsoring and presenting two symposia on biochemical topics as an annual event, now in its seventh year. The two symposia were published as a single volume in 1970, the volumes were expanded to include the discussions that followed each presentation in 1971 and, in 1972, we initiated the publication of the proceedings of the two symposia as separate volumes in the series to allow greater flexibility in the choice of future topics for the joint symposia.

The major emphasis in the selection of the topics for our symposia has been to identify the frontier areas in which progress in biochemistry is leading toward an understanding of the molecular bases of biological phenomena. We follow a pattern in which a common theme is dealt with, in our symposium, on a fundamental basis, and then in the Papanicolaou Cancer Research Institute Symposium, as it relates to an understanding of malignant processes. This volume contains the proceedings of the Biochemistry Department's Symposium on "Molecular Approaches to Immunology" and will be published simultaneously with the proceedings of the Papanicolaou Cancer Research Institute's symposium (Volume 10) on "Critical Factors in Cancer Immunology." The word "Enzym" was first introduced by W. Kühne to describe pancreatic trypsin at a scientific meeting held 4 February, 1876. The proceedings of the meeting were published the following year (W. Kühne, 1877, *Verhandl. Naturhist Medic. Ver. Heidelberg,* 1, 194–198). It is, therefore, appropriate that, one hundred years later, the theme of the Miami Winter Symposia taking place during 12–16 January, 1976, should be enzymology; the topic for the first symposium is the role of proteases in biological regulatory mechanisms and this will be followed by a symposium on cancer enzymology.

Associated with the symposia is a featured lecture, the Feodor Lynen Lecture, named in honor of the Department of Biochemistry's distinguished Visiting Professor. Past speakers were George Wald, Arthur Kornberg, Harland G. Wood, Earl W. Sutherland, Jr., and Luis Leloir. This year the Lynen Lecture was delivered by Gerald M. Edelman. These lectures have provided insights of the history of discovery, and personal and scientific philosophies of our distinguished speakers. As such they appeal also to non-scientific members of the audience, and for ourselves and our colleagues in Miami, remain a source of inspiration. The Lynen Lecturer for 1976 will be Professor A. H. T. Theorell.

PREFACE

This volume opens with the Sixth Lynen Lecture and is followed by an introduction, also by Dr. Edelman, in which he provides, for the benefit of those not directly in the field, some indication of the basic assumptions, approaches and directions of modern immunological research. If others find this overview as helpful as did the editors of this volume, then it will have served its purpose admirably. To bring forward as much of the recent work as possible a session of short communications is included in these meetings. This year, these were presented in a joint poster session for the two symposia. This session proved so successful that we propose to continue with this arrangement in future years. Abstracts of the short communications have been assigned, whenever possible, according to their relevance to each symposium, but in a number of cases an arbitrary decision has been made. Thus, sixteen abstracts appear in this volume and the remainder are published in Volume 10 of the series.

Our arrangement with the publishers is to achieve rapid publication of these symposia and we thank the speakers for their prompt submission of manuscripts and the secretarial staff for their unstinting efforts which enabled us to bring this about. Our thanks also go to the participants whose interest and discussions provided the interactions that bring a symposium to life and to the many local helpers, faculty and administrative staff who have contributed to the success of the present symposium. Our special gratitude goes to the organizers and coordinators of the program: W. J. Whelan, K. Brew, Sandra Black and Olga F. Lopez, and to our two consultants Drs. Gerald M. Edelman and Matthew Scharff for their advice and help in organizing the scientific program.

The financial assistance of the University of Miami Departments of Medicine, Pathology and Radiology, the Howard Hughes Medical Institute, Dermatology Foundation of Miami, Abbott Laboratories, Boehringer Mannheim Corporation, Eli Lilly and Company, Hoffman-La Roche Incorporated, MC/B Manufacturing Chemists and the Upjohn Company, is gratefully acknowledged.

THE SIXTH FEODOR LYNEN LECTURE

THE SHOCK OF MOLECULAR RECOGNITION

GERALD M. EDELMAN

The Rockefeller University

> G: "If the world were not this way then it would be that way."
> E: "Yes, but what way is it?"
>
> "I see nobody on the road," said Alice. "I only wish I had such eyes," the King remarked in a fretful tone. "To be able to see Nobody! And at that distance too!"
>
> Through the Looking Glass
> L. Carroll
>
> "Musicology is to music as ornithology is to the birds."
>
> A Player

It is particularly gratifying to be the Lynen Lecturer this year, not only because of the honor it represents, but because it was my good fortune to have been here with Fritz Lynen on the occasion of the first of these meetings. My being here now prompts warm recollections of that occasion and of this fine tradition.

I hope you will forgive me if I do not indulge myself in recounting autobiographical details. Scientific reminiscence has always struck me as an almost impossible genre. It has none of the juicy quality of gossip and, in any case, the accidental elements of a scientist's life have no necessary relation to the order he hopes to bring out of his work. For these reasons, I do not intend to recollect here at any length my own course of scientific development.

Instead, I hope to take this opportunity to comment in a personal mode upon some psychological aspects of discovery and the nature of scientific insight. The method I have chosen is to compare my present recollections of the state of immunological thinking at a given time with my own recorded scientific guesses at that time, and then to comment with hindsight on those guesses, correct and incorrect. This method has obvious limitations, but I hope it will at least stimulate some of your own recollections. I expect that the results of these efforts will be extremely limited and idiosyncratic, and therefore, I do not hope to draw many general conclusions or give lasting general advice based on my restricted experience. But I do hope to provoke some discussion by reaching some admittedly very personal conclusions.

The concern with creation and form has prompted comparison between art and science. I think it is worth comparing the creative _procedures_ of scientists with those of artists, but it seems to me that although they are very much alike in the beginning, they are very different in the end. I hope that the examples I give will make this clear. But, independent of these acts of creation, there are, of course, great personal and aesthetic similarities between science and art in the act of perceiving or grasping an idea of order in either endeavor.

What I wish particularly to convey here is that in the process of creation, a shock occurs that is very much out of the ordinary when, for example, one recognizes the shape of a molecule or the order of events in a metabolic pathway. The shock is a very complex one, consisting of surprise, wonder mixed with some shame at the simplicity of the picture as compared to one's prior thoughts, and a relief, which I suppose comes from the removal of confusion. Then the shock disappears, the discovery becomes commonplace, is accepted as part of the furniture of the world, and one then goes on hopefully to new subjects. This whole process happens to individuals but it is shared and altered by groups. It seems to me to be the central experience in science.

THE PREVAILING PARADIGM: 1958

In his book on scientific revolutions, T.S. Kuhn (1) has promoted the very useful idea that a period in a particular science is characterized by a paradigm, consisting of the communally shared view of that science, a view made up of both rational and unconscious elements. Following Kuhn, let me take you back to the time that I began to work in immunology and attempt to recollect the paradigm concerning antibody formation and the nature of antibodies.

Although Jerne had published his natural selection theory in 1955 (2), I think it is fair to say that most immunologists then believed in the instructive theory of antibody formation. Linus Pauling (3) was the most lucid and recent expositor of this theory and it was only in the late fifties that his views came under fire. As for antibody structure, what was known came mainly from hydrodynamic and electrophoretic analysis. In accord with the convention of the day, the antibody protein was assumed to be an ellipsoid of revolution. The main point that deserves mention, I suppose, is that this prevailing picture of the antibody was a neutral one, i.e. it was not yet crucial for a choice of a particular theory of antibody formation. And, if I remember correctly, no one seemed to feel that it would be crucial.

I did not share this view. Just after my first glimpse of the multichain structure of antibodies and the gel electrophoretic analysis of their chains, I had occasion to present my work at the Kaiser Foundation Symposium in San Francisco. It was my bad fortune to have to speak after Pauling, whose oratorical gifts matched his scientific brilliance. Because I felt that my data were at variance with his theory, I arranged through a mutual friend to have dinner with him. Although we spent a pleasant evening together, he didn't seem much interested in the chain structure of antibodies and the next day, he presented his original and classical theory with great flair and success. Then I followed with my factual contradictions, which were I am sure, not understood by any of the audience except Pauling, who sent me a terse note with no further comments. It said "Edelman - send reprints." I have not spoken with him about this but I suspect he was the only one in the room who began to see that the jig was up. In any case, at the press conference, he did not talk about antibodies but rather about his new theory of anesthesia and he did not publish anything in immunology after that.

LEEWAY - OR THE ADVANTAGES OF PUBLISHING IN THE WRONG JOURNAL

Independent of theoretical matters, there was a distinguished line of studies establishing the protein nature of antibodies (4), their divalence and binding properties (5) and the suggestion of classes (6). But no one except Pauling insisted very strongly that if you knew what an antibody really looked like, you would know a good deal about the important issues of immunology. Most of the emphasis was upon antigen structure, largely because of the enormous influence of Landsteiner's work and because instructive theories made the antigen crucial in antibody formation.

Not one word about shape, sequence or genetics - but this was hardly surprising. Insulin was just being analyzed by Sanger and ribonuclease by Hirs, Stein, and Moore. These molecules were 25 and 10 times smaller than immunoglobulin G. Nevertheless, we should note the early efforts of Pappenheimer, Petermann and Northrop on the cleavage of antibodies by proteases (7). This work had its natural fruition in the justly acclaimed work of Porter (8).

My own conviction was very strong that antibodies were the key to immunology. I distinctly remember the experiment that led eventually to the conclusion that antibodies consisted of multiple polypeptide chains. Perhaps prompted by Deutsch's work on macroglobulins (9) and Sanger's concern with disulfide interchange, I wanted to correlate the number of disulfide bonds with the shape and activity of antibodies. I proceeded by reducing the immunoglobulin, amperometrically titrating the free SH groups, alkylating them, and examining the products in the ultracentrifuge. At low pH, after cleavage of 6 or 8 S-S bonds, I noticed a peak with a sedimentation coefficient of about 2.3S. My colleagues put it off to conformational change, particularly in view of Porter's paper (10) concluding that rabbit Ig had one polypeptide chain. But it seemed too large a fall in the sedimentation coefficient to me and so I began a systematic study.

These studies led me to publish a paper (against advice, for no one believed the results - who would do ultracentrifugation in weird solvents such as urea-water mixtures?) - in the JOURNAL OF THE AMERICAN CHEMICAL SOCIETY (11). This one page note or letter was terse, dense, and to the point. Its beginning occupied one sentence - "Sir: Reaction of human γ-globulin with sulfhydryl compounds, sulfite, or performic acid resulted in marked diminution in the sedimentation coefficient and molecular weight." Its conclusion was equally as brief:"These findings suggest that human γ-globulin contains subunits linked at least in part by disulfide bonds. The possibility that linkages other than disulfide bonds are involved has not been excluded." No one believed it, it was received lackadaisically by an uninterested chemical audience, and in all I received seven reprint requests.

I am convinced now that being ignored in this way was a stroke of great good fortune. I was working alone, and had any one of the larger protein chemistry establishments taken the problem up, they would have moved it ahead much more swiftly than I could have hoped to do. My estimate is that I had three years of leisurely work given to me by the atmosphere and the paradigm. But I didn't feel this way at the time. I was working in the kind of oscillatory state of excitement and confused despair that comes from being against the paradigm.

CONVICTION AND ACCIDENTS OF NATURE

Although it seemed to me that the instructive theory was inadequate, I had not yet become fully convinced by the selective theory in 1960. I was more obsessed with the notion of fractionating the chains of immunoglobulins. This brought about an impasse in my thinking, not because progress had not been made, but because of the heterogeneity of this class of proteins. I had been able to fractionate chain components with different amino acid compositions by chromotography in 6M urea, but I know that they were likely to be microheterogeneous because electrophoresis in urea showed charge heterogeneity.

At this time, it occurred to me that perhaps myeloma proteins would be valuable to study. A mild controversy was then going on as to whether these proteins were "pathological" or were single normal immunoglobulins. Having various fractions in hand, I discussed this question with M.D. Poulik and suggested to him that we try the new procedure of starch gel electrophoresis in urea. We decided to compare a number of samples of multiple myeloma proteins and Waldenström macroglobulins.

My guess was that each of these would show a different and unique band in the faster moving fractions (now known to be the light chains), and I predicted that these bands would cover the range of diffuse protein staining exhibited by the light chains of normal immunoglobulin. We had labored rather hard to accumulate our samples and with some hesitation, loaded the precious small amounts on one last gel to run overnight.

The next morning, I was confronted by a sad Poulik who told me he had dropped the gel upon staining it. I groaned, at which point he lifted out of a pan a gel that showed just the predicted features topped by his very wide grin. We also noticed a difference in the bands corresponding to heavy chains of myeloma proteins and macroglobulins (12).

At this point, in early 1961, I began to glimpse a general unifying picture of the immunoglobulins. I think it is instructive to examine this picture as revealed in the paper (12) reporting our results, for it has the beginnings of the shock of molecular recognition. I say beginnings because of its obviously general nature and lack of precision:

> "A unifying hypothesis may be formulated for the structure of proteins in the γ-globulin family based on the findings presented above as well as on findings of other investigators. 7S γ-globulin molecules appear to consist of several polypeptide chains linked by disulfide bonds. Bivalent antibodies may contain two chains that are similar or identical in structure. The 19S γ-globulins would be composed of 5 or 6 multichain units of the size of 7S γ-globulin. A provisional explanation for the wide molecular weight range of antigenically related globulins from Bence Jones proteins to macroglobulins is suggested by this model. Heterogeneity and differences in isoantigenicity may arise from various combinations of different chains as well as from differences in the sequence of amino acids within each type of chain.
>
> The finding that γ-globulin contains dissociable subunits has a possible bearing upon the pathogenesis of diseases of γ-globulin production. A primary defect in macroglobulinemia and multiple myeloma may be a failure of specificity and control in production and linkage of the various subunits to form larger molecules. Bence Jones pro-

teins may be polypeptide chains that have not been incorporated into the myeloma globulins because of a failure in the linkage process. Myeloma globulins may consist of combinations of subunits differing from those of the normal γ-globulins, although both types of protein appear to contain subunits that are alike. This may explain in part the antigenic and chemical differences and similarities that have been found between the γ-globulins of disease and normal γ-globulin. The hypothesis outlined above is capable of experimental test, since the products of various chemical treatments may now be separated and compared."

There were still many immunologists who didn't believe that it was of any use to study myeloma proteins "because they didn't have any activity." This belief clearly revealed a hidden faith in instructive theories. I make mention of this because future history was to reveal over and over again the powerful insights to be gained by comparisons of normal Ig and myeloma proteins. Indeed, until very recently, these proteins, provided to us as accidents of nature, have dominated the field. It should be pointed out, in all fairness, that independent of immunological concerns, there were also quite a few people studying these proteins but unfortunately without an hypothesis.

CONVICTION AS A PRELUDE TO SURPRISE

The comment about Bence Jones proteins quoted above grew into a deeper conviction that perhaps the problem of size and heterogeneity could be solved at the same time. This conviction led to one of the more clear-cut (i.e. dramatic) developments in this story of molecular recognition. I became convinced that Bence Jones proteins were polypeptide chains that were synthesized but not incorporated into myeloma proteins. It seemed likely that the chain fraction of lower molecular weight from normal immunoglobulin might simply be a mixture of these proteins.

One day, in a fit of bravado, I announced to Joe Gally, who was then a graduate student, that I would "make" Bence Jones proteins out of my own immunoglobulin. I heated the light chain fraction and was as shocked as he to see the familiar reversible precipitation pattern. But the true shock of molecular recognition came when we then showed the identity of the light chains and Bence Jones proteins from single patients (13).

The shock was great despite the fact that I had predicted the result. I believe to some extent this is true of all hypotheses but that once the corroboration is found, shock is replaced by wonder as all the pieces fall into place. Finally, the prevailing sensation becomes more one of routine expectation until either a new fact or a contradiction is found. But even at that point of the commonplace, there remains a nagging doubt if one does not have a complete picture of a molecule. And even with the Bence Jones story in place, that picture was still vague.

THE PROJECTED VIEW: 1962

By early 1962, a reasonably complete hypothesis on the relationships of immunoglobulin classes and chains was developed on the basis of comparisons between normal and pathological immunoglobulins. The bridge to antibodies was provided when Benacerraf and I decided to examine the chains of specifically purified anti-hapten antibodies of different specificities by gel electrophoresis in urea (14). It became clear that specifically purified antibodies contained a much more restricted population of light chains than normal immunoglobulin. Indeed, these antibodies looked like mixtures of a limited number of myeloma proteins showing 3-5 bands in contrast to the diffuse smear of normal immunoglobulin. This was the first example of truly restricted heterogeneity in elicited antibodies and it permitted a new kind of structural comparison of different antibodies. It soon appeared that each antibody population within a given class was different in its light chain bands; heterogeneity of heavy chains was not revealed as clearly because of their higher molecular weight.

Because we were working on reduced proteins in 6M urea, we concluded that the differences were based on differences in amino acid compositions in the light chains just as in the case of different Bence Jones proteins. Conclusive proof of this was to come later in the work of M. Koshland (15). All of this boded ill for instructive theories even in 1962; the death knell was sounded by Haber's elegant demonstration in 1964 (16) that specific combining sites of antibody fragments can refold after complete denaturation in the absence of antigen.

At this time, my projected view was 1) that all classes of immunoglobulins had light chains but each class had different and distinctive heavy chains, 2) different antibodies had different amino acid compositions, 3) myeloma cells were making single variants of immunoglobulins, 4) Bence Jones proteins were free light chains, 5) heavy chains and light chains both had something to do with specificity. This was one case where there was no chance for a shock because the detailed structure was missing. But we very firmly held to the idea that both chains must contribute on the grounds of conservation: p light chains and q heavy chains of different composition would give a maximum of pq antibodies. But it is now clear to me that only at this time was I becoming a dedicated selectionist and this pq hypothesis, although consistent with theories of selection, was formulated largely in the absence of a clear-cut selective theory.

The findings on Bence Jones proteins and antibody light chains came as a shock that opened up a new chapter - for the first time there was an antibody-related protein small enough, pure enough and available in enough quantity to do structure work. From amino acid compositions (13) and from Putnam's analysis of peptide maps (17), it was clear that each was different in sequence. Exactly how came as another shock when Hilschman and Craig (18) compared two of them and found variable regions at the amino terminal half and constant regions at the carboxyl terminus.

TOTAL STRUCTURE AND THE LEAP FROM ONE TO THREE DIMENSIONS

It was still a guess as to how the immunoglobulin molecule would really look. Valentine and Green's (19) elegant electron microscopic experiment certainly changed the view - from a cigar to a floppy Y or bent T. At that time, I felt that the notion of a freely flapping antibody went too far and remember a pleasant but argumentative afternoon with the late Robin Valentine at the Nobel Symposium in 1964 in which I insisted on limited flexibility and he insisted that hydrodynamics was a pit of iniquity (19). It has turned out that the molecule is indeed not as floppy as he said but the picture of a broad Y that came out of his work did hold up and was important.

None of this could really satisfy though - the critical questions were:

1) What did heavy chains look like in detail?
2) What was the relation of structure to function?
3) Could we ever construct a model that would satisfy that relationship?

The only hope for definitive answers lay in determining the primary structure of a whole immunoglobulin molecule. When Bruce Cunningham and I decided to do this, we concluded that it was going to take about a pound of myeloma protein, a very eclectic strategy of sequence determination, and a climate in which there was no room for any failure of nerve. We reasoned that one total structure would, at the very least, serve as a reference for work in other labs and might, at most, suggest exactly how the molecule was organzed.

In fact, in two areas, the maximum expectation was fulfilled: validation of the evolutionary hypothesis based on Hill's work (20), and construction of a detailed structure - function hypothesis - the so-called domain hypothesis (21). The first was a matter of extending other people's work but the second definitely involved the shock of recognition. The shock expressed itself in some rather unconventional behavior and I vividly remember the look on my colleague's faces when I disappeared into my office with thousands of poppit beads, a small drill, and some piano wire.

The task I had set myself was to see if I could "recognize" what IgG "looked like" at the level of overall and local shape in terms of both structure and function. The facts I started with were:

1) The total sequence, showing homology of V_L and V_H and of C_L and C_H1, C_H2, and C_H3 (21).
2) The finding by Porter (8) that Fab and Fc were functionally distinct - one for antigen-binding and one for effector functions.
3) Valentine's work (19), evidence on relaxation times from fluorescence polarization studies, and some results on X-ray scattering done with Kratky's group (22).

The principles I felt would be guiding ones were:

1) each homology region would fold separately, constrained by its single disulfide bond.

2) each homology region would bear or contribute to one site carrying out a different function. I say contribute, because I was convinced of the p x q hypothesis for V regions. I emerged with bleeding fingers and the poppit bead model, which was built taking advantage of knowledge of the hypervariable regions that came from a great number of labs.

The domain hypothesis (Figure 1) has stood the test of time both for Bence Jones proteins and immunoglobulins. We now have X-ray crystallographic analyses (23,24) confirming the main structural features, and of course, giving us in addition, detailed features of the immunoglobulin fold and the site - features that could hardly be predicted by the method I was using. Still the shock of recognition was there before the X-ray data, and it was strengthened by work on proteolytic cleavage of the molecule into domains (25).

Work on mapping of functions has also tended to support this picture. But it should be pointed out that there remains a good deal to be done to characterize the sites and their functions on each domain before the hypothesis can be considered completely proven. For example, CH3 has a unique feature: a "bottom". Could this be the shared site for linkage to cell surface receptors that bear the immunoglobulin molecule? The main point I wish to emphasize is that the domain hypothesis is not just a structural prediction, but a guess as to the nature of structure-function relations.

This hypothesis ties up and summarizes the relation between antibody binding and effector functions, evolutionary origins and genetics, and class differences of Ig's, all in terms of a succinct structural picture. It seems to me particularly to warrant using the name "molecular immunology" with its connections to selective theories, to genetics, to modern molecular biology and to cell biology. This contrasts with "immunochemistry", the paradigm of 1958, which was largely concerned with antigen and instructive theories. Of course, both paradigms involved chemistry, as all good biology should in the end.

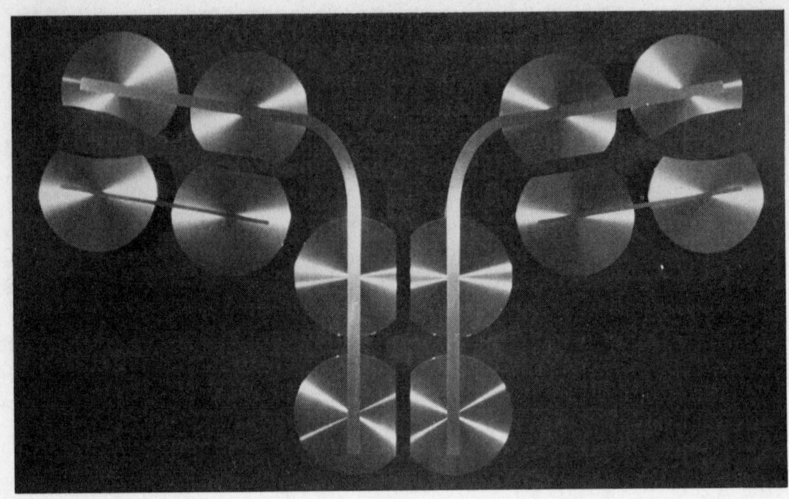

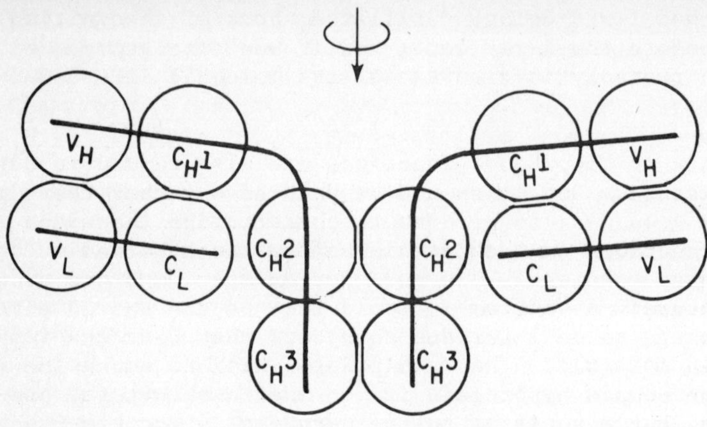

Figure 1. The domain hypothesis. Diagrammatic arrangement of domains in the free immunoglobulin G molecule is shown. The arrow refers to a dyad axis of symmetry. Homology regions that constitute each domain are indicated: V_L and V_H are domains made up of variable homology regions; C_L, C_H1, C_H2 and C_H3 are domains made up of constant homology regions. Within each of these groups, domains are assumed to have similar three-dimensional structures, and each is assumed to contribute to an active site. The V domain sites contribute to antigen recognition functions and the C domain sites to effector functions.

THE PREVAILING PARADIGM NOW

With the domain hypothesis more or less corroborated, it seemed to me that the pursuit of more and more Ig structures of the conventional classes would be a bore - necessary, useful, but not likely to lead to large shocks of recognition. At the risk of being surprised, I still believe that.

The choice was therefore to turn to an analysis of the origin of antibody diversity or of cell triggering after antigen binding. We had toyed with the first problem both theoretically and in a few experiments that were fruitful but not relevant. Gally and I were firm believers in somatic origins of diversity and in gene translocation to construct VC genes (26). We had, in fact, searched for enzymes in bone marrow and thymus to carry these functions out. These studies, carried out by Lindahl, Gally and myself, resulted in the isolation of the first mammalian DNA ligase (27) and several new exonucleases (28,29), but left us no nearer to an answer to the mechanism of translocation or origin of diversity.

I decided that this field should be left to the DNA chemists, but I must say I stuck to my conviction about translocation. Recently, Leder visited me to show me his beautiful experiments. He started off by saying that he thought it was much simpler to assume that there were many complete VC genes because this was a conservative evolutionary model. I almost exploded and said "If that is true, all of formal genetics is wrong." He then smilingly revealed his impressive data showing the presence of a few C genes, and almost guaranteeing the need for some kind of translocation event. Now it also appears that there are very few V genes and that some kind of somatic variation hypothesis is also likely to be correct.

It is much easier to see past paradigms than those of the present but I will hazard a view. The prevailing paradigm now seems to be as follows:

1) Selective theories are correct, in particular clonal selection, although much remains to be understood about control and quantitation.

2) Antibody diversity is likely to be somatic in origin but the mechanism that would tie diversification to translocation has not been worked out in fact.

3) Triggering of lymphoid cells by antigen requires cell cooperation between the T and B cell. But the nature of the T cell receptor and of the detailed interaction remain up in the air. The whole system seems to be connected to the IR genes, which in turn are connected to the complex major histocompatibility locus.

4) The suspicion is bruited about that the immune system may just be a very special evolutionary development of a system of cell-cell recognition that is more general, more fundamental, and more primitive.

The present work in my laboratory is concerned with these aspects of the paradigm and we have not yet run out of shocks or surprises. We have had some success in fractionating immune cells on chemically derivatized surfaces and fibers (30) and have been able to elucidate specificity filtering in clonal selection (31) as well as the appearance of specific binding cells during ontogeny (32,33). But the structural approach has not been abandoned and I should like to mention two examples related to the paradigm.

The first is the analysis of the mitogen, concanavalin A. We felt this to be a kind of "molecular monkey wrench", providing a way into the problems of cell surface recognition and modulation. After determining its structure (34) we have been able to modify it chemically (35) and use it to reveal an entirely new system of modulation of cell surface receptors <u>via</u> microtubules and microfilaments (36,37,38). Using Con A, we also have found that lymphocytes have a responsive state to stimulation that seems to be under autonomous control. Indeed, the cell cycle of lymphocytes as resting cells has a G_0 period which differs from cell to cell (39). These problems certainly bear upon the paradigm and probably will have a general bearing on cell biology.

But perhaps more in the direct immunological tradition has been our work on β_2-microglobulin and histocompatibility antigens. Gally and I have speculated that the gene clusters for immunoglobulins may have arisen by gene duplication of the precursors for the H-2 locus followed by chromosomal translocation (40). The basis for this speculation was the linkage relations of IR genes and the conviction that the immune system must have evolved from a more general cellular system.

At about the time we were toying with this notion, Berggård, (who had worked with me in 1963 and showed the presence of "normal" Bence Jones proteins (41) in our urine, suggested that it would be amusing to do the structure of human β_2-microglobulin, another urinary protein he had isolated. This was of particular interest because of the homology of its first 41 residues with those of immunoglobulin as shown by Smithies and Poulik (42). The complete sequence, determined mainly by Bruce Cunningham in my laboratory strongly confirmed this homology (43). We had found the protein on the surface of lymphocytes but even more amusing were the observations that it was present on and synthesized by tissues other than those of the immune system (44). Indeed, Pressman and his co-workers (45) and subsequently Peterson and co-workers (46) showed it to be associated with HL-A antigens.

Thus, an immunoglobulin-like domain undoubtedly related to Ig in its evolutionary history, is found associated with histocompatibility antigens on the surface of various mammalian cells. Of course, the question is whether an homologous domain exists on the histocompatibility antigen. If so, our hypothesis on the evolutionary origin of the immune system rests more securely. Even if this is not the case, however, the pursuit of this subject cannot fail to enlarge our view of immunology and cell biology. The shock of recognition in immunology now extends itself to the whole of the differentiated organism.

THE ANTI-GUNTHERDÄMMERUNG: AN EPILOGUE ON TASTE, READINESS, AND EASE

My friend, Gunther Stent and I disagree about nearly everything, yet it is a curious feature of our discussions that they are always enjoyable. I attribute this to his scholarship, grace, and tolerance as well as to a mutual lusty appetite for argument He has proposed that creation in science and creation in art are alike (47) and that we may enter into an age in which science shall be post-romantic, post-classical, and post-everything (48). This Guntherdämmerung, which he accepts cheerfully, I find highly unlikely. It seems to me that as one hierarchy of scientific investigation closes, another opens up, whatever the field; indeed, if invention is included, a field is limitless.

In contrast to his views on creation, I believe that scientists, in accepting a single-valued world of order and recurrence, declare themselves, at least as a group, to be servants of the inevitable. If one scientist does not discover or analyze an event, another is likely to seize upon it. While their motives and styles differ, the final reduction by the community will read most of these individual differences out of the work. This is as it should be. It is the strength and the solace of science.

But having said this much, it seems to me of some use to comment on the role of readiness and taste in pursuing a given question. Readiness is not just a question of training and alertness. It seems to me to rest in the willingness to adopt consciously an hypothesis even if the risks of being wrong are high. I believe that Einstein was right when he said "It is the theory that determines what we observe."

Of course, in molecular biology, the type of theory and its general applicability is different than in physics. The great physicist, I. Rabi, once said to me after I gave a lecture, "Now I know what you guys are about - you are engineers. You take things apart and figure out how the parts fit together." When I asked him what physicists did, he lifted his eyes skyward and said "Ah, we speak to God."

In one respect, he was right - a good molecular biologist is a methodological reductionist and he is interested in structure as well as function. But in pursuing his work, he must exercise a kind of taste, mainly by temporarily neglecting facts that he cannot fit into his general hypotheses. And, of course, he risks mistakes if he does this.

In looking back on this account of some of my studies, I see several areas in which I made such errors. One of them was as silly as attempting to isolate antibody chains on Sephadex in 6M urea alone and in acetic acid alone, to no avail, and then failing to mix the two solvents, a procedure which would have worked splendidly, as Porter's work showed two years later (49). Another error was in proposing a model for Ig which was in general too slavishly dependent on hydrodynamics (50). Valentine corrected that. Well before that though, I remember Al Nisonoff saying to me in adopting the model - "Don't you think the Fc region has to stick out more - after all, it must attach to things and have room to interact." I should have listened, but my vision was prejudiced by too much physicochemical formalism.

The main point is: that is what other scientists are for. The exercise of taste is essential and resembles the creative imagination of the artist, but in science it can never be always correct in one individual. The taste and guesses of others fix up the defects. Unfortunately, that rarely satisfies the creative egotism of the individual, even if it gives him strength whether he knows it or not. And there is very little wisdom that can be drawn out of one individual in any easily transferable or communicable fashion. The injunctions are too trite or too general or do not make themselves deeply felt through words. Nevertheless, if I had to write a "Young Molecular Biologist's Vade Mecum" it would contain the following list:

1) In any field, always ask what the central molecule is and does. If it is not in evidence, look for it.
2) Determine its structure.
3) Believe in the results of image-forming methods over hydrodynamic methods.
4) Make models and ask how they relate to the larger prevailing theory of the field.
5) When stuck, look for genetic variants or accidents of nature.
6) Generalize your conclusions by making evolutionary connections.
7) After you have concluded you are right, move up one level higher in physiological organization and see how it all looks from there.

A banal list to be sure. It cannot compare in strength to the implicit, unanalyzed sharing of a conviction about how to attack a scientific problem. But that is the unconscious part of the paradigm and there is nothing to be said or done about it but to enjoy it.

One final word about use: not everything scientists do is useful except to other scientists. The work on antibody structure done in many laboratories throughout the world seems to me to be a good example. It is not easy to document a single great medical advance that has come out of it so far. Nonetheless, the work has eased and rationalized the subject in a fundamental way that is not only beautiful but makes it possible to do many things and think many new thoughts.

A chemist friend of mine, deploring the lack of depth of immunologists, defined an immunological paper as the result of an encounter between an idiot and a rabbit *via* a syringe. Certainly this is unfair - the so-called idiots, including myself, now have a rational basis at their disposal which is the equivalent for immunologists of the periodic table.

In the face of the marvelous challenges of biology, we are all idiots, even chemists. None of the truly fundamental work is easy, but that is not the issue. It is doing science that yields the pleasurable shock of recognition, not talking about it. Still, talking about it is probably the next best thing. It has been my privilege to have done it in the company of remarkable colleagues, and it is an equally great privilege to have been given the opportunity in the Lynen Lecture to talk about it to this distinguished audience, so many of whom have made great contributions to the field.

ACKNOWLEDGEMENT

The work described here was supported in part by grants from the National Institutes of Health and the National Science Foundation.

REFERENCES

1) Kuhn, T.S., The Structure of Scientific Revolutions, Second Edition (University of Chicago Press, 1970).

2) Jerne, N.K. Proc. Natl. Acad. Sci. U.S. 41 (1955) 849.

3) Pauling, L. J. Amer. Chem. Soc. 62 (1940) 2643.

4) Tiselius, A. and Kabat, E. J. Exp. Med. 69 (1939) 119.

5) Karush, F. Advan. Immunol. 2 (1962) 1.

6) Pedersen, K.O., Ultracentrifugal Studies on Serum and Serum Fractions (Almquist and Wiksell, Stockholm, 1945).

7) Petermann, M.L. J. Biol. Chem. 144 (1942) 607.

8) Porter, R.R., Biochem. J. 73 (1959) 119.

9) Deutsch, H.F. and Morton, J.I., J. Biol. Chem. 231 (1958) 1107.

10) Porter, R.R., Biochem. J. 46 (1950) 473.

11) Edelman, G.M. J. Am. Chem. Soc. 81 (1959) 3155.

12) Edelman, G.M. and Poulik, M.D. J. Exp. Med. 113 (1961) 861.

13) Edelman, G.M. and Gally, J.A. J. Exp. Med. 116 (1962) 207.

14) Edelman, G.M., Benacerraf, B., Ovary, Z. and Poulik, M.D. Proc. Natl. Acad. Sci. U.S., 47 (1961) 1751.

15) Koshland, M.E. and Englberger, F.M. Proc. Natl. Acad. Sci. U.S. 50 (1963) 61.

16) Haber, E. Proc. Natl. Acad. Sci. U.S. 52 (1964) 1099.

17) Putnam, F.W. Biochem. Biophys. Acta 63 (1962) 539.

18) Hilschmann, N. and Craig, L.C. Proc. Natl. Acad. Sci. U.S. 53 (1965) 1403.

19) Nobel Symposium, 3rd, (J. Killander, ed.) Almqvist and Wiksell, Stockholm, 1967, 281.

20) Hill, R.L., Delaney, R., Fellows, R.R., Jr., and Lebovitz, H.E. Proc. Natl. Acad. Sci. U.S. 56 (1966) 1762.

21) Edelman, G.M. Biochemistry 9 (1970) 3197.

22) Pilz, I., Puchwein, G., Kratky, O., Herbst, M., Haager, O., Gall, W.E. and Edelman, G.M. Biochemistry 9 (1970) 211.

23) Davies, D.R., Sarma, V.R., Labaw, L.W., Silverton, E.W. and Terry, W.D. in Progress in Immunology, (B. Amos, ed. Academic Press, New York, 1971) pp. 25-32.

24) Poljak, R.J., Amzel, L.M., Avey, H.P., Becka, L.N. and Nisonoff, A., Nature New Biol. 235 (1972) 137.

25) Gall, W.E. and D'Eustachio, P.G., Fed. Proc. 31 (1972) 446.

26) Gally, J.A. and Edelman, G.M. Nature 227 (1970) 341.

27) Lindahl, T. and Edelman, G.M. Proc. Natl. Acad. Sci. U.S., 61 (1968) 680.

28) Lindahl, T., Gally, J.A., and Edelman, G.M. Proc. Natl. Acad. Sci. U.S. 62 (1969) 597.

29) Lindahl, T., Gally, J.A. and Edelman, G.M. J. Biol. Chem. 244 (1969) 5014.

30) Rutishauser, U. and Edelman, G.M. Proc. Natl. Acad. Sci. U.S. 69 (1972) 3774.

31) Edelman, G.M. in Cellular Selection and Regulation in the Immune Response (G.M. Edelman, ed. Raven Press, New York, 1974) pp. 1-38.

32) Spear, P.G., Wang, A.-L., Rutishauser, U. and Edelman, G.M. J. Exp. Med. 138 (1973) 557.

33) Spear, P.G. and Edelman, G.M. J. Exp. Med. 139 (1974) 249.

34) Edelman, G.M., Cunningham, B.A., Reeke, G.N., Jr., Becker, J.W., Waxdal, M.J. and Wang, J.L. Proc. Natl. Acad. Sci. U.S. 69 (1972) 2580.

35) Gunther, G.R., Wang, J.L., Yahara, I., Cunningham, B.A., and Edelman, G.M. Proc. Natl. Acad. Sci. U.S. 70 (1973) 1012.

36) Yahara, I. and Edelman, G.M. Exp. Cell Res. 81 (1973) 143.

37) Yahara, I. and Edelman, G.M. Exp. Cell Res., in press.

38) Edelman, G.M., Yahara, I. and Wang, J.L. Proc. Natl. Acad. Sci. U.S., 70 (1973) 1442.

39) Gunther, G.R., Wang, J.L., and Edelman, G.M. J. Cell Biol., 62 (1974) 366.

40) Gally, J.A. and Edelman, G.M. Ann. Rev. Genet. 6 (1972) 1.

41) Berggard, I. and Edelman, G.M. Proc. Natl. Acad. Sci. U.S. 49 (1963) 330.

42) Smithies, O. and Poulik, M.D. Science 175 (1972) 187.

43) Cunningham, B.A., Wang, J.L., Berggard, I. and Peterson, P.A. Biochemistry 12 (1973) 4811.

44) Nilsson, K., Evrin, P.E., Berggard, I., and Ponten, J. Nature New Biol., 244 (1973) 44.

45) Nakamuro, K., Tanasaki, N. and Pressman, D. Proc. Natl. Acad. Sci. U.S. 70 (1973) 2813.

46) Peterson, P.A., Rask, L. and Lindblom, J.B. Proc. Natl. Acad. Sci. U.S., 71 (1974) 35.

47) Stent, G. Sci. Am., 227 (1972) 84.

48) Stent, G. The Coming of the Golden Age: A View of the End of Progress (Natural History Press, Garden City, New York 1969).

49) Fleischman, J.B., Pain, R.H. and Porter, R.R., Arch. Biochem. Biophys. Supplement 1 (1962) 174.

50) Edelman, G.M. and Gally, J.A. Proc. Natl. Acad. Sci. U.S. 51 (1964) 846.

THE SUBJECT AND STYLE OF MODERN IMMUNOLOGY: AN INTRODUCTION

GERALD M. EDELMAN
The Rockefeller University

Immunology is often viewed by outsiders as both hermetic and baroque. I suppose it was in some anticipation of this view and in the hope that it might be dispelled that I was kindly asked by the organizers of this meeting to provide some introduction to the subject. It is true that modern immunology is eclectic and fast-moving. Its presentation is not simplified by the fact that it serves as both a tool and a model in cell biology and biochemistry, as well as a biological system of great interest in its own right.

I shall attempt here to consider mainly the aims, intrinsic concepts, and terms of the subject and comment only briefly upon its applications. Perhaps the swiftest way to do this is to describe the theory of clonal selection and then pose some of the major questions that concern immunologists at three levels: molecules, cells, and systems of cells. Inasmuch as my purpose here is somewhat didactic, I shall take some liberties and not bother with qualifying my remarks. I am sure that the distinguished group of speakers you are to hear will clarify, extend and correct my comments and I invite them to do so. In this way, I can speak both to the uninitiated and to the cognoscenti in two modes with some hope of positive results.

CLONAL SELECTION AND ITS REQUIREMENTS

Clonal selection is the main guiding theoretical framework of modern immunology. This theory, while vague and incomplete in several respects, has stood the test at various levels of inquiry. I shall try to describe its essential features.

This theory was devised to explain the way in which antigens of a great variety of types could elicit specific cellular or humoral immune responses in a complex system of immune cells and organs. The ontogenetic source of this system rests in certain stem cells of the bone marrow, which in early development seed to central organs known as the thymus and the bursa (or its equivalent in animals other than birds). From these organs, more mature cells are released as T cells (thymus-derived lymphocytes) or B cells (bone marrow-derived or bursa-derived lymphocytes). These cells can circulate in the blood and lymph and can home to a number of secondary organs including lymph nodes, Peyers patches,and spleen. As we shall see, although there is some dispute as to the nature of the main receptor on T cells, T and B cells both contain on their surface molecules capable of specifically binding to antigens. In the case of B cells, these molecules are the various classes of immunoglobulins, and it is fair to say that they are the key molecules of immunity.

The basic premise of the theory of clonal selection (Figure 1) is that an animal already has the information to synthesize all of the necessary T and B cell antibody receptors without using the antigen as a template. The antigen serves only to select those cells containing antibodies having appropriate complementary binding sites for that antigen. The response of the cells then depends upon their prior differentiation; if they are B cells, some of them may be induced to divide and expand into a clone with increased Ig production; if they are T cells, they may carry out helper functions necessary for B cell stimulation in a way not yet completely understood, or they may become "killer cells", releasing a variety of factors that stimulate or inhibit target cells.

Within this system, another unrelated set of cells called macrophages, which do not produce Ig or antibody, may also help stimulation by binding either antigen or antibody. Their role is no clearer in detail than is that of T cells, however, and it may be even more obscure. Let us for the moment not worry about it.

Instead, let us ask what the requirements of clonal selection are. The first requirement is a large repertoire of antibody molecules with different three-dimensional binding sites for different chemical groups or antigenic determinants. As I shall mention later, we now know that the basis for this diversity is variation in the amino acid sequence of amino terminal portions of the polypeptide chains of antibodies. The antibodies must be present on the surface of unstimulated

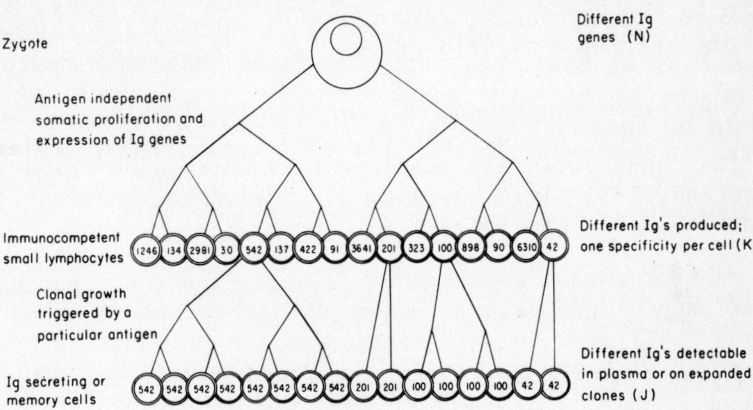

Figure 1. A model of the somatic differentiation of antibody-producing cells according to the clonal selection theory. The number of immunoglobulin genes may increase during somatic growth so that in the immunologically mature animal, different lymphoid cells are formed each committed to the synthesis of a structurally distinct receptor antibody (indicated by an Arabic numeral). A small proportion of these cells proliferate upon antigenic stimulation to form different clones of cells, each clone producing a different antibody. This model represents bone marrow-derived (B) cells but with minor modifications it is also applicable to thymus-derived (T) cells.

cells, and in most cases, there is only one kind of antibody on each cell, present on each cell in about 10,000 copies.

The second requirement for clonal selection is to provide a means of encounter between a specific antigen on a cell with the appropriate antibody. This requirement is complex and depends on circulation and anatomy but, above all, it depends in most cases upon a subtle cooperative relationship between T and B cells of the proper specificity.

The third requirement of clonal selection is that certain of the specific encounters between the antigen and cells with their appropriately complementary antibodies result in maturation, cell division, and, in some cases, antibody production and secretion.

Each of these requirements (diversification, encounter, amplification) generates a major problem in modern immunology and you shall hear in this meeting of the attempts being made to solve these problems. Before considering these problems in more detail, it might be useful to emphasize certain key properties of the system of clonal selection.

I think it is useful to emphasize that the specificity of the system of clonal selection arises from the specificity of binding between antigens and antibodies and from the "triggering" threshold of the cells. In general, only those cells of higher affinity are triggered (Figure 2). Those antibodies of higher affinity are usually also those of greater specificity and therefore this "filtration effect" allows graded specificity to emerge out of an "uninformed" system. By uninformed, I mean that the system does not know in advance which antigenic structure it will encounter. We might say that an immunoglobulin doesn't know it is an antibody until it binds an antigen tightly enough. Another property such a system must have is feedback control: some system of damping and negative feedback must regulate the degree, extent, and quality of response. This occurs *via* intrinsic molecular and cellular pathways.

With this background, we may now introduce three main problems:

1) What is the origin of antibody diversity?

2) What is the nature of encounter between the antigen and cell, and cell and cell?

3) What is the nature of the signal to stimulate or suppress a given cell?

I shall take these up briefly in turn.

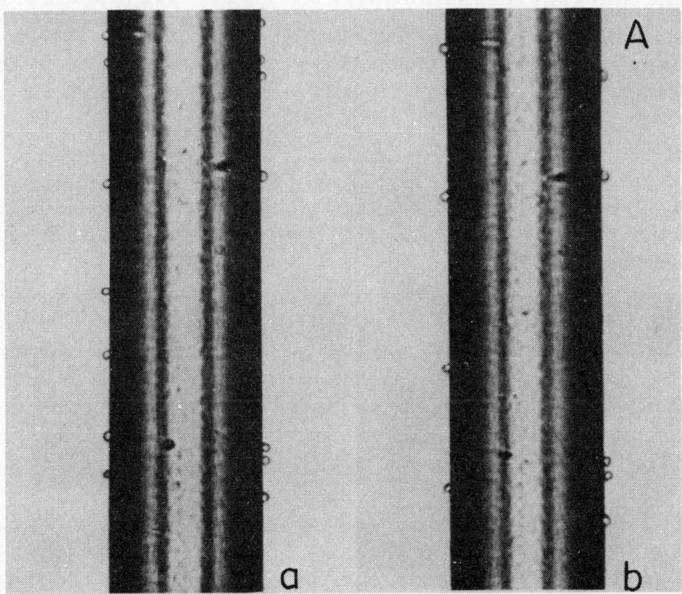

Figure 2A. Lymphoid cells from the mouse spleen bound by their antigen-specific receptors to a nylon fiber to which dinitrophenyl bovine serum albumin has been coupled. Treatment of bound cells in (a) with anti-serum to the T cell surface antigen Θ and with serum complement destroys the T cells, leaving B cells in (b) still viable and attached (X 175).

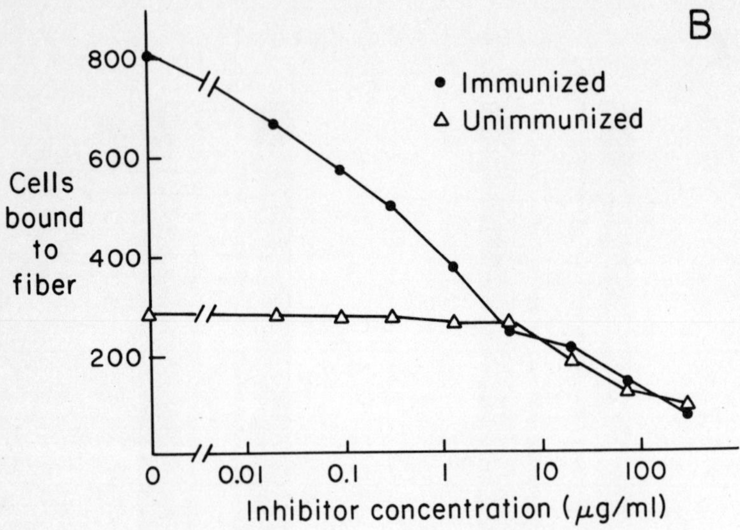

Figure 2B. Inhibition by free Dnp-BSA of spleen cell binding to Dnp-BSA fibers. Cell numbers represent fiber edge counts for a 2.5 cm fiber segment. Spleens from immunized mice were removed at the height of a secondary response to Dnp-BSA and cells from several mice were pooled.

MOLECULES

To ask about the origin of diversity first requires a description of its nature. I cannot do this exhaustively here, but can summarize the key aspects of antibody structure that pose the problem (Figures 3,4).

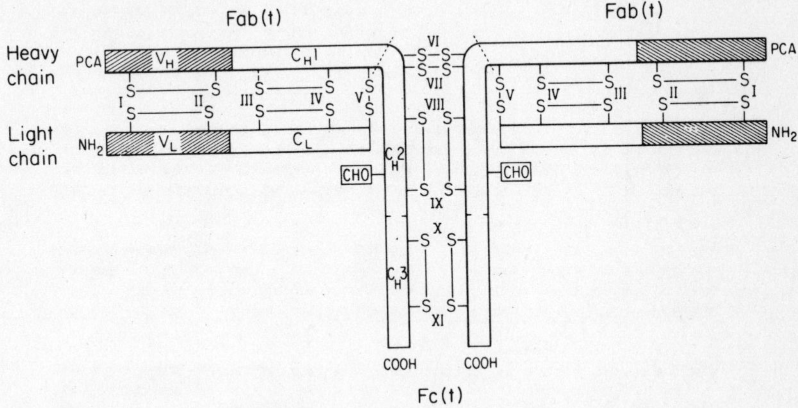

Figure 3. Overall arrangement of chains and disulfide bonds of the human γG_1 immunoglobulin, Eu. Half-cystinyl residues are numbered I to XI; I to V designate corresponding half-cystinyl residues in light and heavy chains; PCA, pyrrolidonecarboxylic acid; CHO, carbohydrate. Fab(t) and Fc(t) refer to fragments produced by trypsin, which cleaves the heavy chain as indicated by dashed lines above half-cystinyl residues VI. Variable regions, V_H and V_L are homologous. The constant region of the heavy chain (C_H) is divided into three regions, C_H1, C_H2 and C_H3, that are homologous to each other and to the C region of the light chain. The variable regions carry out antigen-binding functions and the constant regions the effector function of the molecule.

SEQUENCE HOMOLOGY IN EU CONSTANT REGIONS

		110									120		
EU C_L (RESIDUES 109-214)	THR	VAL	ALA	ALA	PRO	SER	VAL	PHE	ILE	PHE	PRO	PRO	SER
EU C_H1 (RESIDUES 119-220)	SER	THR	LYS	GLY	PRO	SER	VAL	PHE	PRO	LEU	ALA	PRO	SER
EU C_H2 (RESIDUES 234-341)	LEU	LEU	GLY	GLY	PRO	SER	VAL	PHE	LEU	PHE	PRO	PRO	LYS
EU C_H3 (RESIDUES 342-446)	GLN	PRO	ARG	GLU	PRO	GLN	VAL	TYR	THR	LEU	PRO	PRO	SER

										130									
ASP	GLU	GLN	–	–	LEU	LYS	SER	GLY	THR	ALA	SER	VAL	VAL	CYS	LEU	LEU	ASN	ASN	PHE
SER	LYS	SER	–	–	THR	SER	GLY	GLY	THR	ALA	ALA	LEU	GLY	CYS	LEU	VAL	LYS	ASP	TYR
PRO	LYS	ASP	THR	LEU	MET	ILE	SER	ARG	THR	PRO	GLU	VAL	THR	CYS	VAL	VAL	VAL	ASP	VAL
ARG	GLU	GLU	–	–	MET	THR	LYS	ASN	GLN	VAL	SER	LEU	THR	CYS	LEU	VAL	LYS	GLY	PHE

140												150							
TYR	PRO	ARG	GLU	ALA	LYS	VAL	–	–	GLN	TRP	LYS	VAL	ASP	ASN	ALA	LEU	GLN	SER	GLY
PHE	PRO	GLU	PRO	VAL	THR	VAL	–	–	SER	TRP	ASN	SER	–	GLY	ALA	LEU	THR	SER	GLY
SER	HIS	GLU	ASP	PRO	GLN	VAL	LYS	PHE	ASN	TRP	TYR	VAL	ASP	GLY	–	VAL	GLN	VAL	HIS
TYR	PRO	SER	ASP	ILE	ALA	VAL	–	–	GLU	TRP	GLU	SER	ASN	ASP	–	GLY	GLU	PRO	GLU

		160										170							
ASN	SER	GLN	GLU	SER	VAL	THR	GLU	GLN	ASP	SER	LYS	ASP	SER	THR	TYR	SER	LEU	SER	SER
–	VAL	HIS	THR	PHE	PRO	ALA	VAL	LEU	GLN	SER	–	SER	GLY	LEU	TYR	SER	LEU	SER	SER
ASN	ALA	LYS	THR	LYS	PRO	ARG	GLU	GLU	GLN	TYR	–	ASP	SER	THR	TYR	ARG	VAL	VAL	SER
ASN	TYR	LYS	THR	THR	PRO	PRO	VAL	LEU	ASP	SER	–	ASP	GLY	SER	PHE	PHE	LEU	TYR	SER

		180										190							
THR	LEU	THR	LEU	SER	LYS	ALA	ASP	TYR	GLU	LYS	HIS	LYS	VAL	TYR	ALA	CYS	GLU	VAL	THR
VAL	VAL	THR	VAL	PRO	SER	SER	SER	LEU	GLY	THR	GLN	–	THR	TYR	ILE	CYS	ASN	VAL	ASN
VAL	LEU	THR	VAL	LEU	HIS	GLN	ASN	TRP	LEU	ASP	GLY	LYS	GLU	TYR	LYS	CYS	LYS	VAL	SER
LYS	LEU	THR	VAL	ASP	LYS	SER	ARG	TRP	GLN	GLU	GLY	ASN	VAL	PHE	SER	CYS	SER	VAL	MET

		200													210				
HIS	GLN	GLY	LEU	SER	SER	PRO	VAL	THR	–	LYS	SER	PHE	–	–	ASN	ARG	GLY	GLU	CYS
HIS	LYS	PRO	SER	ASN	THR	LYS	VAL	–	ASP	LYS	ARG	VAL	–	–	GLU	PRO	LYS	SER	CYS
ASN	LYS	ALA	LEU	PRO	ALA	PRO	ILE	–	GLU	LYS	THR	ILE	SER	LYS	ALA	LYS	GLY		
HIS	GLU	ALA	LEU	HIS	ASN	HIS	TYR	THR	GLN	LYS	SER	LEU	SER	LEU	SER	PRO	GLY		

Figure 4A. Comparison of the amino acid sequences of C_L, C_H1, C_H2, and C_H3 regions. Deletions, indicated by dashes, have been introduced to maximize homologies. Identical residues are darkly shaded; both light and dark shadings are used to indicate identities which occur in pairs in the same position.

SEQUENCE HOMOLOGY IN EU VARIABLE REGIONS

					1									10
EU V_L	(RESIDUES 1-108)				ASP	ILE	**GLN**	MET	THR	**GLN**	**SER**	PRO	SER	THR
EU V_H	(RESIDUES 1-114)				PCA	VAL	**GLN**	LEU	VAL	**GLN**	**SER**	GLY	–	ALA
									20					30
LEU	SER	ALA	SER	VAL	**GLY**	ASP	ARG	**VAL**	THR	ILE	THR	**CYS**	ARG	**ALA**
GLU	VAL	LYS	LYS	PRO	**GLY**	SER	SER	**VAL**	LYS	VAL	SER	**CYS**	LYS	**ALA**

									20										30
LEU	SER	ALA	SER	VAL	**GLY**	ASP	ARG	**VAL**	THR	ILE	THR	**CYS**	ARG	**ALA**	**SER**	GLN	SER	ILE	ASN
GLU	VAL	LYS	LYS	PRO	**GLY**	SER	SER	**VAL**	LYS	VAL	SER	**CYS**	LYS	**ALA**	**SER**	GLY	GLY	THR	PHE
											40								
THR	–	–	TRP	LEU	ALA	**TRP**	TYR	GLN	**GLN**	LYS	**PRO**	**GLY**	LYS	ALA	PRO	LYS	LEU	LEU	MET
SER	ARG	SER	ALA	ILE	ILE	**TRP**	VAL	ARG	**GLN**	ALA	**PRO**	**GLY**	GLN	GLY	LEU	GLU	TRP	MET	GLY
	50											60							
TYR	LYS	ALA	SER	SER	–	LEU	GLU	SER	GLY	VAL	PRO	SER	ARG	**PHE**	ILE	**GLY**	SER	GLY	SER
GLY	ILE	VAL	PRO	MET	PHE	GLY	PRO	PRO	ASN	TYR	ALA	GLN	LYS	**PHE**	GLN	**GLY**	–	ARG	VAL
		70																	80
GLY	THR	GLU	PHE	THR	–	–	–	–	–	–	–	LEU	THR	ILE	**SER**	**SER**	**LEU**	GLN	PRO
THR	ILE	THR	ALA	ASP	GLU	SER	THR	ASN	THR	ALA	TYR	MET	GLU	LEU	**SER**	**SER**	**LEU**	ARG	SER
									90										
ASP	**ASP**	PHE	**ALA**	THR	**TYR**	TYR	**CYS**	GLN	GLN	–	**TYR**	ASN	SER	ASP	**SER**	LYS	MET	PHE	GLY
GLU	**ASP**	THR	**ALA**	PHE	**TYR**	PHE	**CYS**	ALA	GLY	GLY	**TYR**	GLY	ILE	TYR	**SER**	PRO	GLU	GLU	TYR
100																			
GLN	**GLY**	THR	LYS	**VAL**	GLU	VAL	LYS	GLY											
ASN	**GLY**	GLY	LEU	**VAL**	THR														

Figure 4B. Comparison of the amino acid sequences of the V_H and V_L regions of protein Eu. Identical residues are shaded. Deletions indicated by dashes are introduced to maximize the homology.

Immunoglobulins are a family of molecules produced by lymphocytes. All of them are made up of units consisting of two identical light and two identical heavy polypeptide chains. Each chain carries a variable region with different amino acid sequences and a constant region which is the same in each class of molecule except for minor genetic polymorphisms. Crystallographic analysis has confirmed that each variable region and each of the homologous constant regions is folded in a compact domain (Figure 5). Functional studies indicate that

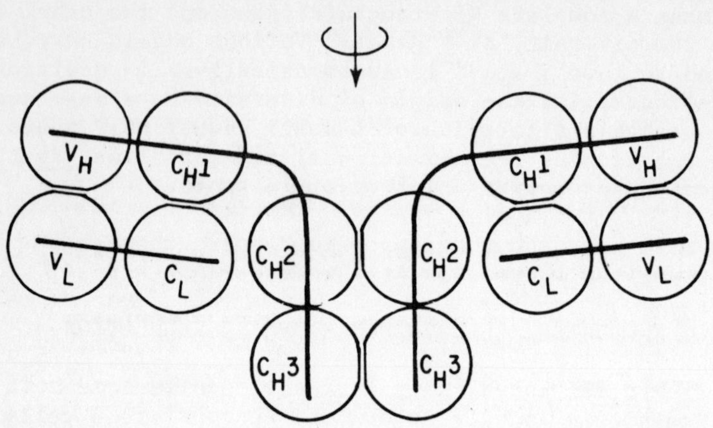

Figure 5. The domain hypothesis. Diagrammatic arrangement of domains in the free immunoglobulin G molecule is shown. The arrow refers to a dyad axis of symmetry. Homology regions that constitute each domain are indicated: V_L and V_H are domains made up of variable homology regions; C_L, C_H1, C_H2 and C_H3 are domains made up of constant homology regions. Within each of these groups, domains are assumed to have similar three-dimensional structures, and each is assumed to contribute to an active site. The V domain sites contribute to antigen recognition functions and the C domain sites to effector functions.

the variable region domains carry out antigen-binding functions and the constant region domains carry out effector functions.

Contrary to prevailing dogma, genetic analysis suggests that Ig chains are specified by two genes, a V gene and a C gene. The evidence is consistent with the presence of at least three unlinked gene clusters specifying two kinds of light chains κ and λ, and the various different kinds of heavy chains whose constant regions are characteristic of a class: μ for IgM, γ for IgG, etc. (see Figure 6).

This arrangement requires two unusual genetic mechanisms, one to make a complete VC structural gene and the other to provide the diversity of V genes. Various models have been suggested to fuse V and C genes somatically. In addition, two main routes for the origin of diversity have been suggested: somatic alteration of a small number of V genes (either mutation or recombinational) and germ line *via* the inheritance and preservation of multiple genes.

You will hear about attempts to resolve these problems by various approaches at this meeting.

ANTIGENIC ENCOUNTER, CELL COOPERATION AND REGULATION

As I have mentioned, many antigens require some sort of processing *via* T cells before the appropriate B cells can be stimulated. The exact nature of this processing or interaction is not clear. This obscurity arises for a number of reasons: 1) the nature of the T cell receptor is in dispute, 2) the response of T cells to antigens appears to be under control of a set of genes other than those for immunoglobulins. These are known as immune response or IR genes and are linked to another immunologically interesting locus, the major histocompatibility locus, which in turn is linked to a gene complex regulating the response of T lymphocytes to each other and foreign cells. 3) The exact sequence of events in processing of antigen by macrophages, and the nature of the various encounters between cell-antigen complexes, antigen-antibody complexes, and cell-antibody complexes are unknown.

This is a most active field of immunology and you will hear about some of the recent attempts to understand these complexities. At this point, I would like to state only one somewhat dogmatic belief - the picture will become clear only if the appropriate molecules are identified, isolated and understood in terms of structure-function relationships. Of course, functional analysis of cellular interactions poses the problem but immunologists will solve it in terms of the molecular interactions. A satisfactory solution will probably require an analysis at all three levels: molecules and their genes, cells and their surface structures, and cell-cell interactions.

MOLECULAR BASIS OF TRIGGERING

Throughout this didactic account, one feature runs as a constant: the cell surface is the nexus for molecular encounter, molecule-cell interaction and cell-cell interaction. Obviously, we must know this terrain better and more and more immunologists are attempting to understand the cell surface-membrane complex in detail. What is required is a picture of the types, numbers, anchorage, specificity, and dynamics of cell surface receptors. Here immunology provides general tools of great power for work on lymphocytes as well as on other cells.

The key problem from the intrinsic point of view has to do with the nature of the signals that stimulate the lymphocyte to mature and divide. Obviously, this problem interacts strongly with that of cell cooperation, and the causal linkage of specific antigen-binding to triggering. A number of other means to analyze this problem exist, however, including the use of mitogenic lectins and the analysis of the effects of lymphocyte factors. Among the key questions are:

1) What is the adequate signal necessary for stimulation - cross-linkage of receptors, conformational change of receptors, or membrane transport of ions? How are cell surface receptors modulated and controlled?

2) What turns the cell off specifically im immune tolerance?

3) What chemical messengers induce maturation and division, and what is their genetic control?

4) What features do lymphocytes share with other differentiated cells? Are the controls a function of population variables in addition to specific signals?

You will hear attempts to dissect out these variables, particularly using lectins, but also by other means.

THE GENERALIZATION OF IMMUNOLOGY

As you can see, the elucidation of clonal selection requires an attack on several fundamental problems of cell biology. These include the nature of cell surface motion, receptor modulation, and the control of cell division. It is not surprising, therefore, to see the lymphocyte being used as a model to study these questions, to some extent independently of intrinsic immunological questions. But even more striking and fundamentally exciting are attempts to relate the evolution, genetics, and molecular functions of immunology to other cellular systems of recognition such as those encountered in developmental biology.

One of the most striking of these efforts relates to the histocompatibility system (Figure 6) that I already mentioned

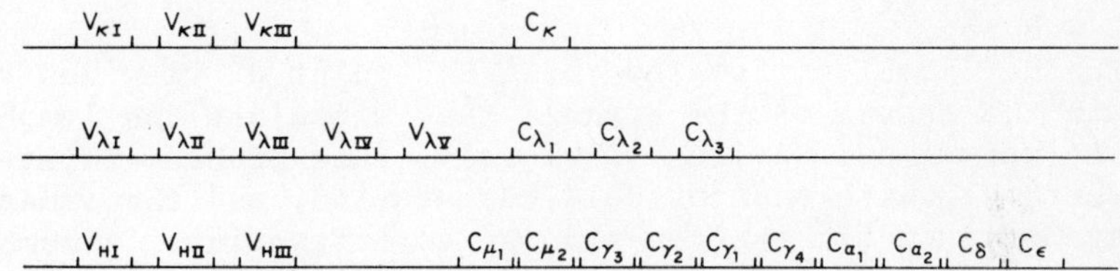

Figure 6A. A diagrammatic representation of the proposed arrangement in mammalian germ cells of antibody genes in three unlinked clusters termed translocons. Light chains κ and λ are each specified by different translocons, and heavy chains are specified by a third translocon. The exact number and arrangement of V and C genes within a translocon is not known. Each variable region subgroup (designated by a subscript corresponding to chain group and subgroup) must be coded by at least one separate germ-line V gene. The number of V genes within each subgroup is unknown, however, as is the origin of intrasubgroup diversity of V regions. A special event is required to link the information from a particular V gene to that of a given C gene. The properties of the classes and subclasses are conferred on the constant regions by C genes.

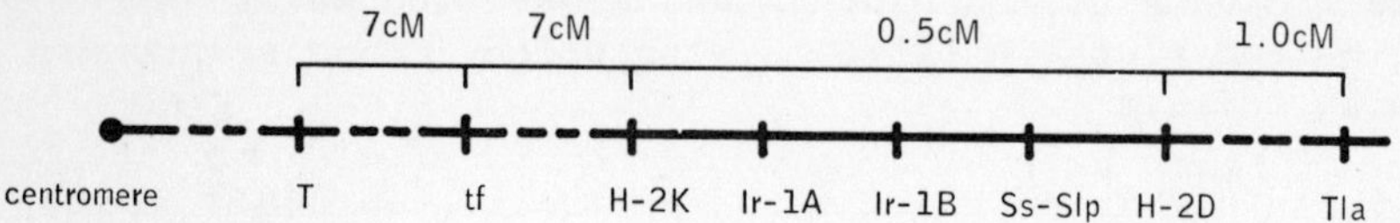

Figure 6B. The major histocompatibility complex of the mouse, including the region defined by the H-2D and H-2K loci. Other loci such as the immune response (Ir) genes and genes coding for a serum protein (Ss) are contained within this region.

in connection with the IR genes. Gally and I have speculated that the Ig structural genes may have arisen by gene duplication from the precursors of histocompatibility genes. Interestingly enough, it is now known that an Ig-like domain, β_2-microglobulin, is synthesized and found on a variety of mammalian cell surfaces, frequently in association with the histocompatibility antigens. We have proposed that the precursor gene for this molecule also gave rise to the Ig's. So there is now the possibility of a connection between at least two (Ig and H-2) and perhaps three gene systems (Ig, H-2, and β_2-microglobulin) depending upon the demonstration of the linkage relationships of the gene locus for β_2-microglobulin.

The immune system arose in true vertebrates and the evidence suggests that immunoglobulins and their classes emerged by gene duplication from a precursor of the size necessary to specify a single domain (100 amino acids). The intriguing question is whether that precursor had to do with more general systems of cell-cell recognition in metazoans. Many of the efforts of immunologists will be devoted to these relationships in the next decade.

A POSTSCRIPT ON LEVELS OF ANALYSIS - THE ANTIGEN AS AN ABSTRACTION AND THE ANTIGEN AS A THING

I cannot terminate this brief account of problems and definitions without saying something about how immunologists approach the universe of antigens. I fear that a misunderstanding of this subject has done as much to frighten away the cell biologist and biochemist as have the metaphysical theories and plethora of terms with which immunologists are casually familiar.

Immunology is a reflexive science. It can study much of its own structure using immunological methods without recourse to standard approaches of other disciplines. This obviously stems from the fact that you can make an antibody to an enormous variety of things and at minute concentrations. Of course, this should be considered a blessing and as an invitation to use immunology as a key approach to unknown structures. But it also generates a bewildering array of abstract serological tabulations and names that are _functionally_ but not structurally defined. It also generates cascaded arrays of assays involving "sandwiches", cytotoxicity, blocking, and indirect inhibitions, the number of which is only limited by the imagination and lexicographical patience of the researcher. Thus, there are antibodies to antibodies, cell surface antigens, differentiation antigens, tumor antigens, etc. Until we define the chemical structure of these entities we must make do, but it does not hurt to remember, for example, that a cell surface antigen is a protein, or a glycoprotein, or a glycolipid, whose structure-function relations remain to be defined. Immunology will not have discharged its task or recognized its proper alliances until those tasks are completed.

And with that injunction, I turn you over to the practitioners and aficionados of an exciting science.

SELECTED GENERAL REFERENCES

1) G.M. Edelman (ed.), Cellular Selection and Regulation in in the Immune Response (Raven Press, New York, 1974).

2) G.M. Edelman, Scientific American 223 (1970) 34.

3) N.K. Jerne, Scientific American 229 (1973) 52.

4) M. Sela, Science 166 (1969) 1365.

5) J.A. Gally and G.M. Edelman, Ann. Rev. Genet. 6 (1972) 1.

6) G.J.V. Nossal and G.L. Ada, Antigens, Lymphoid Cells, and the Immune Response (Academic Press, New York, 1971).

7) M.F. Greaves, J.J.T. Owen and J.C. Raff, T and B Lymphocytes: Origins, Properties, and Role in Immune Responses (American Elsevier Publishing Co., New York 1973).

8) G.J.V. Nossal, Antibodies and Immunity (Basic Books, Inc., New York, 1969).

CURRENT CONCEPTS IN CELLULAR IMMUNOLOGY

H.N. CLAMAN
Departments of Medicine and Microbiology
University of Colorado Medical School

Abstract: The current framework of cellular immunology distinguishes two large universes of immune responses -- cell-mediated immunity (CMI) and humoral antibody (immunoglobulin) production. Each universe is complex and involves a variety of cells and cellular products, both specific and non-specific. In CMI, the specific cells are thymus-derived (T) lymphocytes, which, upon interaction with antigen attached to nonspecific macrophages, become activated to produce soluble non-immunoglobulin products called lymphokines. These substances are responsible for a variety of biological processes including "delayed" inflammatory reactions, cell killing, etc. T lymphocytes appear to recognize largish antigenic determinants, but we are not sure of the chemical nature of their antigen-recognizing surface receptors.

Immunoglobulins are produced by bone marrow-derived (B) lymphocytes and their descendants. B cells also have antigen-specific surface receptors capable of recognizing small haptenic antigens, and these receptors appear to be samples of the antibodies they are destined to manufacture in quantity. In some cases, B cells need "help" from T lymphocytes and macrophages, but the nature of this "help" is not clearly understood. It is also not clear what the "signals" are which activate resting B cells to become antibody producers.

Equally important is the problem of turning immune responses "down" or "off." Under certain circumstances, antigen-specific responses can be specifically inhibited to induce immunological unresponsiveness or "tolerance." It is now becoming clear that there are a variety of mechanisms by which tolerance can be induced. These include clone deletion, cell inhibition and active blocking factors produced by either T or B cells.

INTRODUCTION

The current knowledge explosion has hit immunology, and it is only fitting that the number of experiments being reported is growing close to the number of kinds of immunoglobulin molecules. Reviews are also proliferating. In taking an overview of the current situation, it is still useful to distinguish two large universes of the immune response -- that of cellular immunity (formerly called delayed hypersensitivity) and that of humoral immunity. These two universes have distinguishing characteristics and yet are linked to each other in both positive and negative pathways.

The "action" is now at the cellular and subcellular level where investigators are pursuing concepts of specificity and diversity which were learned during the investigation of immunoglobulin structure. In general, the two universes are strongly associated with two classes of lymphoid cells -- cell-mediated immunity with thymus-derived (T) cells and humoral immunity with B cells derived from the Bursa of Fabricius in birds and from the bone marrow in man. Before discussing cellular aspects of these universes, there are a number of caveats to point out.

- Cell membranes are fluid -- they change.
- Cells are mobile in the body -- they move around.

- Something that binds to a cell may - or may not - turn it on. In fact, it may turn it off.
- Things that happen *in vitro* may not happen *in vivo*.
- Differences which are statistically significant may be biologically trivial.

B CELLS AND IMMUNOGLOBULIN PRODUCTION

The clonal theory appears to be nicely illustrated at the B cell level. B lymphocytes are the precursors of immunoglobulin - (Ig) producing cells. In general, each B cell carries immunoglobulins on its surface of only one class and one allotype of light and heavy chain. This immunoglobulin molecule is both the receptor for the appropriate antigen and a sample of the antibody which the cell may later produce for export. Recently, antiidiotypic immunoglobulins specific for a given antibody have been shown to block the binding of the antigen corresponding to that antibody (4). Precursor B cells have relatively abundant Ig on their surface, about 10^5 molecules per cell. After cell triggering and differentiation towards Ig-producing plasma cells, the number of Ig molecules on the B cell surface drops off and indeed they may be difficult to find on mature plasma cells. Ig surface markers may be induced to move into "patches" and "caps" on the cell surface, but the relation of this to cell activation is not clear (5).

What can "trigger" the B cell to proliferate and mature? In some cases, antigen alone appears sufficient -- no other lymphoid cells (e.g. T cells) or accessory cells (e.g. macrophages) need participate. Antigens capable of doing this -- "T independent antigens" -- and the corresponding antibody responses show unusual characteristics. The antigens are primarily polymeric, such as dextran, levan, PVP, and the antibody responses are generally IgM with little anamnestic responses and easy induction of unresponsiveness if too much antigen is given. Thus the "signal" for the B cell in these cases seems to be only a matrix arrangement of antigenic determinants. The response of B cells to nonpolymeric antigens will be discussed later.

T CELLS AND CELLULAR RESPONSES

T cells are activatable by antigen, but the nature and specificity of the T cell receptor for antigen is open to more controversy than is the case with B cells. The ability to destroy functionally a specific T cell population with radioactively "hot" antigen appears to indicate that T cells have specific antigen receptors (6). The most specific antigen receptors known are immunoglobulins and the results of analyses of whether T cells have surface immunoglobulins has been answered in various laboratories in various ways, from none detectable (7) to some (8) to easily detectable (9). The whole area is further clouded by the recent finding that activated T cells may nonspecifically bind immunoglobulins to their surfaces (10). Therefore, if Ig's are found on a T cell, it becomes highly desirable to show that indeed, they are produced by that T cell if one wants to complete the analogy to B cells of clonally restricted antigen-specific cell receptors.

The problem remains vexed but important, because if T cells recognize antigens by some receptor which is _not_ immunoglobulin, then what is the molecule and in what does its specificity lie? One possibility is that the difference is merely one of quantity -- T cells have fewer receptors than B cells and so they are harder to demonstrate. Or perhaps parts of the T cell receptor is "buried" in a thicker sialomucin membrane covering and is therefore less accessible to analytic reagents.

There are reasons for believing that these simple reasons may not suffice. The antigenic determinants recognized in delayed hypersensitivity (and hence recognized by T cells) seem to be larger determinants than those recognized by B cells (11). Hapten specific B cells may be stimulated by haptenic determinants (together with a "second signal" -- see below) while the concept of a hapten-specific T cell is still controversial (12).

It is likely that while there are DNP-specific B cells, T cells recognize DNP-tyrosyl residues and not DNP alone (13). Because genetic control of immune responses is located primarily at the T cell level, and because of the intimate relation between IR gene products and B_2 microglobulin (highly analogous to constant regions of Ig molecules) it is becoming possible to conceive that the T cell receptor has similarities to immunoglobulins and possibly to histocompatibility antigens. This still leaves unsolved the problem of the molecular basis for the specificity of the receptor.

Even if we do not know the precise nature of the T cell receptor for antigen, we can still investigate the mechanism of T cell triggering by antigen. A number of models of T cell activation are available. One involves the stimulation of *in vitro* DNA synthesis when primed lymphoid cells are exposed to the appropriate antigen. Previous *in vivo* experiments indicated that macrophage-associated antigen is highly immunogenic -- far more efficient than equivalent amounts of soluble antigen. While previous work on macrophage "handling" of antigen focussed on some "processing" which the macrophage might do, the work of Unanue and colleagues indicated that it is the small amount of native antigen on the surface of the macrophage which is highly immunogenic, not the majority of the antigenic molecules which are processed and degraded by the macrophage into non-immunogenic pieces (14). Furthermore, Rosenthal and his colleagues indicated that not only were macrophages obligatory in T cell triggering (15) but also *any* macrophage would not do -- histoincompatible macrophages were very ineffective (16). These experiments are reminiscent of the fact that in the mixed leukocyte reaction (MLR) (another kind of T cell activation), the stimulator cell may be treated with mitomycin but must not be killed if it is to stimulate. These facts indicate that T cells can best be triggered if the antigen is presented "by the right diplomatic pathways" and that the pathway may be via attachment to a cell surface (e.g. a macrophage membrane). What the relation may be between the antigen on the macrophage surface and the T cell is not yet clear.

T-B CELL COOPERATION

It has been known for ten years that for most complex antigens, including proteins and foreign erythrocytes, the production of antibody by B cells requires "T cell help." What is not clear is the nature of the help. At one time, the function of T cells was felt to be that of an antigen-focusser. That is, carrier-primed T cells might help B cells produce anti-hapten antibodies by focussing the antigen on the T cell surface so that what the B cell actually "saw" was a matrix of haptenic determinants to which it could respond as it would to a polymeric antigen such as dextran or PVP. This model has the virtue of simplicity, but it seems to require that a T cell specific for one antigenic determinant (the right carrier) find itself touching a B cell specific for a certain other antigenic determinant (the right hapten). Since the clonal selection theory indicates that the probability that two cells with the "right" specificities would be adjacent is the product of the frequency of each cell in the general lymphoid population (perhaps $1/1000 \times 1/1000 = 1$ in 10^6) this would appear to be an unlikely event. Therefore, many investigators favored the idea that T cells and B cells collaborated by means of a diffusable T cell factor which would obviate the necessity for the specific T cell and B cell to be in opposition. Indeed, the ability to get T cells to cooperate with B cells which were located across a cell-impermeable membrane (17) made such a factor a more likely possibility.

For some time, a large number of experiments were done to show ways in which T cells could help B cells make antibody. Then there was considerable interest in finding ways in which B cells could make antibodies to T cell dependent antigens *without* T cells. Such methods include the induction of a graft-versus-host reaction ("the allogeneic effect") (18), substitution of T cells by B cell mitogens such as lipopolysaccharide (LPS)(19) or by adjuvants in general. *In vitro*, activated T cells were shown to release soluble factors which could substitute for intact T cells. Some of these factors seem to be non-specific for the B cell triggering antigen (20) while others appear to be specific (21). Feldmann and his colleagues believe that their specific molecule mediating T-B cell collaboration is monomeric IgM which is the antigen-specific T cell receptor. Upon stimulation by the appropriate antigen, this receptor is released by T cells and passively attaches to a macrophage surface which becomes the site for B cell triggering.

SIGNALS FOR B CELL TRIGGERING

These experiments on the mechanism of T-B cell cooperation bring us back to the question -- how are B cells triggered? Before the distinction between T and B cells was made, Dresser proposed that to be immunogenic, molecules must possess both the specific antigenic determinants and a nonspecific and ill-defined quality which he called "adjuvanticity" (22). If the molecule contained only the specific trigger, he proposed that cells would not be turned on -- in fact they would be turned off or tolerized. The materials he used were plain bovine gamma globulin (BGG) which was a good immunogen and the supernatant of ultracentrifuged BGG which was not immunogenic but was tolerogenic; i.e., it blocked the response to immunogenic BGG. He felt that plain BGG containing aggregates had both antigenicity and adjuvanticity and thus was immunogenic while removing aggregates removed adjuvanticity leaving ultracentrifuged BGG as a tolerogen. Further work showed that bacterial endotoxin (LPS) administered separately could provide adjuvanticity to ultracentrifuged BGG, thus converting it from a tolerogen to an immunogen (23). This experiment showed that the "two signals" for immunogenicity could be physically separated.

These concepts have been discussed in detail by Bretscher and Cohn (24) and integrated into the current framework of T and B cell physiology. Most antigens carry their own adjuvanticity, which, for T cell-dependent antigens, is probably what we call T cell "help." T-independent antigens have little adjuvanticity and hence, in general, are weak immunogens and good tolerogens. There is not full agreement on the mechanism of B cell triggering, and G. Möller and his colleagues have provided a somewhat different model (25).

TURNING CELLS OFF -- TOLERANCE

Over the last 35 years, a large number of experiments have been done indicating that specific immunologic unresponsiveness can be induced in a variety of ways. That is, antigen can be presented in a form which is not only not immunogenic but which in fact makes the system unresponsive to the same antigen in a form which is ordinarily immunogenic (see Dresser experiments above).

The "mechanism" of tolerance has been a puzzle to immunologists and in general, procrustean attempts to squeeze all experiments into a single model have been unsuccessful. Today it is recognized that there are several mechanisms involved in producing unresponsiveness, and it is likely that more than one process may be going on in a single system (26). In retrospect it is hardly surprising to find that the phenomenon of specific immunologic unresponsiveness is multifactorial. In a system as complex as the immunological system, one might expect that multiple pathways of activation would be mirrored by multiple pathways of repression or negative control.

Experiments in whole animals are relatively easy to do, but necessarily are often difficult to analyze -- a "black box" situation. On the other hand, *in vitro* work is easier to analyze but must constantly be applied to *in vivo* situations. At the level of the whole animal, it has been possible to selectively induce tolerance in either CMI or antibody-producing systems by modifying the antigen (27). At a cellular level, tolerance to protein antigens can be induced in T cells, B cells or both (28). When one tries to move to events at the cell membrane, where tolerance is certainly induced, there may be difficulties.

T CELL TOLERANCE

T cell-dependent protein antigens can induce temporary tolerance, and this tolerance is prolonged if the thymus is removed (29). This strongly implies that the waning of tolerance depends on the emergence of new responsive cells under the influence of (and presumably via migration from) the thymus. The results do not tell us what the tolerogen did to the clone of T cells. It might have destroyed them ("clone loss") or inactivated them. (In this case the inactivation is rather prolonged.) The molecular events have to be interpreted in terms of T cell triggering and by analogy to the situation in B cells (see below), excessive epitope density at the cell membrane might well be involved. But since the fine mechanism of T cell triggering is not known, conclusions are only tentative at this point.

Recently, work has been done showing that tolerance at the T cell level can be an active process (30,31,32,33). The mechanism of this phenomenon is also unclear, but may be related to the presence of antigen-antibody complexes or specific suppressor molecules. So far, active suppression has not been found in tolerance to protein antigens such as human gamma globulin (HGG), but as one prominent immunologist put it so well -- "absence of proof is not the same as proof of absence" (34). Active suppression has been found with other carriers (34a).

B CELL TOLERANCE

In the case of B cell tolerance, explanations are simpler. With T-independent antigens, one can get reversible tolerance (pneumococcal polysaccharide) or irreversible tolerance (levan) (26). These phenomena are best interpreted by the model of Diener and Feldmann (35) where tolerance *in vitro* was induced either by polymerized flagellin (POL) or by monomer flagellin (MON) together with critical amounts of antibody. The "turning off" of the B cell seems to be correlated with high levels of epitope density which can be produced either by POL alone or by MON plus antibody. In the latter case, the authors believe that the antibody produces a stable matrix of epitopes which prevents cell activation. Presumably, in the "two-signal" model of B cell triggering, an excess of the specific signal will prevent activation by both signals.

In the case of T dependent antigens, it is known that haptens on nonimmunogenic carriers are not only nonimmunogenic but may be tolerogenic. This is best seen in models using haptens on autologous carriers. At least one report indicates that the hapten-specific receptor is blocked by the hapten-carrier. Presumably one again has an excess of the specific signal (hapten) and since the carrier is nonimmunogenic, one has no T cell help as the carrier is not recognized as foreign. This interpretation is not agreed to by everyone (37).

BLOCKING FACTORS

Finally, there is extensive work on the presence of serum blocking or enhancing factors which may be responsible for the appearance of immunologic unresponsiveness. This problem is particularly acute in the areas of transplantation and tumor immunology. There is no question that blocking factors exist in some systems (26), but whether they are antibodies or antigen-antibody complexes is not clear, and will have to be determined in each system.

MISCELLANEOUS

This review has outlined some of the recent concepts and current problems in cellular immunology. It has not even mentioned large areas which are nonetheless fascinating in spite of their omission at this point (they will be covered later on in the Symposium). I mean concepts of thymic hormones and stimuli to cell differentiation as well as transfer factor. Also it is being increasingly recognized that the entire lymphoid system is mobile, and that antigens and mitogens not only move receptors around on cell surfaces but that alterations of cell surfaces may change the migration patterns of cells (38,39).

There is much to be done.

REFERENCES

(1) D.H. Katz and B. Benacerraf. Adv. Immunol. 15 (1972) 1.

(2) N.L. Warner. Adv. Immunol. 19 (1974) 67.

(3) M.F. Greaves, J.J.T. Owen, and M.D. Raff. T and B Lymphocytes. (American Elsevier, N.Y., 1973).

(4) J.L. Claflin, R. Lieberman and J.M. Davie. J. Exp. Med. 139 (1974) 58.

(5) E.R. Unanue and K.A. Ault, in: Immunological Tolerance, ed. D.H. Katz and B. Benacerraf. (Academic Press, N.Y., 1974) p. 301.

(6) A. Basten, J.F.A.P. Miller, N.L. Warner and J. Pye, Nature New Biol. 231 (1971) 104.

(7) E.S. Vitetta, C. Bianco, V. Nussenzweig and J.W. Uhr. J. Exp. Med. 136 (1972) 81.

(8) J.J. Marchalonis, J.L. Atwell and R.E. Cone. J. Exp. Med. 135 (1972) 956.

(9) V. Santana, N. Wedderburn and J.L. Turk. Immunol. 27 (1974) 65.

(10) J.F.A.P. Miller. Ann. N.Y. Acad. Sci. (in press).

(11) S.F. Schlossman. Transpl. Rev. 10 (1972) 97.

(12) S.S. Alkan, E.B. Williams, D.E. Nitecki and J.W. Goodman. J. Exp. Med. 135 (1972) 1228.

(13) C.A. Janeway, Jr. Personal Communication.

(14) E.R. Unanue. Adv. Immunol. 15 (1972) 95.

(15) J.A. Waldron, Jr., R.G. Horn and A.S. Rosenthal. J. Immunol. 111 (1972) 58.

(16) E.M. Shevach and A.S. Rosenthal. J. Exp. Med. 139 (1974).

(17) M. Feldmann and A. Basten. Nature New Biol. 237 (1972) 13.

(18) D.H. Katz, W. Paul, E.A. Goidl, and B. Benacerraf. J. Exp. Med. 133 (1971) 169.

(19) J.R. Schmidtke and F.J. Dixon. J. Exp. Med. 136 (1972) 392.

(20) R.M. Gorczynski, R.G. Miller and R.A. Phillips J. Immunol. 110 (1973).

(21) M. Feldmann, R.E. Cone and J.J. Marchalonis. Cell. Immunol, 9(1973) 1.

(22) D.W. Dresser. Immunol. 5 (1962) 378.

(23) H.N. Claman. J. Immunol. 91 (1963) 833.

(24) P. Bretscher and M. Cohn. Science. 169 (1970) 1042.

(25) A. Coutinho and G. Möller. Eur. J. Immunol. 3 (1973) 608.

(26) J.G. Howard. Immunological Tolerance and Immunosuppression . in: M.T.P. International Review of Science, Biochemistry Series One, Vol. 10. Defense and Recognition. Ed. R.R. Porter. (University Park Press, Baltimore) p. 103.

(27) C.R. Parish and F.Y. Liew. J. Exp. Med. 135 (1972) 298.

(28) W.O. Weigle, J.M. Chiller and J. Louis. Transpl. Proc. 4 (1972) 372.

(29) H.N. Claman and D.W. Talmage. Science. 141 (1963) 1193.

(30) R.K. Gershon and K. Kondo. Immunology 21 (1971) 437.

(31) G.L. Asherson and M. Zembala. Proc. Royal Soc (B) 187 (1974) 329.

(32) P. Phanuphak, J.W. Moorhead and H.N. Claman. J. Immunol. 113 (1974) 1230.

(33) J.A. Kapp, C.W. Pierce, S. Schlossman and B Benacerraf. J. Exp. Med. 140 (1974) 648.

(34) D.W. Talmage. Personal Communication

(34a) T. Tada in ref. 5, p. 471.

(35) E. Diener and M. Feldmann. Transpl. Rev. 8 (1972) 76.

(36) M. Aldo-Benson and Y. Borel. J. Immunol. 112 (1974) 1793.

(37) Discussion in D.H. Katz and B. Benacerraf, eds. Immunological Tolerance, (Academic Press New York, 1974) p. 343.

(38) J.J. Woodruff. Cell. Immunol. 13(1974) 378.

(39) A. Bernstein and A. Globerson. Cell. Immunol. 14 (1974) 171.

DISCUSSION

W. THILLY: I question the experiment in which spleenic lymphocytes were exposed to high specific activiity ^{3}H-thymidine. You concluded that, since clone forming ability was reduced by 50% in a one hour exposure, 50% of the cells must be in the division cycle. I suggest that such levels of ^{3}H-thymidine may create a condition toxic to cells whether they are cycling or not. Secondly, were 50% of the spleenic lymphocytes actually in S-phase then their mass would be doubling in about sixteen hours, unless large numbers of apparently healthy, dividing lymphocytes are leaving the body. Margarita Krause examined this question of ^{3}H-thymidine effects and found that high concentrations induced a tritium uptake not associated with replicative DNA synthesis. On another level, Pelc has interpreted the results of a series of in vivo auto-radiographic studies to indicate a spontaneous degradation and resynthesis of DNA that is not related to division cycling (metabolic DNA).

H.N. CLAMAN: The experiment shows that cells exposed to thymidine suicide do not give strong PHA stimulation, but the same population gives increased GVH. This is odd and suggests that cells which suppress GVH reactions are cycling.

R.W. LONGTON: Have you noticed any association between molecular size and charge in the T- and B-cell mitogenesis?

H. N. CLAMAN:That is a good question but I have not done any work in that area. I will be delighted if somebody else will comment. Are the T- or B-cells dependent on molecular size or charge for mitogenesis?

R.W. LONGTON: At the Naval Medical Research Institute, Dr. Knudsen, Dr. Sell and I have preliminary evidence that the T-cell mitogen is a large polyanionic mitogen whereas the small molecular weight and perhaps cationic molecule will stimulate the B-cells.

E. A.KABAT: I don't think there is a real difference between the size of the determinants for cell mediated immunity and for antibody formation. The determinant of Leskowitz's arsenilic acid azomonotyrosine is quite small and it produces only cell mediated immunity. Also, Joel Goodman's data on glucagon, in which the first half of the molecule gives immediate hypersensitivity and the second half gives cell mediated immunity, again shows a similar size range. I think that the problem is that when you are dealing with various determinants in proteins you really don't know what the determinants are, and there is a tendency to think that things are bigger than they actually are.

H.N. CLAMAN: I can't disagree with you. You are giving us the two most common examples of very low molecular weight antigens which seem to be able to stimulate T-cells instead of B-cells. Whether they are exceptions or critical experiments indicating the real size of the antigen determinants for T- and B-cells, cannot be definitely stated right now.

E.W.LAMON: The scheme you just drew on the board (that is, that B-cells could be the initial antigen receptor cell) could work if a T-cell subpopulation had receptors for IgM when it is complexed to antigen, since the initial IgM response by B-cells is largely thymus independent. Recently in our laboratory we have found that unprimed thymocytes have IgM-complex receptor There are 10-15% IgM-complex receptor bearing cells in normal thymi. Furthermore, tumor specific IgM coated on tumor cells will induce normal thymus cells to be cytotoxic. We haven't yet tested for helper-functions but I think these are things that have to be kept in mind in the interpretation of all these experiments.

H.N. CLAMAN: Yes, that could fit this scheme. The B-cell might be triggered a little without any T-cell function. The IgM then may activate the T-cell which activates other B-cells or perhaps switch B-cells from IgM to IgG production. This would fit a B-cell→ T-cell → B-cell sequence.

C. BELL: Are you assuming then that T-independent antigens activate B-cells directly to produce IgM which may adsorb onto T-cells which then, in turn, will activate more B-cells? In other words the products of B-cells may later immunoregulate their further biosynthetic products? If so, how in your model do T-cells play an immunosuppressive role on the response of B-cells to T-independent antigens? Do you envisage the existence of T-cells?

H.N. CLAMAN: Suppression may depend upon the way in which the cells are activated.

RECOGNITION OF ANTIGEN BY T LYMPHOCYTES

G.E. ROELANTS
Basel Institute for Immunology

It is generally accepted that lymphocytes are pre-committed to interact with one antigenic determinant. The hypothesis put forward to explain how a predetermined clone of lymphocytes recognizes its corresponding epitope was that the cells bear at their surface, as receptor, a sample of the immunoglobulin they will produce after activation (1). The demonstration of surface Ig of restricted specificity on precursors of antibody secreting cells ("B lymphocytes") supported this hypothesis (2-6).

Surface Ig is not detected on another major type of lymphocyte ("T lymphocytes") involved not in antibody secretion, but in various aspects of cellular immunity, by methods which easily detect Ig on B lymphocytes (7). For this and other reasons discussed below, it was suggested that the mode of antigenic recognition of T cells was completely different from that of B cells (8). In the present paper I would like to briefly discuss the heretofore available experimental evidence and conclude that this is not the case. Indeed:

a) T lymphocytes also are precommitted and have specific receptors for antigen

b) T lymphocytes also have a high power of discrimination i.e. specificity, comparable to that of B lymphocytes

c) The T receptor is also of immunoglobulin nature although it could represent a new Ig class.

Moreover, it will be evident that binding of antigen to the surface receptor is not sufficient to activate the cell. Activation mechanisms are far more complex and not understood but some in vitro correlates of T cell functions appear to be blocked by perturbing the membrane distribution of surface antigens controlled by the main histocompatibility region.

The data selected are by no means exhaustive but try to present a fair cross section of various viewpoints.

A. ANTIGEN BINDING T LYMPHOCYTES

Antigen binding lymphocytes can readily be visualized by a variety of techniques (reviewed in 3-6), the most commonly used being immunocytoadherence detecting "rosette forming cells" (RFC) and autoradiography detecting radioactive "antigen binding cells" (ABC). The mere existence of antigen binding T lymphocytes was at some point controversial mainly for technical reasons e.g. the greater fragility of T-RFC (9) or the greater antigen concentration dependence of T-ABC (10). The presence of RFC or ABC in lymphoid populations greatly enriched in T lymphocytes or their depletion in populations deprived of T lymphocytes gave strong support for the existence of T antigen binding cells (reviewed in 3-6, 11). More recently the formal demonstration of antigen binding T lymphocytes was provided by the immunofluorescent detection of the Thy-1 (θ) antigen — a surface marker of T lymphocytes absent on B lymphocytes (7) — on ABC (12) and RFC (13).

Among others T antigen binding cells have been demonstrated for particulate antigen: erythrocytes (11,13-14), proteins: Maia Squinado haemocyanin (12), fowl γ-globulin (15), horse γ-globulin, keyhole limpet haemocyanin, bovine serum albumin (Roelants, unpublished), synthetic polypeptides: native and heavily iodinated (Tyr, Glu)-Ala--Lys (10,12,16,17), Tyr-Glu (18), and small molecular weight haptens: NNP (19,20), DNP, TNP, NIP, NAP, ABA (21 and Roelants, unpublished).

When studied under saturating antigen concentration T-ABC are shown to have as many receptors for antigen as B-ABC (up to about 50,000/cell) (Fig. 1) (10). The low frequency of antigen specific T binding cells (in the order of 200 x 10^{-6}) in any given lymphocyte population and the presence of large numbers of receptors with identical specificity on a single cell demonstrate the antigen commitment of T lymphocytes.

The effect of antigen dilutions below saturation levels on the label density (Fig. 1) is far more pronounced for T-than B-ABC indicating that the apparent avidity of T lymphocytes for antigen is lower (10). It does not necessarily follow that T receptors are of lower affinity, it may reflect a different disposition of the T receptor in the cell membrane.

Analysis of regression of B- and T- ABC frequencies at antigen concentrations below the saturation level (10) as well as hapten inhibition of RFC to NNP (19,20) show that the avidity of B cells, but not of T cells, increases after priming (Fig. 2). This increase appears to be due not only to selection of B cells with higher affinity receptors but also to maturation of cells acquiring a larger number of receptors (10).

By analogy with the specific suppression of the B cell antibody response by exposure of lymphocytes suspensions to radioactive antigen of high specific activity (22,23), the relevance of T-ABC to the immune response was demonstrated by showing that T lymphocyte functions could also be specifically "suicided" by ^{125}I-antigen in both unprimed and primed situations (24-26). This confirms the antigen commitment of T lymphocytes and shows that the study of the antigen binding moiety on the specific T-ABC discussed so far is relevant to the problem of functional T lymphocytes receptors.

B. SPECIFICITY AND DICTIONARY OF T LYMPHOCYTES

Having shown that T lymphocytes are antigen specific, I now would like to establish (a) that the discriminatory power i.e. the specificity of the T receptor is as refined as that of the B receptors and (b) that the dictionaries of recognition of T and B lymphocytes are largely similar. However, some determinants or some forms of presentation activate preferentially one or the other cell class.

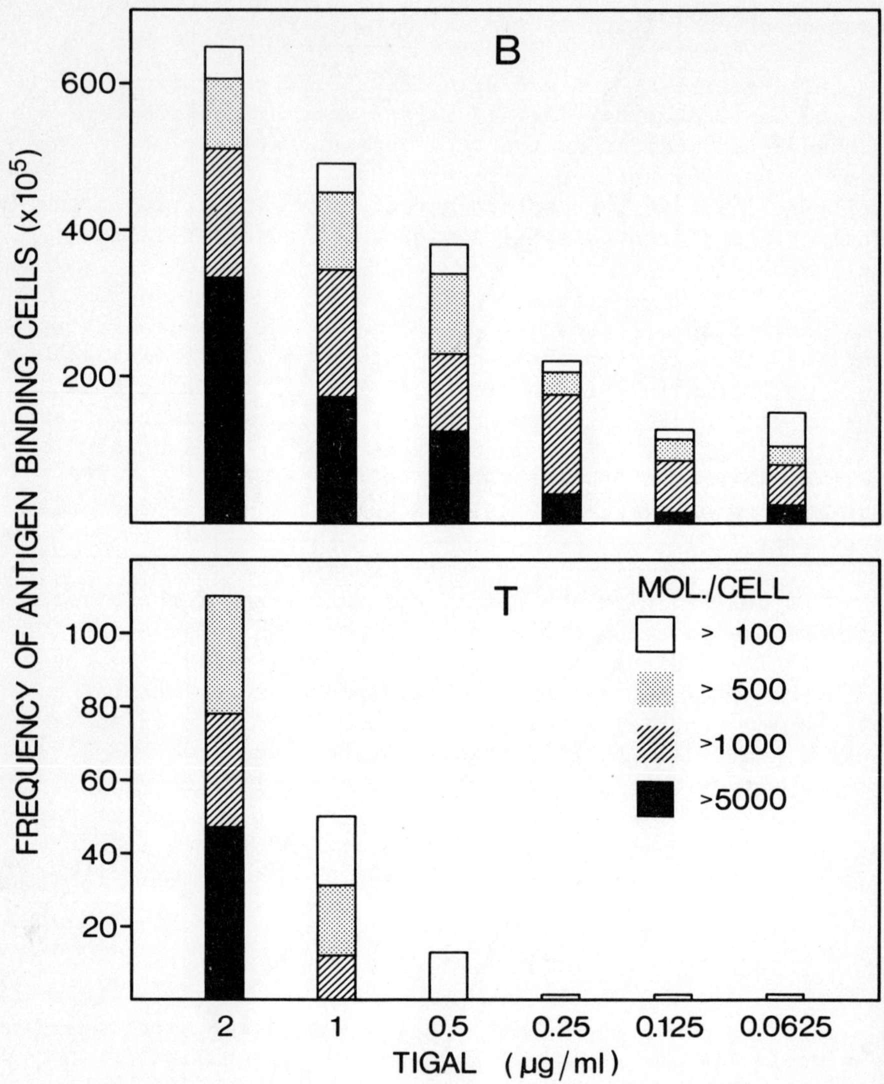

Fig. 1. Degree of labelling of TIGAL-primed (a) B-ABC and (b) T-ABC at various antigen doses. With permission from Nature.

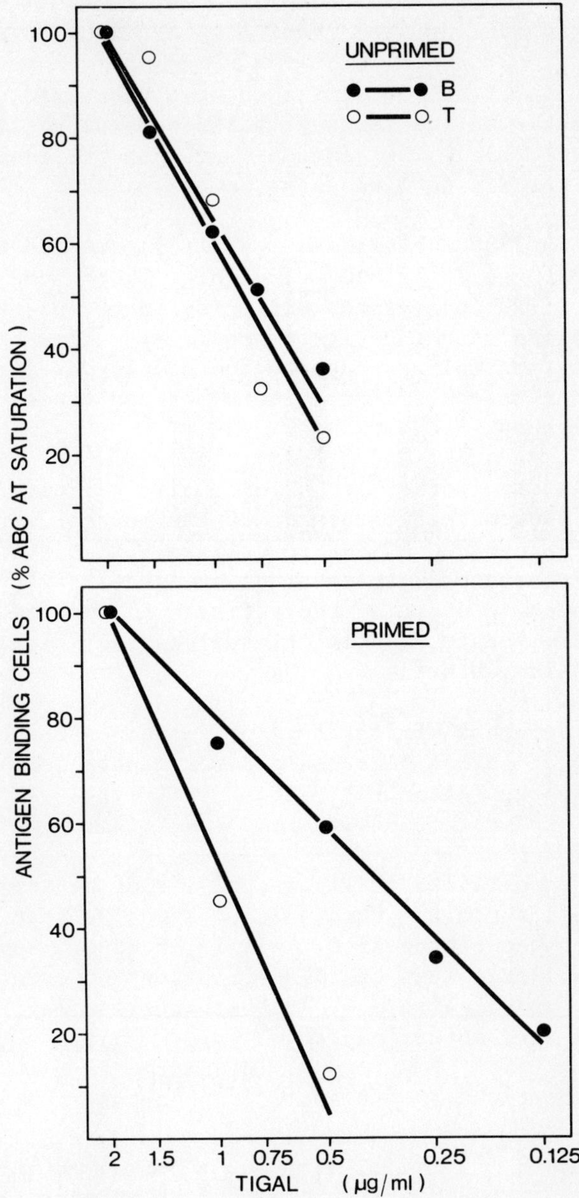

Fig. 2. Titration of (a) normal and (b) TIGAL primed ABC at antigen doses below the plateau level. ●---● B, o---o T lymphocytes. With permission from Nature.

(a) Specificity studies with chemically defined determinants

Chemically defined determinants have been used extensively to characterize the immunoglobulin combining site (reviewed in 27,28). The same approach has provided the most salient results on T receptor specificity.

Already in 1969 Schlossman et al. (29) studied the proliferative response of primed guinea-pigs lymph node cells to a series of DNP-nonalysines differing in the position of the DNP group and of one D- lysine residue. They show that there was maximal response to the homologous immunogen, thus T lymphocytes could discriminate between those very subtle differences.

Goodman and co-workers in an extensive series of experiments (30), showed that compounds of the general structure L-tyrosine-p-azobenzene-R induced cellular immunity in guinea-pig. There was little or no cross-reactivity between compounds containing the radicals R: arsonate, carboxylate, sulfonate, acetamide, sulfonamide, nitro- or trimethylammonium chloride.

Using a somewhat similar type of immunogen Becker et al. (31), found that guinea-pigs could discriminate between p-azobenzenearsonate (ABA)-L-Tyr, ABA-Tyr $(L\text{-}Tyr)_3$, ABA-L-Tyr $(L\text{-}Ala)_3$ and $(L\text{-}Tyr)_3$ ABA-L-Tyr.

Studies on detailed chemical analysis of determinants inducing T cell functions remain less extensive than those on the antibody combining site. It is, however, apparent from those available that the discriminatory power of B and T lymphocytes is comparable. Another question is if they recognize the same determinants.

(b) Compared dictionary of B and T lymphocytes

Rajewsky and co-workers (32,33) studied in great detail the cross-induction and cross-tolerance of various albumins at the level of B and T lymphocytes, both primed and unprimed. They concluded that B and T cells have the same highly refined specificity, recognize the same determinants and have the same system of antigen binding receptors.

On the other hand, when cross-reactivity was examined at the B and T level in other systems e.g. lysozyme and carboxymethyl-lysozyme (34), flagellin and acetoacetylated derivatives (35), flagellins of various serological specificities (26), native and methylated BSA (36) it appeared that the T cell specificity is not as refined and is different from B cells.

Investigations using better defined antigens of characterized structure lead to similar conclusions. Bovine glucagon, a polypeptide of 29 amino acids, is immunogenic in guinea-pig (37). Using tryptic and synthetic peptides, a functional dissection of the immunogen was demonstrated into an amino-terminal part against which most antibody was elicited and a carboxy-terminal part mainly responsible for cellular immunity reactions. Poly-γ-D-glutamic acid (MW 35,000) is unable to elicit cellular immunity reactions but will elicit antibody production when coupled to an appropriate carrier molecule (38,39). Conversely L- tyrosine-p-azobenzene-arsonate (RAT) and analogues elicit by themselves only delayed hypersensitivity reactions (30). Conjugates of poly-γ-D-glutamic acid and RAT will again elicit antibody to the former and cellular immunity to the latter (40). The same type of result was obtained using small bifunctional molecules e.g. DNP-6 amino-caproic acid - RAT (30). Cellular immunity is induced to RAT, antibody to DNP. This can be compared to the well established hapten-carrier dichotomy (41,42).

(c) Discussion: Fundamental distinction between binding and activation

The latest results could be interpreted to show a distinction between B and T determinants and a difference in the B and T recognition units. However, on closer analysis, they do not bear on the B and T receptors combining sites at all but on the activation of B and T lymphocytes, which is obviously a far more elaborated process. Already in the case of lectins it was clearly demonstrated that binding does not necessarily lead to activation (43). Concanavalin A (Con A) and phytohemaglutinin (PHA) bind equally well to B and T lymphocytes but activate only the latter. However, B lymphocytes are stimulated by those lectins on a solid surface.

Thus what those experiments really show is that antigenic determinants presented to the cells in a certain way may trigger preferentially B or T lymphocytes, presented in another way they may act differently. Indeed, the functional dichotomy of glucagon is not absolute: some antibody is directed against the carboxyterminal part, the aminoterminal part induces some cellular reactions (37). When glucagon is conjugated to a carrier, good antibody is produced against both moieties and delayed hypersensitivity is not elicited (44). In the RAT system anti-ABA antibody is obtained by ABA conjugated to tyrosine residues of proteins or even by a small bifunctional molecule containing two RAT residues separated by a rigid spacer: RAT-$(pro)_{10}$-RAT (30,45). Thus in the situations described earlier B or T cells able to recognize a given determinant were not missing, they were just not activated under the conditions used. This is confirmed in the RAT system by the demonstration of both B- and T-ABC (Goodman and Roelants, unpublished).

Likewise, we saw in section A that T cells binding conventional haptens can be demonstrated. Helper activity by those haptens was reported (46) as well as various other T functions when these haptens are administered to the animal conjugated to mycobacteria (28,47,48) showing again that both B and T cells specific for a given determinant are present but that the mode of administration of that determinant activates preferentially one or the other.

(d) Conclusion

In conclusion of this section it appears that T receptors have the same discriminatory power and the same dictionary i.e. the same range of specificity than B receptors. This argues strongly "a priori" but does not prove their identical nature. We will see that this problem, treated in the next section, has also been confused by the lack of distinction between binding (= initial recognition) and activation or inactivation (= induction or tolerance).

(e) Remark about evaluating cross-reactivity

As seen in subsection (b) cross-reactivity at the T level is often reported broader than at the B level. However, B cross-reactions are often assayed with soluble antibody, not B cells, while assays on cellular T reactions involve the T cells themselves. The lattice of receptors on the T lymphocyte surface may stabilize low affinity binding due to weak cross-reactions; this is not the case for antibody in solution, hence the broader specificity of some T responses may be more apparent than real.

C. NATURE OF THE T LYMPHOCYTE RECEPTOR

The controversy about the nature of the T lymphocyte receptor is even ampler than the debate about B and T compared specificities. Two main concepts are opposed, either that the T receptor is immunoglobulin, may be of a new class, or that it is a molecule unrelated to immunoglobulin, coded in the main histocompatibility complex, possibly the histocompatibility antigens themselves or else the Ir-gene product. I will briefly discuss the main approaches on both sides and show that the two positions can be largely reconciled provided that here again one carefully makes the distinction between antigen binding and cell activation.

(a) The T lymphocyte receptor is immunoglobulin

Initial results on inhibition of antigen binding to T lymphocytes by anti-Ig reagents has been reviewed in detail (5,6). Although these results were variable depending on the antisera and assays used, a general trend emerged: binding of antigen to T cells can be inhibited by anti-κ sera and some anti-μ sera in mice. "Enriched" populations of T or B lymphocytes were used in these studies and any given antigen binding cell could only indirectly be characterized as a T cell.

Antigen binding T cells can be directly visualized using combined fluorescence and autoradiography techniques with fluorochrome conjugated anti-Thy 1 (θ) reagent (TRITC-AKR-IgG-α-θC3H) and ^{125}I-antigen (10,12). The influence of anti-Ig reagents on T-ABC characterized in this way was investigated using two parameters (a) the inhibition of antigen binding (b) the polar redistribution of receptors for antigen (12). It was found that binding of Maia squinado haemocyanin (MSH) and the heavily iodinated synthetic copolymer (Tyr, Glu)-Ala--Lys (TIGAL) was inhibited by pretreatment of the cells with the anti-Ig, anti-κ and anti-μ reagents used. Binding to T cells was more readily inhibited than to B cells. Furthermore, when lymphocytes were pretreated with subinhibiting concentrations of anti-Ig reagents, under conditions inducing B cells to display superimposed polar redistribution of fluorescent Ig and antigen grains, a comparable proportion of T cells also bound the antigen in a cap. This effect was not obtained when the anti-Ig reagent was used after absorption with a purified preparation of mouse Ig, different from the preparation that had been employed to raise the antiserum. The conclusion reached at that point was that the antigen binding moiety on the surface of both B and T lymphocytes is Ig.

A similar but modified approach was used to investigate whether the T Ig receptors were the synthetic product of the T lymphocytes themselves (49). The experimental procedure is described in Fig. 3. Normal lymph node lymphocytes are put in culture in "capping conditions" with subinhibitory doses of FITC-RIgG-α-MIg. Samples were taken after variable length of incubation and the receptors position on TIGAL specific cells revealed by incubation with ^{125}I-TIGAL in "non capping conditions". Some samples were also stained with TRITC-RIgG-α-MIg to reveal the Ig position on B cells; others with TRITC-AKR.IgG-α-θC3H to visualize T cells. The results are schematized in Fig. 4: 10 min after starting the culture the FITC-anti-Ig reagent has redistributed receptors in caps on both B and T cells. After 1 h. no receptors are left on either B nor T cells and no antigen is bound. Starting at 3 h. and completed between 6 and 18 h. there is a resynthesis of receptors on both cell types.

It is crucial for the interpretation of the experiment to realize that only lymph nodes of normal mice, not previously exposed to TIGAL, are used and that TIGAL is not present during the culture period. It is only used afterwards to reveal the position of the receptors and could not by itself induce any redistribution nor trigger TIGAL specific cells. From all this it would seem far-fetched that, in this normal lymph node cell population, rare T cells (frequency 23-43 x 10^{-5}) would bear at their surface enough passively adsorbed specific antibody to bind up to 50,000 molecules of TIGAL and even less likely that during the

Fig. 3. Basic experimental procedure (with permission from Nature).

(1) Normal lymph node cells in RPMI 1640 medium 0.03 M HEPES, 10% foetal calf serum (FCS), 2 mM glutamin, penicillin streptomycin, pH 7.2.

+ FITC-RIgG-α-MIgG 250 μg ml^{-1} + FITC-RIgG-α-TMV (control) 250 μg ml^{-1}

0^oC, 10 min) 50 x 10^6 cells ml^{-1},
37^oC, 50 min) medium without NaN_3

wash 3 x

(2) (Optional) + Sser-α-RL
1/40 final dilution
37^oC, 15 min, 50 x 10^6 cells ml^{-1},
medium without NaN_3

wash 3 x

(3) Incubate at 37^oC, for variable lengths of time, 0.5 x 10^6 cells ml^{-1}, medium without NaN_3, 4 ml in Falcon Tissue Culture Flasks 3012.

wash 2 x in medium with NaN_3 (1.5 mM
0^oC.

(4) + ^{125}I-TICAL (200-468 μCi μg^{-1}) 2.5 μg 25 x 10^6 cells ml^{-1}

0^oC, 30 min, medium with NaN_3 (1.5 mM)

wash through FCS gradients

(5) + TRITC-RIgG-α-MIgG 250 μg ml^{-1} + TRITC-anti-θ 250 μg ml^{-1}

0^oC 30 min
50 x 10^6 cells ml^{-1}
medium with NaN_3 (1.5 mM)

(6) Wash 3 x, smear on gelatine coated slides, fix in absolute ethanol (5 min), process for autoradiography (Ilford K5 emulsion).

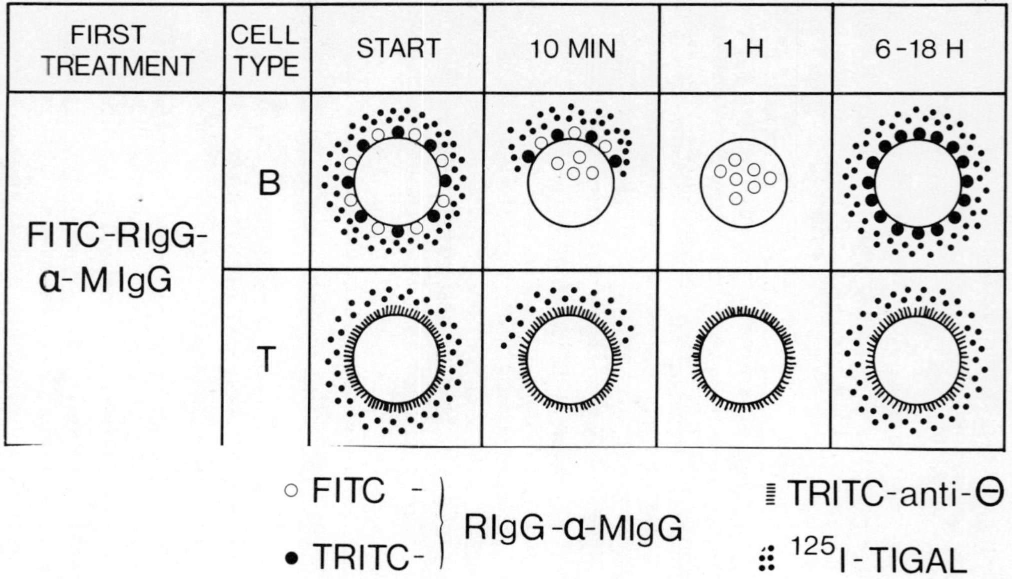

FIRST TREATMENT	CELL TYPE	START	10 MIN	1 H	6-18 H
FITC-RIgG-α-M IgG	B				
	T				

○ FITC - } RIgG-α-MIgG
● TRITC- }

TRITC-anti-Θ

^{125}I-TIGAL

Fig. 4. Capping and resynthesis of Ig receptors for antigen on T and B lymphocytes. For experimental protocol see Fig. 3 and text. With permission from Nature.

in vitro incubation after capping, TIGAL specific B cells (frequency 54 to 108 x 10^{-5}) would have been triggered, in the absence of antigen, to secrete enough anti-TIGAL antibody which would bind only to those rare T-ABC to bring their number back to their initial level. To ascertain that the resynthesized receptors were indeed Ig the cells were treated again with FITC-RIgG-α-MIg and another round of capping, disappearance and resynthesis achieved.

In my opinion these experiments demonstrate the Ig nature of the receptor for antigen on T lymphocytes and also that those receptors are the active product of the T cells themselves.

One can't help but wonder why T cell receptors are not readily detected by immunofluorescence. It should be noted that this problem remains, whether the receptor is Ig or not and does not really pertain to it. Indeed in the experiment just described, T cells are not stained by FITC-RIgG-α-MIg. If one would hold the position that it is a contaminant "anti T receptor" antibody and not anti-Ig which was active on T cells in this preparation, the fact remains that this contaminant FITC conjugated antibody does not stain T cells either. Several possible explanations of this paradox have been discussed in detail (50). It becomes more and more apparent that the most likely one is the different relationship of T and B receptors between themselves and toward other membrane constituents under physiological conditions. This area requires further investigation.

The final answer to this problem depends of course on the biochemical isolation and characterization of T receptors. Reports from several laboratories (51-54) indicate that an immunoglobulin molecule, slightly different from known Igs, can be isolated from T lymphocytes; however, other laboratories have reported their inability to do so (55,56, R.M.E. Parkhouse, personal communication). This is not so surprising considering that the technical conditions required appear to be extremely rigorous and that the different groups do not use exactly the same procedures. Biochemical characterization of IgT still requires the elaboration of an easily reproducible isolation technique.

(b) Blockade of T lymphocyte activation by anti-histocompatibility antisera

Based mainly on the difficulty to find Ig on T lymphocytes and on the discovery and characteristics of immune response (Ir) genes (57) it was suggested that the T receptor is not Ig but the Ir gene product (8,58). The initial finding that some T cell functions could be inhibited by anti-histocompatibility antisera gave some support to this view (allo-antisera prepared by injecting ground lymphoid cells in Freund's adjuvant could contain anti Ir gene products as well as many other specificities). Alternatively they could mean that histocompatibility antigens themselves are involved in antigen recognition.

Thus Shevach *et al.* (59,60) using Ir controlled responses to synthetic copolymers in guinea-pigs, reported that the antigen induced lymphocyte proliferation and macrophage migration inhibitory factor production by sensitized cells from responder guinea-pigs could be abolished by alloantisera. Geczy and de Weck reported similar observations (61). The results obtained in F_1 hybrids first appeared of particular interest: alloantisera raised against one of the parents inhibited, in the hybrid, mainly the antigen response controlled by the Ir gene of that parent. However, the proliferative response to an antigen controlled by the Ir gene of the other parent, or even to an unrelated antigen or to PHA, as well as background thymidine incorporation were also reduced and it was later shown (62) that the apparent specificity for strain associated immune responses was dependent on the concentration of antiserum used.

Further investigations in outbred and backcrosses of strain 2 and 13 guinea-pigs, where responsiveness controlled by Ir and histocompatibility type were dissociated, showed that the inhibitory activity of alloantisera was directed against the histocompatibility antigens and not Ir products (62-64). For example the response of sensitized responder lymphoid cells lacking strain 2 histocompatibility antigens was not inhibited by 13- anti-2 serum.

Keeping in mind the discussion, in the preceeding section, of the difference between binding and activation, it is apparent that these studies bear on the activation of primed T cells by antigen and not directly on the primary recognition i.e. the binding of antigenic determinants by T lymphocytes. This is confirmed by a recent report of Bluestein (65) showing that inhibition by alloantisera in the system described above requires bivalent antibody, suggesting the necessity for redistribution of membrane components rather than simple steric hindrance, and quite significantly that the alloantiserum is still active when added to the cells several hours after the antigen.

These results do not compel one to postulate a new type of specific receptors, with the difficult theoretical problems it introduces about a new generation of diversity; indeed they are not contradictory with the evidence presented in subsection (a) that the T receptor is Ig, but only show that anti-histocompatibility antisera inhibit some *in vitro* T lymphocyte activity.

This conclusion is amply supported by autoradiography studies of T-ABC. In guinea-pigs T lymphocytes of strain 2 (non-responder), strain 13 (responder) and F_1 hybrids (responders) bind Glu-Tyr copolymer equally well (18). In mice there is no difference in B- and T-ABC for (Tyr, Glu)-Ala--Lys in high and low responder strains at saturation (66) and even below saturating concentrations of antigen (17). Upon priming the frequency of ABC increase only in the high responder strain (17) indicating again a control at the level of activation not binding.

(c) Molecular mechanisms of activation

The mechanisms of lymphocyte activation are still obscure. No clear direct data on the molecular phenomenon accompanying the process of lymphocyte stimulation by antigen are available to date. Loor discussed in detail why conclusions based on analogies with stimulation by lectins have to be taken with great caution (43). In this respect it should be remembered that triggering of the unfecondated zygote by a variety of methods leads to division and aberrant differentiation which were studied in great detail but had finally nothing to do with the events following true fecondation.

One fact is, however, quite apparent: antigen binding is only a first step, certainly not sufficient for cell activation. In addition to the examples given earlier it is interesting that T lineage lymphocytes (probably pre-thymic T precursors) in nude and T deprived mice bind antigen but appear to lack the capacity to be activated (50, 67-70).

D GENERAL CONCLUSION

The present paper is an attempt to analyse and reconcile the available conflicting data on T lymphocytes receptors. Provided one carefully distinguish the analysis of antigen binding to receptors from that of cell activation it appears convincingly, at least to me, that T lymphocytes recognize and bind antigen via an Ig receptor and that this initiates but is by no means sufficient for cell activation. The exact nature of this Ig and its relationship to known Ig classes both in structure and in phylogenetic apparition is still a matter of conjecture.

REFERENCES

(1) N.A. Mitchison, in: Differentiation and Immunology ed. K.B. Warren, (Academic Press, New York and London, 1968). p. 729.

(2) B. Pernis, M. Ferrarini, L. Forni and L. Amante, Progress Immunol. 1 (1971) 95.

(3) G. L. Ada, Transplant. Rev. 5 (1970) 105.

(4) D. Sulitzeanu, C.T. Microbiol. Immunol. 54 (1971). 1.

(5) G. E. Roelants, C. T. Microbiol. Immunol. 59 (1972) 135.

(6) N.L. Warner, Adv. Immunol. 19 (1974) 67.

(7) M. C. Raff, Transplant. Rev. 6 (1971) 52.

(8) B. Benacerraf and H. O. McDevitt, Science 175 (1972) 273

(9) J. Charreire, M. Dardenne and J-F. Bach, Cell. Immunol. 9 (1973) 32.

(10) G. E. Roelants and A. Rydén, Nature 247 (1974) 104.

(11) M.F. Greaves, Transplant. Rev. 5 (1970) 45

(12) G. E. Roelants, L. Forni and B. Pernis, J. Exp. Med. 137 (1973) 1060.

(13) R. F. Ashman and M.C. Raff, J. Exp. Med. 137 (1973) 69.

(14) J. S. Haskill, B. E. Elliott, R. Kerbel, M.A. Axelrad and D. Eidinger, J. Exp. Med. 135 (1972) 1410.

(15) A. D. Bankhurst and J.D. Wilson, Nature New Biol. 234 (1971) 154.

(16) G. J. Hämmerling and H.O. McDevitt, J. Immunol. 112 (1974) 1726.

(17) G.J. Hämmerling and H.O. McDevitt, J. Exp. Med. 140 (1974) 1180.

(18) G.E. Roelants, reported in the Basel Institute for Immunology, Annual Report (1973) 52.

(19) E. Möller, W.W. Bullock and O. Mäkelä, Eur. J. Immunol. 3 (1973) 172.

(20) E. Smith, L. Hammarström and E. Möller, Scand. J. Immunol. 3 (1974) 61.

(21) L. Polak, A. Rydén and G.E. Roelants, Immunology, in press.

(22) G.L. Ada and P. Byrt, Nature 222 (1969) 1291.

(23) J.H. Humphrey and H.U. Keller, in: Developmental aspects of antibody formation and structure. eds. J. Sterzl and I. Riha, (Publ. House of the Czechoslovak Acad. Sci. Prague, 1970) 485.

(24) A. Basten, J.F.A.P. Miller, N.L. Warner and J. Pye, Nature New Biol. 231 (1971) 104.

(25) G.E. Roelants and B.A. Askonas, Eur. J. Immunol. 1 (1971) 151.

(26) M.G. Cooper and G.L. Ada, Scand. J. Immunol. 1 (1972) 247.

(27) J.W. Goodman, Immunochemistry 6 (1969) 139.

(28) J.W. Goodman, in: The antigens. eds. M. Sela (Academic Press, New York and London) in press.

(29) S.F. Schlossman, J. Herman and A. Yaron, J. Exp. Med. 130 (1969) 1031.

(30) S.S. Alkan, E.B. Williams, D.E. Nitecki and J.W. Goodman, J. Exp. Med. 135 (1972) 1228.

(31) M.J. Becker, H. Levin and M. Sela, Eur. J. Immunol. 3 (1973) 131.

(32) K. Rajewsky and H. Pohlit, Progress in Immunology 1 (1971) 337.

(33) K. Rajewsky and R. Mohr, Eur. J. Immunol. 4 (1974) 112.

(34) K. Thompson, M. Harris, E. Benjamini, G. Mitchell and M. Noble, Nature New Biol. 238 (1972) 20.

(35) C.R. Parish, J. Exp. Med. 134 (1971) 21.

(36) V. Schirrmacher and H. Wigzell, J. Exp. Med. 136 (1972) 1616.

(37) G. Senyk, B. Williams, D.E. Nitecki and J.W. Goodman, J. Exp. Med. 133 (1971) 1294.

(38) J.W. Goodman and D.E. Nitecki, Immunology 13 (1967) 577

(39) G.E. Roelants, G. Senyk and J.W. Goodman, Israel J. Med. Sci. 5 (1969) 196.

(40) S.S. Alkan, D.E. Nitecki and J.W. Goodman, J. Immunol. 107 (1971) 353.

(41) N.A. Mitchison, Eur. J. Immunol. 1 (1971) 10.

(42) N.A. Mitchison, Eur. J. Immunol. 1 (1971) 18.

(43) F. Loor, Eur. J. Immunol. 4 (1974) 210.

(44) G. Senyk, D.E. Nitecki, L. Spitler and J.W. Goodman, Immunochemistry 9 (1972) 97.

(45) M.E. Bush, S.S. Alkan, D.E. Nitecki and J.W. Goodman, J. Exp. Med. 136 (1972) 1478.

(46) R.B. Taylor and G.M. Iverson, Proc. Roy. Soc. (London) Ser. B. 176 (1971) 393.

(47) B. Benacerraf and P.G.H. Gell, Immunology 2 (1959) 219.

(48) P. Trefts, S.S. Alkan, H.S. Koren, D.E. Nitecki, J.W. Goodman and R.I. Mishell, manuscript in preparation.

(49) G.E. Roelants, A. Rydén, L-B. Hägg and F. Loor, Nature 247 (1974) 106.

(50) F. Loor and G.E. Roelants, in: The immune system. Genes, receptors, signals. eds. E.E. Sercarz, A.R. Williamson and C.F. Fox. (Academic Press, New York and London, 1974) 201.

(51) J.J. Marchalonis and R.E. Cone, Transpl. Rev. 14 (1973) 3.

(52) J.J. Marchalonis, in: The immune system. Genes, receptors, signals. eds. E.E. Sercarz, A.R. Williamson and C.F. Fox. (Academic Press, New York and London, 1974) 141.

(53) R.E. Cone, ibid. (1974) 217.

(54) C. Moroz and N. Lahat. ibid (1974) 233.

(55) E.S. Vitetta and J.W. Uhr, Transpl. Rev. 14 (1973) 50.

(56) H.M . Grey, R.T. Kubo and J-C. Cerottini, J. Exp. Med. 136 (1972) 1323.

(57) H.O. McDevitt and B. Benacerraf, Adv. Immunol. 11 (1969) 31.

(58) H.O. McDevitt and M. Landy.(eds.). Genetic control of immune responsiveness. (Academic Press, New York and London, 1972).

(59) E.M. Shevach, W.E. Paul and I. Green, J. Exp. Med. 136 (1972) 1207.

(60) S.Z. Ben-Sasson, E.M. Shevach, I. Green and W.E. Paul, J. Exp. Med. 140 (1974) 383.

(61) A.F. Geczy and A.L. de Weck, Eur. J. Immunol. 4 (1974) 483.

(62) H.G. Bluestein, J. Immunol. 113 (1974) 1410.

(63) E.M. Shevach, W.E. Paul and I. Green, J. Exp. Med. 139 (1974) 661.

(64) E.M. Shevach, I. Green and W.E. Paul, J. Exp. Med. 139 (1974) 679.

(65) H.G. Bluestein, J. Exp. Med. 140 (1974) 481.

(66) G.E. Roelants, reported in the Basel Institute for Immunology Annual Report (1973) 53.

(67) F. Loor and G.E. Roelants, Nature 251 (1974) 229.

(68) F. Loor and G.E. Roelants, Ann. N.Y. Acad. Sci., in press.

(69) G.E. Roelants, F. Loor, H. von Boehmer, J. Sprent, L-B. Hägg, K.S. Mayor and A. Rydén, Eur. J. Immunol, in press.

(70) G.E. Roelants, K.S. Mayor, L-B. Hägg and F. Loor, submitted.

DISCUSSION

L. HERZENBERG: Dr. Roelants that was a very fine presentation of one particular point of view. Would you agree with the idea, that antigen binding T-cells are relevent to the immune response as helpers, is based essentially on very indirect evidence derived from the deletion of biological activity by antigen binding suicide experiments.

G. ROELANTS: Yes, that is right.

L. HERZENBERG: This in my mind leaves things in a rather unsatisfactory state because one has rather a complex system in which on one side activity is removed by putting in a very hot antigen,and on the other side, there is your evidence that T-cells do bind antigen, even in large amounts. It would be very nice if someone could tie the two together as has been done with B-cells. B-cells which bind antigen can be shown to be the precursors of antibody forming cells. The reverse has not been shown for T-cells, as I understand it.

G. ROELANTS: Important in those suicide experiments is that they are, of course, specific for the antigen. The addition of radioactive antigen to a lymphocyte suspension does not kill helper activity to all antigens. This indicates a relationship between the antigen binding cells, which are the only ones exposed to highly radioactive antigen and the specific deletion of a clone. Would it be possible to isolate the first type of cell in a pure form using your machine and then to show that it can be turned into an active cell?

L. HERZENBERG: Yes for B-cells but we are only now trying it for T-cells. Let me comment on what you said. I think that the key question at this point is whether the specific deletion of an activity is related to the production of some factor by the B-cells, that is where we know there is direct specificity. One deletes an activity when we refer to helpers T-cells. In the case of B-cells one deletes or enriches for clones, and that is indeed what we have done with our FACS machine.

In the experiment where you cap the receptor on T-cells with anti-immunoglobulin, as evidenced by the capping with radioactivity, and hen cap off and allow resynthesis of receptor, you emphasized that you find 50,000 molecules of antigen binding to some of those T-cells. Why is it not possible to show immunoglobulin directly by either fluorescent or anti-immunoglobulin in those cells.

G. ROELANTS: That is puzzling but one does not know if the receptor is immunoglobulin or something else, because when cells are first treated with anti-immunoglobulin reagent labelled with fluorescein, you do not see anything on the surface of T-cells whereas you do see something on the surface of B-cells. Thus, you do not see the immunoglobulin with your anti-immunoglobulin reagent but you do something to the receptor. If the reagent possessed an anti-receptor activity even though it is not immunoglobulin, the receptor would also be labelled because the anti-receptor antibody in the reagent would be labelled with fluorescein. The fact that the cells are negative for fluorescence is puzzling and probably has something to do with the structure of the T-cell membrane.

L. HERZENBERG: I think if that could be explained we might be closer to an answer. Since we have been bedazzled by overviews and more overviews, I would like to make one more point. I think the speaker has to remain puzzled and that it is good for the audience in this sort of a group also to remain puzzled with respect to the nature, number and characteristics of receptors on the cooperator and other immunologically functional T-cells. I point to one finding in the literature which does not fit anyone's party line, except for those who are interested in keeping people open minded until some definite evidence comes along. I refer to the experiments of Webb and Cooper (J. Immunol. 1974) in which antigen binding T-cells are not found in agammaglobulinemic chickens. In these birds, which do not make an antibody response, you do not find antigen binding T-cells,but if you inject these chickens with antibody, you do find antigen binding T-cells. The frequencies are similar to those in normal birds.

G. ROELANTS: Yes, there is about 3% of antigen binding cells, which is far higher than any specific cells you would expect. However, Cooper agrees that those cells have never been identified positively as T-cells.

R.K. GERSHON: You pointed out the importance of distinguishing recognition from a response. Many people try to measure recognition by determining if a response takes place. You showed very clearly that this is not valid, and this is also relevant to what Len Herzenberg was talking about. The question is whether all the antigen binding we see has anything to do with the receptor, if we think of the receptor as the site at which the cell is triggered. The B-cell has a lot of immunoglobulin on its surface which naturally is called the receptor, but does it follow that any of this immunoglobulin has anything to do with the triggering site? In one of your slides the major portion of the immunoglobulin was in a cap. On the side of the B-cell, where staining immunoglobulin could not be seen, there were a few grains demonstrating some antigen binding in the absence of immunoglobulin.

G. ROELANTS: Yes, but iodine goes on the side of the cells as well and the label is never only on top of the cell.

R. K. GERSHON: What do you think of possibility that the real receptors on the T-cell and on the B-cell are identical and that the only reason that a difference is seen in all the assays is that B-cells, because they produce immunoglobulin, have large amounts on their surface. This may have nothing to do with the triggering receptor. The same may be true of the passive immunoglobulin on T-cells. We should keep this possibility in mind.

G. ROELANTS: Yes, Francis Loor and myself have often discussed that possibility , but we have not dared to state it publicly.

THE LOGIC OF CELL INTERACTIONS IN DETERMINING IMMUNE RESPONSIVENESS

MELVIN COHN
Salk Institute of Biological Studies

I. PRINCIPLE OF THE ARGUMENT

The immune system faces two problems of regulation:

1. the self-nonself discrimination
2. the determination of class.

These two problems are hierarchical in that the model one proposes for the self-nonself discrimination limits the way in which the mechanism determining the class of the response can be viewed.

The easiest way to deal with regulation is to present one possible model before considering details of mechanism and Watt Knott.

The unit of interaction is the antigen-sensitive cell. This cell is postulated to have two properties.

1. It expresses an antibody-receptor unique in its combining site.

2. Upon interaction of the antibody-receptor with antigen, the cell has two pathways open to it, paralysis or induction.

The various antigen-sensitive cells differ in the function of their induced end-cell which is neither paralyzable nor inducible.

A. THE SELF-NONSELF DISCRIMINATION

Antigen-sensitive cells of all classes directed against self and nonself components are generated continuously throughout life. This is an inevitable consequence of the generation of diversity (1). In an animal with a mature immune system the anti-self cells are irreversibly eliminated as they appear; a steady state known as maintenance of paralysis. The anti-nonself cells accumulate to another level and are induced. In other words there is competition between paralysis and induction at the level of the antigen-sensitive cell upon interacting with antigen (Fig. 1).

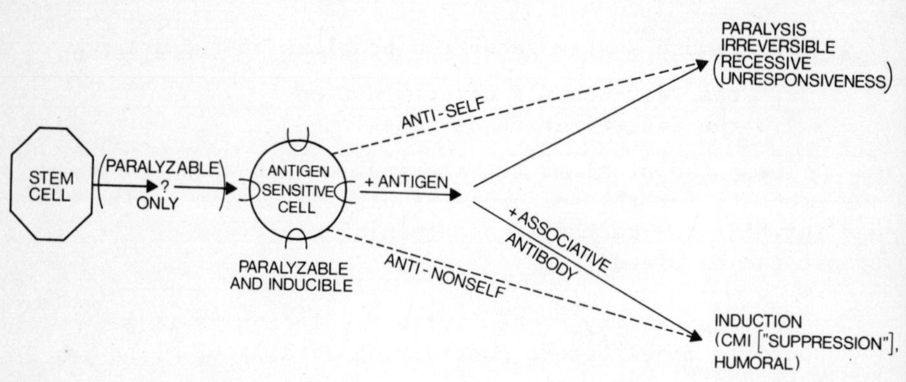

Fig. 1. The genesis of antigen-sensitive cells and their fate, paralysis or induction.

We have proposed a <u>minimum</u> associative recognition model for the self-nonself discrimination.

1. Paralysis: The interaction between the antibody receptors on an antigen-sensitive cell and antigen leads to a Signal ① to that cell which results in its being irreversibly inactivated (rendered irreversibly non-inducible).

2. Normal induction: If in addition to Signal ①, the antigen is recognized by another specific receptor (termed associative antibody) which acts via an independent cell system, a second signal (Signal ②) is delivered to the antigen-sensitive cell. The two signals delivered sequen-

tially or simultaneously results in differentiation of that cell to produce more antigen-sensitive cells as well as "effector" end cells.

The justification of this model has been discussed in detail (1-4). We originally termed this the associative recognition model because normal induction is postulated to require the associative recognition of at least two determinants physically linked on an antigen, one by the antibody receptor on the antigen-sensitive cell and the second by associative antibody which experiment has established to be expressed on a special class of cooperating thymus-derived cells.

The minimum elements of the model are illustrated in Fig. 2 without any details of mechanism (see Section II).

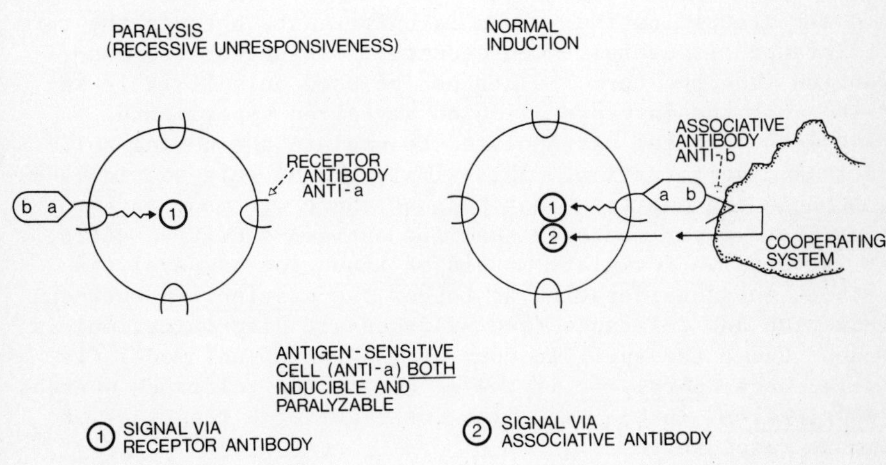

Fig. 2. A minimum associative recognition model of normal induction and paralysis.

For purposes of clarity the term unresponsive will be

used to describe an animal whose prior experimental treatment with a given antigen renders it specifically unable to respond to that antigen when delivered in a form immunogenic for the untreated control animal. Unresponsiveness takes two forms, recessive or dominant. Paralysis or recessive unresponsiveness is revealed by mixing "paralyzed" cell populations, e.g. from spleen, with untreated or "responsive" cell populations and showing that the introduction of the specific immunogen leads to an immune response. Paralysis is recessive because it is the result of the irreversible, specific inactivation of the antigen-sensitive cell itself. "Suppression" or dominant unresponsiveness is revealed similarly by demonstrating that the "suppressed" population inhibits the response to the specific immunogen by the untreated population. "Suppression" is dominant because it is the result of the reversible, specific inhibition of induction of the antigen-sensitive cell by an induced inhibitor cell.

The term "tolerance" is being used more and more to mask an incomplete formulation of the problem of the self-nonself discrimination. This is unfortunate because the term "tolerance" is useful. Consequently, we suggest the convention that the term "tolerance" be used only if it is implied that the interpretation of any given experimental situation is being extrapolated to explain the normal self-nonself discrimination. This simple ground rule should make untenable the position that because there are many ways to inactivate experimentally specific antigen-sensitive cells, it is valid to formulate models of induction or paralysis without any consideration as to how the distinction between induction and tolerance (the self-nonself discrimination) is made. Under the specific form of the two signal model discussed here, paralysis is the mechanism for tolerance whereas "suppression" is the mechanism for regulating the class of immune response.

The associative recognition or "two-signal" model is based on a minimum of four considerations which have been analysed in detail (1-4) for it would be well to have a competing model which accounts for all of them.

1. The determinants recognized by the receptor and associative antibodies must be physically linked for normal induction (see Section I D).

2. The establishing of paralysis is antigen-concentration dependent whereas the maintenance of paralysis is antigen-concentration independent.

3. There is competition between paralysis and induction at the level of the antigen-sensitive cell.

4. The self-nonself discrimination must be learned by exposure of the newly arising immune system to self components during ontogeny.

B. THE CELLS AND THEIR INDUCTION

Responsiveness of all antigen-sensitive cells is determined by the cooperating system. The self-nonself discrimination is regulated by the "presence" or "absence" of cooperating activity. The level of cooperating activity as we will see later (Section I C) determines the class of the response. The pathway of induction is illustrated in Fig. 3.

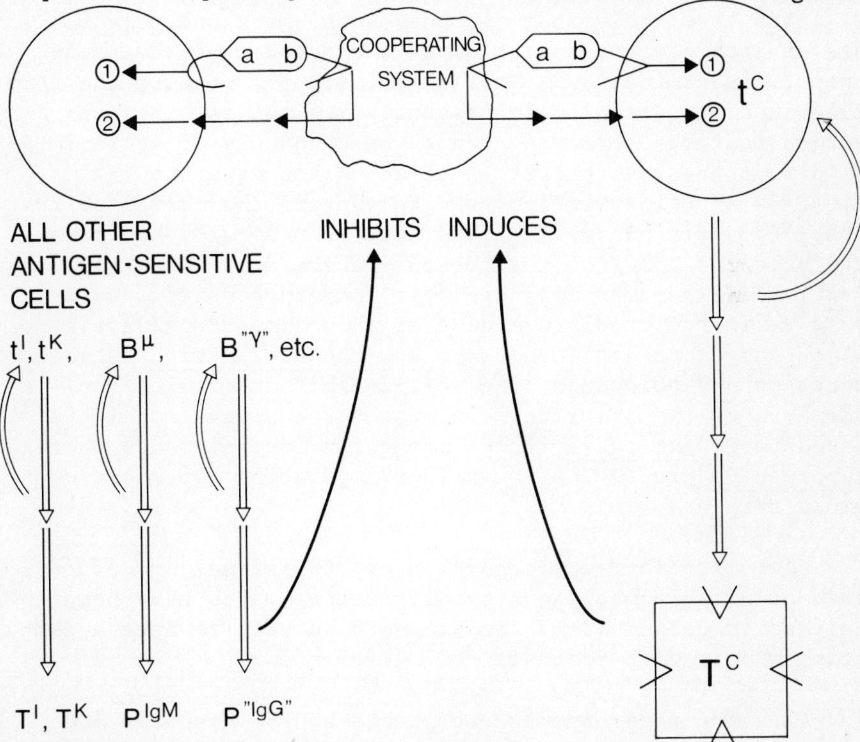

Fig. 3. The pathway of induction of all antigen-sensitive cells.

Thymus-derived antigen-sensitive cells of the cooperating system (t^C) are induced by an associative interaction with antigen both to become end cells (T^C) and to produce more (t^C) cells. T^C cells may act directly as the cooperating cell or secrete their associative antibody which is bound cytophilically to a third party effector cooperating cell.

The induction of "effector" antigen-sensitive cells, i.e. B^{μ}, B^{γ}, B^{α} etc. or t^K (thymus-derived cell-mediated "killer" antigen-sensitive cells), follows the same induction pattern requiring associative recognition. The induction of the antigen-sensitive cells t^C, t^K, $B^{\mu,\gamma,\alpha}$, etc is more X-ray sensitive because division is involved than the functioning of the corresponding "effector" end cells, T^C, T^K and $p^{IgM, IgG, IgA\ etc}$, because division is not involved.

There is an asymmetry in the relationship of the cooperating system to the remainder of the immune system. T^C-cells are required for the induction of all antigen-sensitive cells (B or t) whereas no other antigen-sensitive cell or its induced end-cell is required for the induction of t^C-cells. In general, they inhibit induction by a variety of mechanisms.

It should be stressed in discussions of regulation at this level that it is the function of the cell which counts not whether it is "T" or "B". Confusion is hidden under the term "T-cell", if it is not stated whether cooperating, killing or inhibitory activities are being considered.

C. REGULATION OF THE CLASS OF RESPONSE

A wealth of experimental data can be summarized (5,6) as follows (Fig. 4).

Response to antigen is correlated with the effective level of the associative antibody system. Fig. 4 illustrates this relationship.

At a "zero" effective level (i.e. below a given value) of associative antibody, receptor interaction with antigen leads to paralysis (Signal ①).

At all effective levels (i.e. above a given value) of associative antibody, from very low to high, the antigen-sensitive cooperating thymus-derived cell (t^C) is induced.

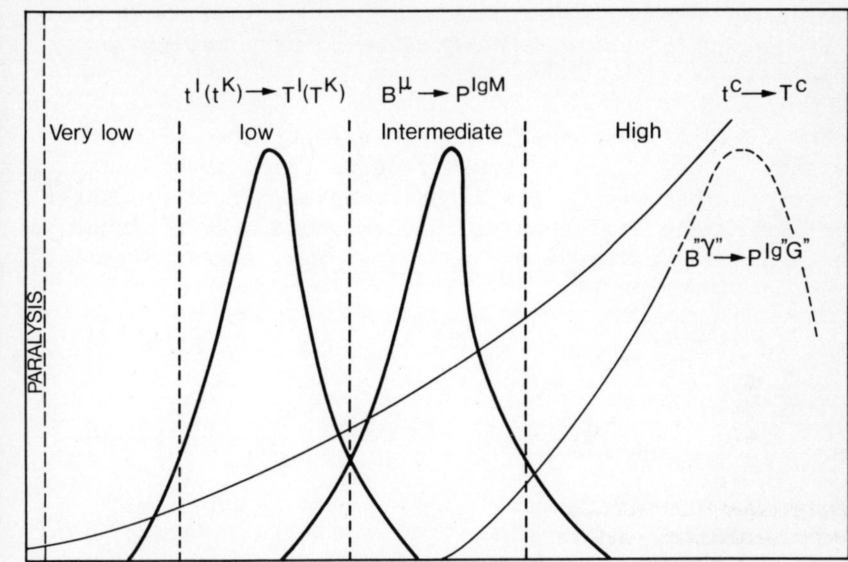

Fig. 4. A qualitative summary of the relationship between the class of response and the level of cooperation.

At low effective levels the antigen-sensitive cell-mediated killer cell (t^K) is induced.

At intermediate effective levels induction of the antigen-sensitive "cell-mediated killer" cell (t^K) is suppressed but the antigen-sensitive IgM bone marrow-derived cell (B^μ) is induced.

At high levels the induction of B^μ (as well as t^K) is suppressed but the antigen-sensitive Ig"G" bone marrow-derived cell ($B^{"\gamma"}$) is induced.

The induction of more antigen-sensitive cells (Fig. 3) seems to be possible at a slightly lower level of Signal ② per receptor than the induction of differentiated end cells e.g. P^{IgM}. Thus for "memory" cells one might draw a series of identical curves as those shown in Fig. 4 displaced slightly to the left (6).

Bretscher (5) has made the following proposal as to mechanism.

The class of response is not just correlated with but is actually determined by the effective level of cooperating activity (number of Signals ② per receptor per cell). At a given level, one cell type is induced whereas at a higher level the same cell type is <u>suppressed</u> i.e. excess Signal ② suppresses (Section II).

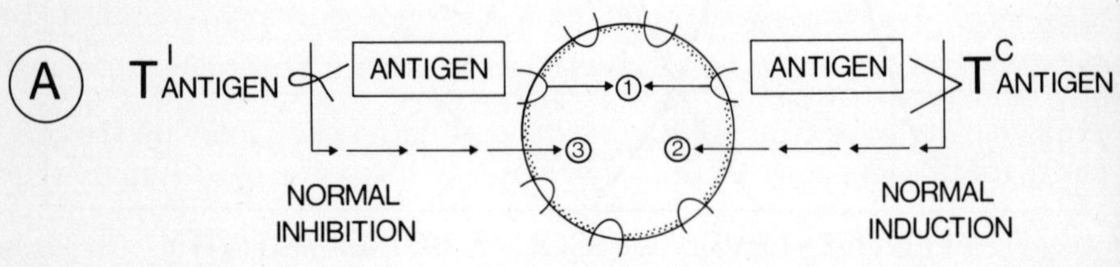

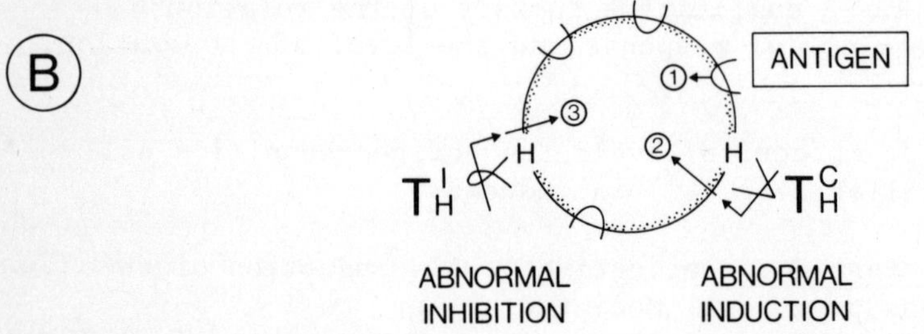

Fig. 5. The interactions of normal and abnormal induction and inhibition.

The second part of the problem of regulation of class is the mutual exclusivity between CMI and humoral responsiveness. Stable states of either CMI or humoral responsiveness can be established. Here again Bretscher (5) has made a proposal which I will extend as follows:

The T^K-cell itself or one induced in parallel with it (T^I-cell) inhibits the induction of the t^C- and B-cell by associative delivery of Signal ③ to them (Fig. 5A). Thus the effective level of cooperating activity is maintained too low (Fig. 4) to induce humoral antibody. The inhibition of induction of the B-cell has no role in maintaining the steady state of CMI. However, T^I-inhibition at the level of the B-cell does prevent any low levels of blocking humoral antibody from leaking through. Thus the effector level of CMI is maximized. If the effective level of cooperating activity is intermediate to high, the induction of the t^I-cell is suppressed and a stable state of humoral antibody synthesis is achieved.

The important point is that there is a tug-of-war between the T^I- and T^C-system, the former pulling the response towards CMI and the latter pulling the response towards humoral immunity (Fig. 6).

D. NORMAL AND ABNORMAL CELL-CELL INTERACTIONS DETERMINING INDUCTION AND INHIBITION.

The associative recognition model predicts the existence of a phenomenon called <u>abnormal</u> induction or inhibition (Fig. 5). Normally for induction or inhibition, two determinants on the antigen must be recognized, one by the receptor on the antigen-sensitive cell and the other by the receptor of the T^C-or T^I-system (Fig. 5A). However, the antigen-sensitive cell itself cannot tell that two determinants on an antigen are being associatively recognized. It only responds to the signals it receives. Therefore it is possible to uncouple the delivery of Signals ①, ② and ③. This occurs when the T^I- and T^C-systems recognize surface determinants on the antigen-sensitive cell, not on the antigen (Fig. 5B). These surface determinants could be histocompatibility antigens, lectins, viral antigens, BCG,

LPS, foreign mammalian membrane constituents, idiotypic or allotypic determinants etc. This is abnormal only in that the uncoupling of the associative recognition of antigen sabotages the specificity of both the self-nonself discrimination and the regulation of class. The Signals 1, 2, and 3 delivered to the antigen-sensitive cell are normal. Of course if one knew what were the extra-and intracellular mediators of the signals, all antigen-specific steps could be bypassed.

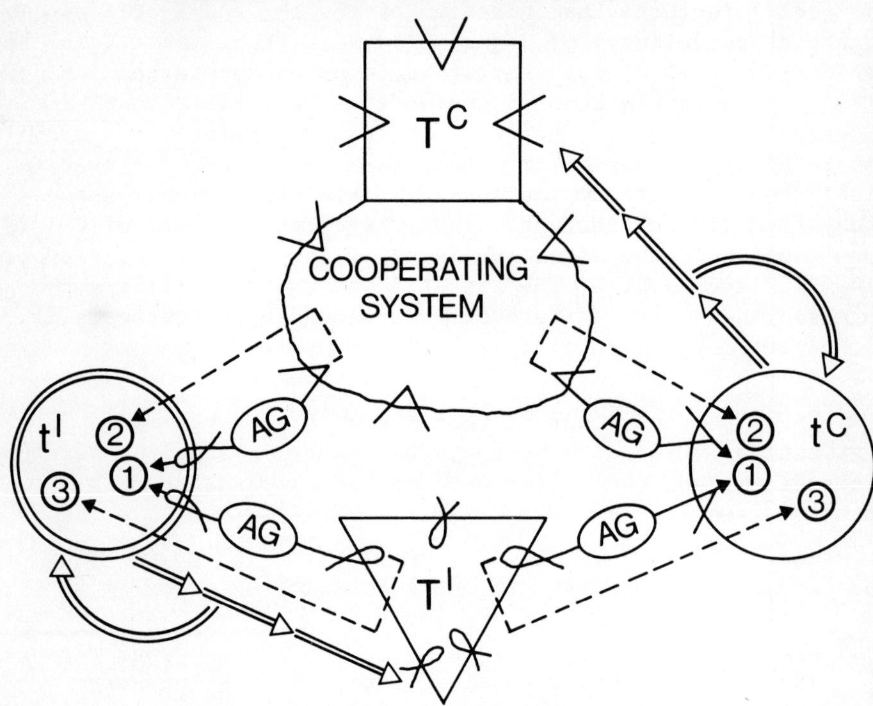

Fig. 6. The interaction between the cooperating and inhibitory system in determining responsiveness.

E. THREE EXPERIMENTAL EXAMPLES OF ABNORMAL INDUCTION AND INHIBITION USED TO ANALYZE THE NORMAL RESPONSE.

1. The *in vitro* regulation of a response to SRBC by the T^C- and T^I-systems recognizing major histocompatibility antigens (7).

A BALB/c spleen induced *in vitro* to C57Bl/6 antigens under conditions which optimize cell-mediated reactivity, will inhibit the response of normal C57Bl/6 or F1(C57Bl/6 x BALB/c) spleen to SRBC (Fig. 7). This inhibitory response requires specific recognition by the induced BALB/c spleen of C57Bl/6 histocompatibility determinants.

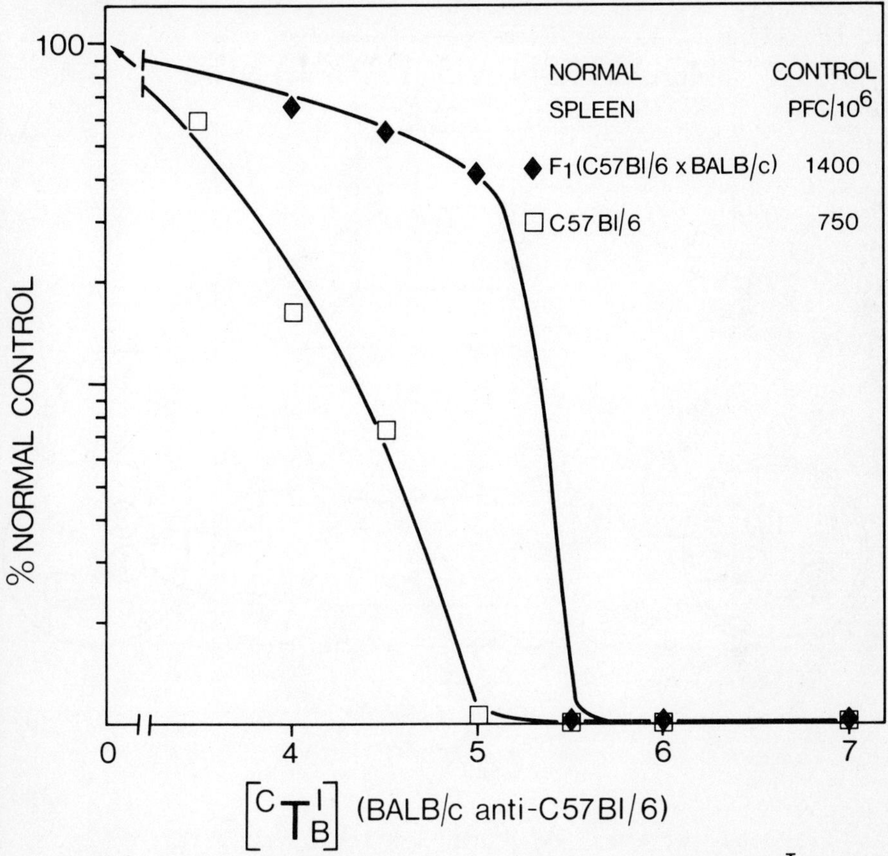

Fig. 7. The inhibition of a response to SRBC by T^I cells induced to histocompatibility antigens.

The inhibitor cell acts on both the t^C- and B-cell and its effect is reversed in each case by cooperating activity (Fig. 8).

The inhibitor cell is thymus-derived in that its activity is destroyed by treatment with anti-θ serum and complement, is not retained on Sephadex and nylon wool columns, and cannot be induced in spleens from nude and mice.

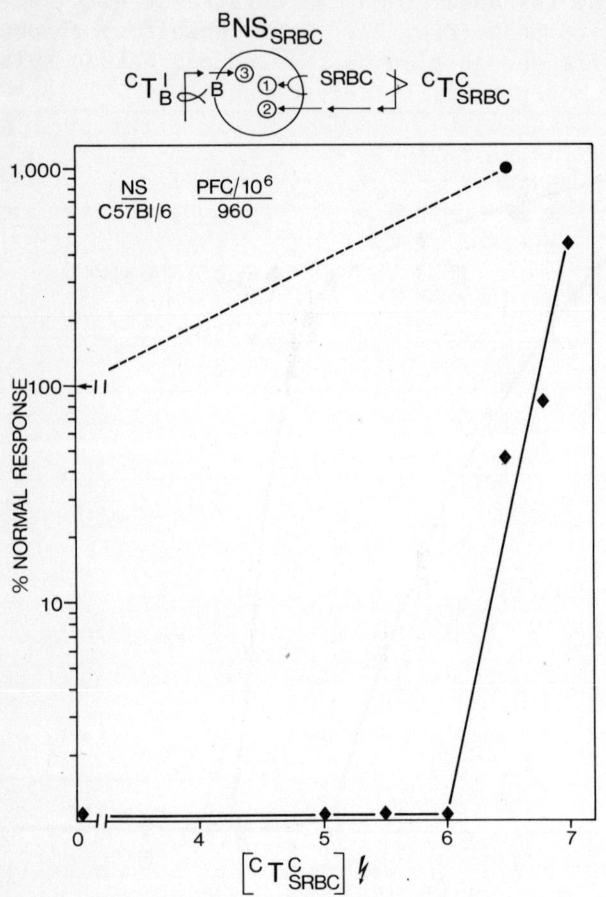

Fig. 8. Reversal of T^{I} inhibition by cooperating activity (${}^{C}T^{C}_{SRBC}$). Response with (—♦—) and without (-- ● --) T-inhibition.

2. The <u>in vitro</u> induction of inhibitory activity by treatment of spleens. with LPS (7).

A spleen induced by LPS develops inhibitory activity analogous in behavious to that of one induced by allogeneic cells. The addition of LPS-treated to normal spleen inhibits the response to SRBC (Table 1). This inhibition is reversed by cooperating activity and is mediated by a θ-bearing cell, nonadherent to Sephadex or nylon wool i.e. a

T^I-cell.

TABLE 1

Reversal of LPS induced inhibition by cooperating activity

Preculture ($2x10^6$ cells)	Normal spleen ($1x10^7$ cells) PFC/10^6	T^C_{SRBC} ($1x10^7$ cells) PFC/10^6
- LPS	1400	2300
+ LPS	260	1200
NONE	1100	1600

Mouse strain: C57Bl/6

T^C_{SRBC} = cooperating activity induced by adoptively transferring thymus plus SRBC into irradiated recipients. The spleens were used 7 days later

3. The in vivo induction of inhibitory activity by treatment of the animal with BCG and cyclophosphamide (Cy) (7).

The spleen of an animal from a BCG-Cy treated animal (8) will inhibit the response of a normal spleen to SRBC (Table 2). The inhibitory activity is not induced in BCG-Cy pretreated spleen from nude mice and is not retained by Sephadex or nylon wool. This argues for its being a thymus-derived cell (T^I). However, this far it has resisted an anti-θ and complement treatment which inactivates the inhibition by the allogeneic and LPS treated cells.

Of these three examples, the first is the best worked out. In any case, they all can be understood by assuming

TABLE 2

Reversal of BCG-CY induced inhibition by cooperating activity

Normal spleen 10^7 cells	BCG-CY treated spleen $3x10^6$ cells	T^C_{SRBC} $3x10^6$ cells	Direct PFC/10^6
+	-	-	550
+	-	+	1100
+	+	-	<10
+	+	+	750

Mouse strain: F1(C57B1/6 x BALB/c)

T^C_{SRBC} = cooperating activity induced by adoptively transferring thymus plus SRBC into irradiated recipients. The spleens were removed from BCG-CY treated mice as per (8)

that the preinduction induces T^I-cells specific for histocompatibility determinants or LPS or BCG. The reason is that the cooperating activity directed to these antigens under the conditions of the preinduction is low. These T^I-cells interact abnormally via the surface determinants (histocompatibility, LPS or BCG) on both t^C- and B-cells as illustrated in Fig. 5B to inhibit induction of humoral antibody to any antigen. In example 1 the cell-mediated response of the preculture as measured by ^{51}Cr release from a sensitive target is very high (7). In example 2 the cell-mediated response of the BCG-Cy treated mouse to SRBC as measured by delayed hypersensitivity is very high (8). In these, as in all studied cases, inhibitory and cell-mediated activity are induced together.

II. DETAILS OF MECHANISM.

Signal (1) could comprise the following steps (4):

1. A conformational change in the receptor on binding ligand.

2. A polymerization (aggregation) of the bound receptor via F_{AB} interactions.

3. Activation of adenylcyclase followed by a series of cAMP initiated reactions leading to paralysis.

Since monomeric antigens e.g. BSA, lysozyme, flagellin MON, fragment A can paralyze, a conformational change in the receptor on binding ligand is suggested as a first step. Since all known antibody activities are mediated by aggregation e.g. complement activation or histamine release from basophils, the second step is postulated by analogy only. The third and fourth steps are based on the inhibitory effects of cAMP on induction of antigen-sensitive cells and their reversal by cGMP (see Signal ②). Step 1 can in principle be bypassed by aggregating the receptor via non combining site interactions and Step 2 by raising the intracellular level of cAMP.

Signal ② could comprise the following steps (1-5, 9-12):

1. The induced T^C-cell secretes its associative antibody.

2. The associative antibody is cytophilic for a third party cooperating cell.

3. The antigen-associative antibody complex triggers the cooperating cell to synapse with the antigen-sensitive cell receiving Signal ①.

4. A short-lived transmitter acting at high concentration is released across the synapse to initiate the intracellular events comprising Signal ②.

5. One of the early steps is activation of guanyl cyclase and raising of cGMP levels.

6. The combined reading of the levels of intracellular mediators of Signals ① (cAMP) and ② (cGMP) determines induction.

In principle, the T^C-cell itself (neither inducible or paralyzable) could act as the cooperating cell. The original prediction (10-12) that a third party cell was involved came from a consideration of how the immune system gets started in ontogeny i.e. where does the first T^C-cell come from?, a question outside of our present discussion. The evidence for this at the worst has remained controversial and at the best "no-easy-to-work-with" system has emerged. The proposal is simply reasonable.

It is not necessary to postulate a conformational change in associative antibody acting as the cytophilic receptor of the cooperating cell because in any case an antigen-antibody complex is required to trigger it as in the case of all immune-related cells, macrophages, basophils, K-cells etc., which derive their receptors passively. This is a consequence of the competition for Fc receptors between a given specific antibody population under analysis and the other immunoglobulin of the same class. The dissociation constant of the Fc-Ig interaction must be greater than or equal to the average concentration of the given Ig class so that an antigen-antibody complex has no difficulty interacting with the effector cell.

The cell-cell interaction leading to induction must be arranged so that the result is a specific response. The original model describing this (10) was drawn by analogy with the nervous system. If the cooperating cell poured out its transmitter into the surrounding medium, non-specific induction would occur, the worst being induction of anti-self cells. This non-specific effect is minimized if the cooperating cell requires two events to trigger it to release transmitter; first an aggregation signal from the antigen-antibody complex and second a "synapse" signal from the antigen-sensitive cell receiving Signal ①. If now as in the nervous system the transmitter is short-lived and acts at high concentration specificity of the connection is maximized. Given these considerations, there is reason to doubt the relevance of most of the non-antigen specific supernatant factors which have been isolated from various "cell mixtures", as the actual mediators of the cooperative interaction.

It is evident under this model that in addition to antibody-receptors which recognize antigen, various other surface receptors must be postulated to be on antigen-sensitive cells for the interactions involving transmitters and synapses (10).

What is not so evident is that these non-antigen recognizing receptors should be highly polymorphic and all coded between the K and S region of the major histocompatibility complex. The experiments of Katz <u>et al</u> (13) claiming to show this are based on the failure of allogeneic cells to cooperate to give an IgG response in an adoptive transfer system. Since these studies do not distinguish between population and cell level events they will not be convincing until they are repeated using allogeneic cell populations mutually tolerant (paralyzed) of each other as in allophenic (14) or tetraparental chimeras(15). This question as to which genes code <u>non-antigen specific</u> cell-cell interactions is open. The existence of abnormal induction and inhibition (Sections I D and E) across histocompatibility barriers makes it likely that mutually tolerant populations will co-operate allogeneically or even xenogeneically.

The possible role of intracellular mediators cAMP and cGMP as part of the Signal ① and ② systems has been reviewed recently (9). What should be stressed is that under the two-signal model Signal ① plus Signal ② are required for induction. This implies that no cell can be induced which in principle could not have been paralyzed. Since there is a strong somatic selection pressure for a cell to escape paralysis (death?) by mutation, if the mutant non-paralyzable cells were inducible, a lethal autoimmunity would result. This implies that the totality of the paralytic pathway is included in the inductive one.

This model for delivering Signal ② is one of the two originally proposed mechanisms (ref. 10 pg 270). The other one was a membrane-membrane interaction signal following associative recognition. The two models are still viable.

Signal ③ could comprise the following steps:

1. The T^I-cell itself interacts across an antigen-bridge with the antigen-sensitive cell, t^C or B.

2. The inhibitor antibody-antigen-receptor antibody complex triggers the T^I-cell to render the antigen-sensitive cell unresponsive to Signals ① and ② either by 1) a membrane-membrane interaction or 2) secreting an inhibitory transmitter or 3) injecting an inhibitor across a cytoplasmic bridge.

It is a reasonable guess that the T^I-cell is the T^K-cell responsible for effecting cell-mediated immunity. This cell acts as far as is known as such without secreting its receptors. The antigen-sensitive cell must be resistant to killing activity and respond only by being inhibited. The fact that the inhibition is reversible by increasing the cooperative activity can be understood either as an intracellular or extracellular event. As an example of the former, Signal ③ need only block activation of the adenyl and guanyl cyclases or inhibit a step common to the Signal ① + ② induction. As an example of the latter, the inhibitory event at the cell level must be of a duration which frees the cell occassionally to respond to an inductive encounter. As the level of cooperating activity increases, induction becomes more probable than inhibition and the population escapes inhibition.

The effective level of cooperating activity drives the class of response. The sensitivity to level of cooperating activity shows the following order: $t^C > t^K > B^{\mu} > B^{"\gamma"}$ etc. (Fig. 4). It is not necessary to postulate an intracellular mechanism with differential sensitivity for the intracellular mediators or for their production. All classes of cell could have identical intracellular mechanisms and differ only in the number of functional receptors per cell (assuming of course that the distribution of binding constants of the various classes is similar). This number then should reflect the sensitivity to induction, $t^C > t^K > B^{\mu} > B^{"\gamma"}$. Implied also is that <u>in the absence of cooperating activity</u> [T^C] the sensitivity to <u>paralysis</u> by Signal ① would follow the same order. On the other hand, the sensitivity to inhibition by T^I would appear to follow the reverse order $B^{"\gamma"} > B^{\mu} > t^C$ because a higher effective level of cooperation is required to induce $B^{"\gamma"}$ than t^C.

In general it is believed that paralysis of the t^C-cell is acheived at a faster rate and at lower concentrations of antigen than that required for the B-cell. While this may be true, it is not derivable from the qualitative experiments which are done because of the asymmetry in the relationship between t^C and all other antigen-sensitive cells (see discussion ref. 2,4,16). Further, differences in the "sensitivity" of antigen-sensitive cells to paralysis during their ontogeny is claimed (17). Here too, this difference could reflect a difference in the level of cooperating activity in the various cell populations, fetal liver, bone marrow, spleen etc., not a difference in the inherent sensitivity of the antigen-sensitive cell to paralysis.

In summary, studies on rates of paralysis of given cell types must take into account the effective level of co-operating activity and be carried out quantitatively. Nevertheless, there are *a priori* reasons for accepting a hierarchy of sensitivity to paralysis $t^C > t^K > B^\mu > B^\gamma$.

It is generally believed that T^I-cell *inhibition* is more easily acheived for B^γ than for B^μ.

Since this is a competitive system involving the opposing activities of T^I and T^C it is not possible at the moment to be certain whether the greater sensitivity to *inhibition* of the $B^{"\gamma"}$ cell is a property of the cell or of the level of cooperating activity necessary to reveal or reverse the inhibition. In any case, at the level of the population (which is the experimental finding), sensitivity to T^I-inhibition follows a hierarchy $B^{"\gamma"} > B^\mu > t^C$ certainly in part because a higher level of T^C-activity is required to induce $B^{"\gamma"}$ than B^μ or t^C.

Two models for the suppression of each class in the hierarchical order $t^K > B^\mu > B^{"\gamma"}$ as the level of cooperating activity rises, could be proposed.

1) The cell might become unresponsive to excess Signal ② for which an intracellular mechanism could be envisaged based upon the cell reading the correct ratio of ①/② which differes from the t^K to the $B^{"\gamma"}$ cell.

2) The product of the induction of one cell type might feed back and turn off the induction of the cell type higher in the hierarchy.

Thus far I have discussed the problem of regulation of class assuming essentially the first model. The second model at the moment has not yet been formulated in a way which accounts for the determination of class

III. WATT KNOTT

A. ENGLISH PRAGMATISM

Howard and Mitchison (18) have proposed that antigen-sensitive cells need not distinguish two signals, one for paralysis and the other for induction. They argue that the antigen-sensitive cell is programmed for induction only. An appropriate interaction of antigen with the receptor leads to induction. Paralysis is essentially the "gumming-up" of the receptors on the cell so that no inductive signal can be delivered. The "permanently-gummed-up" cell is gradually eliminated either by normal turnover or by antibody-mediated destruction i.e. autoimmune reaction.

Their argument is based on the *in vitro* experiments of Diener and Feldmann in which large polymeric antigens e.g. POL or antigen-antibody complexes can render cells specifically unresponsive.

There is no doubt that imprisoning cells in an antigen-antibody cage so that immunogenic encounters are not possible will make them unresponsive. With time, such cells will be eliminated ("paralyzed") at a rate dependent on the culture conditions *in vitro* compared to *in vivo*. It would be tempting to argue that this proposal is a detail of mechanism involving the precise meaning of the word "signal" but the issue is not here. It resides in how this *in vitro* Diener-Feldmann finding is extrapolated to explain the self-nonself discrimination or even *in vivo* experimental paralysis. It should be recalled that in the Diener-Feldmann system, the *in vitro* and *in vivo* findings are at variance. *In vivo* the order of establishing unresponsiveness is fragment A > MON > POL whereas *in vitro* the order is POL > MON > fragment A and in the latter two cases, the addition of antibody is required to establish unresponsiveness in B-cells.

The problem is clear. Which set of phenomena mirror the central mechanism of paralysis and induction, the *in vitro* or the *in vivo* findings?

We have argued (2,4) that the *in vivo* findings reflect the fundamental paralytic mechanism i.e. Signal ①, and that the *in vitro* result reflects a superimposed secondary process. This is obvious under the two-signal model because the fewer the number of foreign determinants per antigen particle, the lower the *effective* level of cooperating activity and the more the response tends towards paralysis. The Diener-Feldmann *in vitro* result can be explained by assuming that the half-life of a cell receiving a maximum level of Signal ① *in vivo* is of the order of 5-10 hours, while *in vitro*, due to poorer culture conditions, it is of the order of 20-30 hours. Monomers would be bound to the cell "reversibly" whereas polymers or antigen-antibody complexes would be bound "irreversibly". Thus several hours of contact with a putative paralytogen, subsequent washing and incubation with immunogen, could not possibly reveal paralysis by "reversibly" bound monomers whereas the "irreversible" blocked cell would remain unresponsive. This "gummed-up" state might be revealed by presenting the blocked B-cells with an *abnormal* inductive stimulus (Section I D) in which case they might respond. If they did, then it would be clear that a paralytic signal (Signal ①) is being delivered to them but the time constant of inactivation *in vitro* is long. More important would be to show that *in vitro* the non-immunogenic fragment A could be rendered immunogenic by abnormal induction, thus proving a monomer-receptor interaction signal.

The point being made is that the Diener-Feldmann experiments are telling us what we know already. The interaction between a polymeric antigen and the receptors on a cell can be essentially "irreversible" because of multiple binding. However, these experiments do not permit the extrapolation that no signal passes via the receptor when it interacts with a monomer.

Howard and Mitchison disagree and argue that the *in vitro* result is the fundamental one and the *in vivo* data reflect a secondary process because "it is entirely possible that some alternative mechanism exists *in vivo* for the presentation of monomeric antigens in a repeating form (18)".

At first glance this argument looks like a "piège à con" but on reflection it is sufficiently challenging to be worth trying to get the cheese without springing the trap. In order to do this, I must try to complete their model as they would see it because no mechanism of induction is actually proposed by them.

If the assumption were *incorrect* that monomers can paralyze, the two-signal model would be unaffected. What would have to be changed is a detail of mechanism namely that it would become unnecessary to assume a conformational change in the receptor as the initiating step of the paralytic

Signal ① (Section II). As Howard and Mitchison point out, in vivo, monomers could aggregate by some process and the aggregate would initiate the paralytic Signal ① by lattice formation as previously discussed (ref. 4 pg 548). Signal ② would remain unchanged.

The Howard-Mitchison formulation does not fare as well. Since they are challenging the two-signal model, I would imagine that we can put aside as unacceptable to them either as associative recognition inductive signal via the cooperating ("helper") system or a simple monomer-receptor inductive signal. This leaves only the conclusion that induction requires some kind of lattice signal (aggregation) not sufficiently extensive to completely encage the cell (freeze the membrane) and lead to paralysis. In other words, if it is assumed that monomers are inert in that they can neither induce nor paralyze (freeze the membrane) then the inductive signal delivered by an aggregate under the Howard-Mitchison formulation would be a paralytic signal under our formulation. The paralytic event under the Howard-Mitchison formulation is a blocking of induction most often by a "gumming-up" interaction and the inductive signal under our formulation is a consequence of associative recognition of antigen by the cooperating system. [It is possible to argue under the Howard-Mitchison formulation that monomers at saturating concentrations would block all receptors and create a state definable as "paralysis" but this would apply to a small number of self-monomers e.g. serum albumin, and to very few cases of experimental paralysis by monomers].

The Howard-Mitchison formulation of paralysis and induction applies to B-cells, not to t^C-cells, because, as they stress, B-cell paralysis is dependent on a "gumming-up" interaction while t^C-cell paralysis can result from a monomer-receptor interaction (Signal ①). This is very untidy because under the Howard-Mitchison formulation, 1) the same inductive events cannot operate in t^C- and B-cells as the former may be paralyzed by monomers when the latter are induced by aggregate; 2) the in vivo findings reflect the basic mechanism of t^C-paralysis while the in vitro findings reflect that of B-paralysis; and 3) t^C-paralysis is the consequence of an intracellular signal initiated by a conformational change in the bound receptor whereas B-paralysis is a ridding of cells which have no internal clue as to why they are "effete".

However, it is possible to accept untidiness and to insist that the *in vitro* result reveals the fundamental paralytic process in B-cells. This requires that one explain the *in vivo* findings by proposing mechanisms for properly aggregating monomers *in vivo* to make them immunogenic at one concentration and paralytic at another i.e. establishing paralysis.

There are two classes of mechanism; those which are antibody-dependent and those which are non-antibody dependent.

As a general mechanism non-antibody-dependent aggregation processes are ruled out under the Howard-Mitchison formulation because they would have to distinguish between inducing and paralyzing aggregates as well as between self and non-self monomers. In addition there is the general experience that *in vivo*, fragmentation, monomerization or deaggregation of antigens favors a paralytic response whereas polymerization of antigens favors an inductive response (19). Such a rule would not be expected if a random *in vivo* aggregation process were obligatory to establish paralysis because sometimes it would be more or less efficient than the experimental aggregation process.

Antibody-dependent aggregation mechanisms are ruled out also because this assumption requires that B-cell induction precede paralysis and monomers under the Howard-Mitchison hypothesis cannot induce B-cells. Further, maintenance of paralysis conditions are precisely those where anti-self B-cells arise and are paralyzed in the absence of humoral antibody as well as cooperating activity. Put with Dizzynessland clarity by Britton (ref. 19 pg 298) the Howard-Mitchison formulation implies that, "the T-cell independence of the induction of B-cell tolerance is reflecting the T-cell dependence of synthesis of the antibody which will combine with the antigen in such a form that it becomes tolerogenic".

B. TRY IT YOURSELF.

If one tries to develop a model in which a low level of Signal ① is inductive whereas an excess is paralytic, then it is not possible to account for the competition between the paralytogen and the cross-reacting immunogen in the breaking of paralysis. This is in essence the Diener-Feldmann-Nossal-Cohen and "under predictable protest" the Howard-Mitchison formulation.

If one tries to develop a model in which a low level of Signal ② is inductive whereas an excess is paralytic, then it is not possible to account for the difference between establishing and maintenance of paralysis.

If one tries to develop a model in which Signal ① only is used by t^C-cells and Signal ② only is used by B-cells then it is not possible to account for B-cell paralysis by non-immunogenic antigens i.e. maintenance of B-cell paralysis (ref. 3 for discussion). This is the Coutinho-Möller formulation.

In general any models in which the paralytic and inductive events follow independent pathways (18) require that t^C- and B-cells be induced and paralyzed by different mechanisms (3) and lead to situtations in which non-paralyzable cells are inducible. This latter would lead inevitably to autoimmunity. Key to the Two-Signal model described here is that the paralytic Signal ① is included in the inductive Signal ① + ② so that no cell can be induced which could not have been paralyzed.

C. T^C vs T^I.

The present formulation of regulation of class is based on there being two populations of cells, t^I and t^C. This has been sharply under dispute (ref. 19 pg 137) because markers other than function are not available. However, an argument can be made on function alone. First, when T^C-activity is high, IgG synthesis is induced and cell-mediated immunity and IgM synthesis are <u>suppressed</u>. When the T^C-activity is low, cell-mediated immunity is induced and humoral antibody synthesis is <u>inhibited</u>. This inhibition is due to the T^I-cell. Since the two activities are antithetical and induced under different conditions, the simplest assumption is that they are derived from the induction of two different t-cell populations, t^I and t^C. In fact at the moment it is possible to assume that <u>inhibition</u> and cell-mediated reactivity are properties of one cell population, $t^I(t^K)$, and suppression and cooperative activity are properties of the other cell population, $t^S(t^C)$.

It is well to stress at this point that only too often one type of immune response is measured e.g. IgM synthesis, and this response can be inhibited by the T^I-system which drives the response towards cell-mediated reactivity or suppressed by the T^C-system which drives the response towards Ig"G" synthesis. In order to analyze this feedback system CMI, IgM and IgG responsiveness must be studied.

D. A CAUTION.

The terms self and nonself are ambiguous and are used tautologously. There is no harm in this as long as we understand it. A major constituent of membranes is lecithin which has glycerophosphorylcholine as a component. Mice respond to various antigens to produce anti-phosphorylcholine which reacts to agglutinate lecithin in suspension. They are therefore not "tolerant" to this self-component because the phosphorylcholine determinant is internal in the cell and only exposed on breakdwon of cells. In fact much of what is described as autoimmunity with no clinical symptoms could be an immune response to dying cells which in fact might be the mechanism of elimination of breakdown products from cell turnover. This could involve cell mediated lysis and via the present model of regulation introduce an "inhibition" of humoral responsiveness to cryptic "self-components".

E. MORE HEAT THAN LIGHT.

A leading Ivy League pathologist, performing a Newtonian transplant, (ref. 20 pg 471) refers to T cell regulation as the immune system's "Second Law of thymodynamics"; "that is to say for every T cell dependent augmentation there is an equal and opposite T cell suppression".

If the biological role of this regulatory system is to determine the class of response, then it could not be true that increased T^C-activity automatically engenders increased T^I-activity. These activities must be antithetical to permit mutually exclusive stable states of CMI, IgM or Ig"G" to be established i.e. high T^C-activity means low T^I-activity and vice versa.

F. END GAME.

To my mind the real strength of the present formulation is that paralysis-induction decisions are the main pathways of the self-nonself discrimination while "suppression"-induction decisions are the main pathway of the regulation of the class of response. Thus biological sense is put into the phenomenology.

The Two-Signal hypothesis as discussed here has the same relationship to immunology as the ideal law "PV = nRT" has to physical chemistry. Deviations from it enable one to understand the secondary or superimposed phenomena which are constantly encountered. The hypothesis itself is obeyed only under limiting conditions.

REFERENCES

(1) M. Cohn. Cell. Immunol., 5(1972) 1.

(2) P. Bretscher. Transplant. Rev., 11(1972) 217.

(3) M. Cohn and B. Blomberg. Scand. J. Immunol., in press.

(4) M. Cohn. Ann. N.Y. Acad. Sci., 190(1971) 529.

(5) P. Bretscher. Cell. Immunol., 13(1974) 171.

(6) M. Cohn, in: Immunobiology of the Tumor-Host Relationship, eds. R. Smith and M. Landy (Academic Press, New York, 1974) p. 268.

(7) M. Cohn and R. Epstein, manuscript in preparation.

(8) G.B.Mackaness and P.H. Lagrange, J. Exp. Med. 140(1974) in press.

(9) J. D. Watson, Transplant. Rev., in press.

(10) M. Cohn, in: Control Processes in Multicellular Organisms, eds. G.E.W. Wolstenholme and J. Knight (J. and A. Churchill Ltd, London, 1970) p. 255.

(11) P. Bretscher and M. Cohn, Nature 220(1968) 444.

(12) P. Bretscher and M. Cohn, Science 169(1970) 1042.

(13) T. Hamaoka, D.P. Osborne and D.H. Katz, J. Exp. Med. 137(1973) 1393;
D.H. Katz, T. Hamaoka and B. Benacerraf, J. Exp. Med. 137(1973) 1405;
D.H. Katz, T. Hamaoka, M.E. Dorf and B. Benacerraf, Proc. Nat. Acad. Sci. U.S.A. 70(1973) 2624;
D.H. Katz, T. Hamaoka, M.E. Dorf, P.H. Maurer and B. Benacerraf, J. Exp. Med. 138(1973) 734;
D.H. Katz, T. Hamaoka, M.E. Dorf and B. Benacerraf, J. Immunol., 112(1976) 855.

(14) T. Meo, T. Matsunaga and A.M. Rynbeck, Transplant. Proc. V (1973) 1607.

(15) H. von Boehmer, J. Sprent and M. Nabholz, J. Exp. Med. in press.

(16) M. Cohn, in: Genetic Control of Immune Responsiveness eds H.O. McDevitt and M. Landy (Academic Press, New York, 1972) p. 370.

(17) G.J.V. Nossal and J.W. Schrader, Transplant Rev., in press.

(18) J.G. Howard and N.A. Mitchison, Progr. Allergy, in press.

(19) Immunological tolerance, eds D.H. Katz and B. Benacerraf (Academic Press, New York, 1974) p. 645.

(20) The Immune System, eds E.E. Sercarz, A.R. Williamson, C.F. Fox (Academic Press, New York, 1974) p. 632.

Under pressure from a deadline, this paper was written when I was far away from my usual sources of bibliography and reprints. Consequently, I must apologize for the casual references. I depended on some favorite reviews and papers which I carry everywhere (but to bed).

The work was supported by N.I.H. Grant A-105875.

DISCUSSION

R. CITRONBAUM: I have one suggestion and one question. I suggest that in this last experiment you add BCG X-ray treated cells; this would help to show that the T-cooperating system was involved because T^c-cells are X-ray resistant. My question involves a chicken and egg-type situation which I believe I have asked you before, but perhaps in the year since then you have come up with an answer. Where does the first T^c-cell come from?

M. COHN: At the first Brook Lodge symposium on "Tolerance" the same question was asked by Gerry Edelman and I answered "Well I really don't know". He commented "Then you are in an infinite regress" which was published as "infinite mess" and I will never forget that phrase. This is obviously a key question, by the way, for any theory you may have. How does the immune system get started? In this model the best guess is that during ontogeny as anti-nonself t^c cells accumulate there is a small leakage of associative antibody from them which reaches a level sufficiently high to permit induction by polymeric antigens (high affinity interactions). This induction of T^c cells primes the system.

C. BELL: You mentioned that the increase in the level of the cooperating activity leads to a decline in IgM and to a switch from IgM to IgG. Can the IgM also be regarded as the associative antibody leading to an increase in the IgG production? How does your model reconcile with the possibility that the IgM synthesized by the few B-cells that can be activated directly by antigen may cytophilically bind to receptors on T-cells which then have an immunoregulatory effect on the remaining cells. According to Dr. Claman's model some T-independent antigens may directly act on B-cells and induce them to produce a small amount of surface IgM or secrete some IgG molecules.

M. COHN: Essentially, you are asking two questions "why do so-called T-independent antigens give you only an IgM response?" and "what is the signal driving the switch from IgM to IgG?"

C. BELL: I would like to know the answer to both questions.

M. COHN: You switch classes when you increase the level of cooperating activity. For example, lets take a Benacerraf experiment. He immunizes mice with S III which is a so-called "thymus-independent" antigen. He gets an IgM response only. He couples the S III to bovine gammaglobulin, and shows that immunization results in an IgG response. Effectively he has increased the level of the cooperating activity by use of an immunogeneic carrier. Now to the first question: Why do so-called thymus independent antigens induce an IgM response only? The generalization is not correct. So-called thymus-independent antigens for the mouse:1) may induce an IgM response in the mouse and an IgG response in man (for example, S III) or be immunogenic (that is thymus-independent) for mouse and nonimmunogenic (that is thymus-dependent) in the rabbit (for example S III) and 2) may induce in mice a IgM response only (for example dextran) or an IgG response (for example ficoll). The reason that certain antigens induce an IgM response only (S III or dextran) in mice must be related to their inducing and maintaining an intermediate effective level of cooperating activity. This would be an expected property of repeating non-metabolizable antigens which treadmill antibody. Essentially what I am saying is that the concentration of free antigen (immunogen) is kept so low during treadmilling that the effective activity of the cooperating system is maintained at a level below that required to induce an IgG response.

THE USE OF MUTANT MYELOMA CELLS TO EXPLORE THE PRODUCTION OF IMMUNOGLOBULINS

M.D. SCHARFF, B. BIRSHTEIN, B. DHARMGRONGARTAMA, L. FRANK, T. KELLY, W.M. KUEHL, D. MARGULIES, S.L. MORRISON, J.-L. PREUD'HOMME and S. WEITZMAN
Department of Cell Biology
Albert Einstein College of Medicine

Abstract: A method has been developed for identifying and quantifying mouse myeloma cells which have undergone mutations in immunoglobulin production. Such variants arise at a very high rate both spontaneously and with mutagenesis. Mutagenesis results in primary sequence variants which are blocked in a variety of steps in the synthesis, assembly, glycosylation, and secretion of H chains. These mutants can be used to investigate the production and genetic control of immunoglobulins.

INTRODUCTION

Studies carried out in a number of laboratories have provided a good general description of the synthesis, assembly, and secretion of mouse immunoglobulin (1,2,3). These studies have been done both with mouse myeloma and normal lymphoid cells. The molecular events involved in the production of IgG immunoglobulins are presented schematically in Figure 1. The immunoglobulin messenger is transcribed and processed in the nucleus, and transported into the cytoplasm where it becomes associated with membrane bound ribosomes to form the rough endoplasmic reticulum. There it is translated into heavy (H) and light (L) chains (1,2), which in mouse myeloma cells together represent 20 to 40% of the newly synthesized protein (4). These H and L chains are released into the cisternae of the endoplasmic reticulum and assembled through a variety of covalently linked intermediates into the fully assembled H_2L_2 IgG molecule. The H chains, and in some cases the L chains, are glycosylated in both the rough and smooth endoplasmic reticulum (5,6,7). Most of the immunoglobulin molecules are secreted relatively rapidly, but a small percentage is inserted into the plasma membrane and remains there for many hours (5,8).

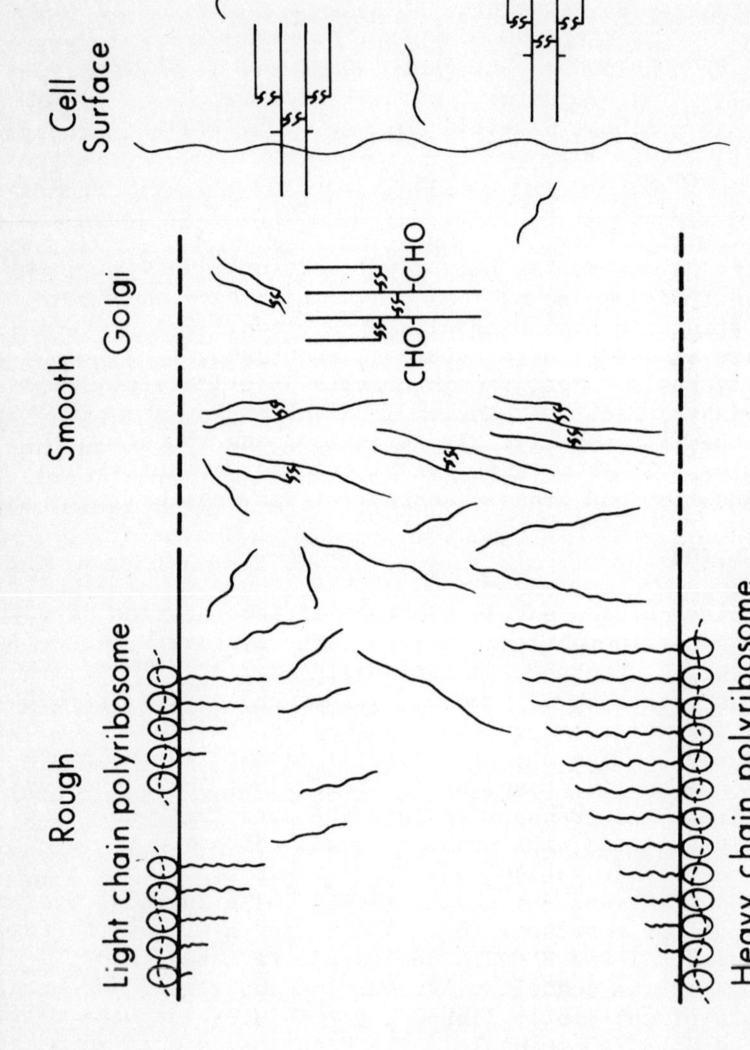
Rough
Smooth
Golgi
Cell
Surface
Light chain polyribosome
Heavy chain polyribosome
CHO-
-CHO

Figure 1

The events depicted in Figure 1 raise a number of interesting questions. Since the genes coding for H and L chains are unlinked (9), are approximately equimolar amounts of the two polypeptide chains synthesized? If so, what is the mechanism of coordinated control? We would also like to know what determines the kinetics, pathways, and completeness of assembly, whether the carbohydrate plays any role in assembly or secretion, and why some molecules remain associated with plasma membrane while others are secreted? Most importantly, is there some way that we can use the highly differentiated and malignant myeloma cells which synthesize large quantities of a homogeneous immunoglobulin to learn something about the unique aspects of the genetic control of immunoglobulin production. For example, can we learn how two genes code for one polypeptide chain, why only one of the two alleles is expressed, or if there is any somatic contribution to the generation of antibody diversity?

Attempts to answer these and other questions and to understand the detailed mechanism responsible for each of the steps in production of immunoglobulin would be greatly facilitated if a series of mutants blocked at each step in the process could be isolated and characterized. Additionally, myeloma cells with mutations in the H or L chain genes would be very useful in studying the somatic cell genetics of animal cells since large amounts of the mutant gene products could be purified and characterized chemically.

THE ISOLATION OF VARIANTS

Mouse myeloma cells growing in continuous culture are cloned in soft agar. In order to obtain high cloning efficiency, nearly confluent monolayers of primary, secondary, or tertiary rat embryo cells are used as feeders. These are overlayed with agarose in growth medium after which a single cell suspension of myeloma cells in very soft agar is layered on top of the base layer (Figure 2). With most cell lines

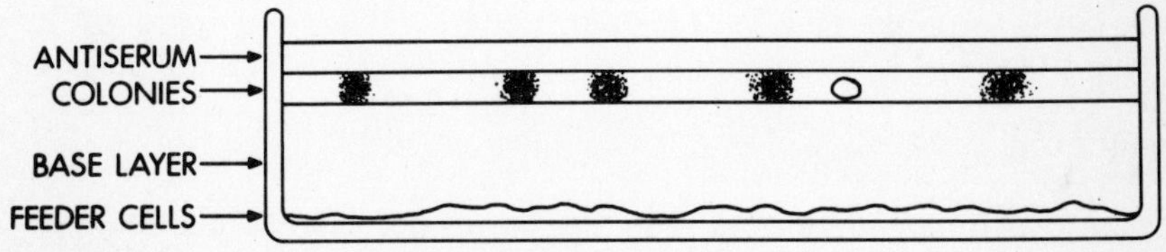

Figure 2

50-100% of the myeloma cells form clones. When the growing clones contain 4-16 cells, a third layer of agarose containing high titre rabbit antiserum against mouse heavy chains is placed over the clones (Figure 2). Two to three days later the plates are screened under medium power with an inverted microscope. Cells producing normal heavy chain containing molecules secrete them into the surrounding agar. The antibody diffuses down into the agar to form a visible antigen-antibody precipitate which surrounds and obscures the clone (10). All colonies which are not surrounded by precipitate are presumptive variants and can be recovered from the agar, grown up to mass culture, and characterized biochemically and serologically.

Such presumptive H chain variants could have three different sets of defects: 1) loss of ability to synthesize H chains; 2) defects in assembly or secretion; and 3) the synthesis and secretion of defective heavy chains which no longer react with the antiserum used. If antiserum against L chains is used, then cells with similar defects in L chain production can be identified.

TYPES OF SPONTANEOUS VARIANTS AND THE FREQUENCY WITH WHICH THEY OCCUR

When freshly isolated clones from the MPC-11 (IgG_{2b}), P3 (IgG_1), MOPC-31 (IgG_1) or C1 (IgG_{2a}) cell lines were examined for variants with antibody against H chains, 0.5 - 1% of the clones were unstained. Because of the unexpectedly high frequency of variants, fluctuation analysis (11) was carried out to determine if the variants arose spontaneously and the exact rate at which they were being generated. All three lines lost the ability to produce H chains at the rates of $1\text{-}2 \times 10^{-3}$/cell/generation, or one in every thousand cell divisions resulted in a "mutation" (10). This enormous instability of immunoglobulin production is also found in IgA and IgM producing mouse myeloma cell lines and seems to be peculiar to immunoglobulin production. The same cells became resistant to four different drugs at a frequency of 10^{-6} - 10^{-7}/cell/generation, which is many orders of magnitude lower than the spontaneous instability of immunoglobulin production (12).

Over a hundred MPC 11 and P3 variants which had spontaneously lost the ability to secrete H chains have been examined by incubating with radioactive amino acids for intracellular H chains. Short labelling times were used to rule out synthesis and subsequent degradation. Antiserum raised against denatured H chains was used to increase the chance of precipitating fragments or molecules which had lost many of the normal antigenic determinants. No detectable H chains were found. We concluded that such spontaneously occurring variants were synthesizing less than 1/50 - 1/100th of the amount of complete H chains produced by the parental H plus L chain producing cells (10,13). Eleven P3 variants synthesizing only H chains and over thirty P3 and MPC 11 variants which no longer secreted either H or L chains were also studied and the missing chains were not detected intracellularly.

One of the non-producing variants has been examined in detail for L chain messenger RNA translatable in heterologous cell free systems or hybridizable to cDNA (14). No messenger for complete L chains was detected. Revertants have also been sought and not found. Without revertants or mutant gene products it has not been possible to determine the mechanism responsible for these spontaneously occurring variants.

VARIANTS ARISING THROUGH MUTAGENESIS

In an attempt to find variants making defective gene products which could be characterized chemically, we have examined the effect of a number of mutagenizing agents on the types and frequency of variants. Ethylmethane sulfonate did not increase the frequency of variants. Nitrosoguanidine caused a 2-3 fold increase in variants. However, ICR 191, which is an acridine half mustard that causes frame shift mutations in microorganisms, caused a very significant increase in variants (12) (Table 1). Melphalan, a phenylalanine mustard used in the treatment of human multiple myeloma, is also an effective mutagen (15) (Table 1). Most of the mutagen induced variants resembled those that occur spontaneously in that they have lost the ability to synthesize one or both of the immunoglobulin polypeptide chains. However, 30-40% of the unstained clones continued to synthesize H chains which were chemically and serologically different from those produced by the parental cells. Twenty such mutants with changes in the primary sequence of their heavy chains have been studied in more detail (16,17). The general serological and chemical characteristics of three representative primary sequence mutants are summarized in Table 2.

TABLE I

Effect of mutagens on the incidence of variants

	Mutagen (μg/ml)	% Cell survival	Incidence of variants	% Variant	p
ICR 191	0	100	18/2104	0.86	
	1	60	56/3635	1.54	0.016
	2	25	110/3404	3.24	<0.001
	4	<1	15/229	6.55	<0.001
Melphalan	0	100	17/3777	0.45	
	.2	32	31/2336	1.33	<0.001
	.4	28	100/5926	1.65	<0.001
	.6	16	55/2961	1.86	<0.001
	.8	9	31/1298	2.39	<0.001

Briefly summarized, the variants fall into two groups. The first set synthesize short H chains ranging in different variants from 39,000 to 50,000 daltons compared to 55,000 daltons for the parent. Those presented in Table 2 all have the same variable region antigenic determinants (idiotype) as the parent but others not shown are either less reactive or not reactive with idiotypic antibody (18). When examined with antibody against denatured H chains, all of the short chain variants lack some of the antigenic determinants found on the parent and this is confirmed by their lack of reactivity both with antibody against the Fc region of the parent and with antibody against the IgG_{2b} subclass specific determinants of the parent (Table 2)(16). Comparison of tryptic-chymotryptic digests of the variant and parental H chains reveals that most of the 35 peptide peaks visualized are identical but that 4-6 of the peaks present in the parent are missing from the variant and a few new peaks are detected in the variant (16). When a 39,000 dalton H chain is compared to a 50,000 one, they both lack some of the same peaks but fewer are missing from the larger chain. Furthermore, we have observed the conversion of a variant synthesizing a 50,000 dalton H chain to one synthesizing a 39,000 dalton H chain. Dr. Birshtein is currently carrying out detailed structural studies on these variants and one possible interpretation is that these short chain variants are missing the C-terminal portion of their H chains. A similar type of variant has been reported to have arisen spontaneously in the P3 cell line (20).

TABLE II

Mutagen	Molecular weight of H chain	Cytoplasmic lysates					Secretion	Tryptic chymotryptic peaks in common with parent
		denatured H chain	idiotype	Fc	IgG_{2b}	IgG_{2a}	denatured H chain	
0	55,000	+	+	+	+	-	+	
Melphalan	39,000–44,000	+S	+	-	-	-	+	27/35
ICR	50,000	+S	ND	-	-	-	-	26/30
Melphalan	55,000	+S	+	+S	-	+	+	18/34
ICR	75,000	+S	+	+S	-	+	-	18/34

Cells were concentrated by centrifugation, lysed with Nonidet P-40 and the cell lysates examined with the indicated antisera by double diffusion in agar. "S" indicated a spur with the parent containing antigenic determinants not found in the variant. Idiotypes were examined by R. Lieberman and M. Potter of the NIH using hemagglutination inhibition. Peptide analysis was carried out by mixing ^{3}H amino acid labelled parental H chains with ^{14}C amino acid labelled variant H chains, digesting and then chromatographing the digest as described previously (16).

The second set of variants synthesize normal size or large (75,000 dalton) heavy chains. Again the ones described in Table 2 have the same idiotypic determinants as the parent but others are less reactive (18). Like the short chain mutants, these lack antigenic determinants thought to be located in the C-terminal portion of the H chain. However, the distinguishing characteristics of these mutants is that they have not only lost the IgG_{2b} subclass specific determinant found in the parent but have also acquired antigenic determinants distinctive for the IgG_{2a} constant region gene which was not expressed in the parent. Instead of lacking only a few of the tryptic-chymotryptic peptides of the parent, less than half of the parental peptides are found in these "2a positive" H chains. Amongst the many new peptides seen, at least five are present in another IgG_{2a} but not in other IgG_{2b} heavy chains (Table 2)(17). Different 2a positive mutant H chains all differ from each other by peptide analysis. The L chains of all of the variants so far studied are identical with parent by peptide maps.

The phenotypes of all of these primary sequence variants as well as of all of the other MPC 11 and P3 variants characterized so far are presented in Table 3. These variants can be used to begin to answer some of the general questions raised earlier.

COORDINATION OF H AND L CHAIN SYNTHESIS

As already noted, H and L chains are synthesized in large amounts by the mouse myeloma cells. For example, the MPC 11 IgG_{2b} producing cell line devotes 20-25% of its protein synthetic activity to the production of H and L chains. In absolute terms, these cells are synthesizing 3.6 pg of immunoglobulin/cell/hr or approximately a million H and L chain molecules/cell/min. (21). Since there are a limited number of constant region genes in each cell (see elsewhere in this volume) and probably only one constant region gene is being expressed, this amplification of H and L chain synthesis is not due to gene reiteration. Although the H and L chain genes are not linked (9), relatively equal numbers of the two chains are synthesized. For example, when 18 mouse myelomas were examined, 13 synthesized a significant excess of L chains while 5 produced exactly equimolar amounts of H and L chains (4,22). A heterogeneous population of normal lymph node cells synthesized 1.6 times as many L chains as heavy chains. Since cloned populations of myeloma cells produce the same excess of L chains as the whole population it is unlikely that the excess L chains are produced by cells that are not synthesizing H chains. In fact we have ruled out this possibility by directly measuring the number of cells producing only L chains in the culture (21).

TABLE III

Types of variants of IgG producing mouse myeloma cells

	inducing agent	number P3	MPC-11
1. Synthesis variants			
a. loss of heavy chain (L chain producer)	spont. NTG ICR 191	hundreds	
b. loss of light chain (H chain producer)	spont. NTG ICR 191	11	0
c. loss of heavy & light chain (non producer)	spont. NTG ICR 191	30+	
d. selective decrease of heavy or light chains	spont.	1	1
2. Primary sequence variants			
a. short chain	ICR 191 Melphalan		12
	spont.		1
b. change in subclass	ICR 191 Melphalan		5
3. Assembly and secretion variants			
a. secondary to 1 and 2			
1. decreased rates of assembly			
2. blocks in assembly			
3. blocks in secretion			
4. changes in carbohydrate			

These findings raise the question of whether the synthesis of either chain depends upon the synthesis of the other chain. In the P3 cell line this is certainly not true since we have been able to isolate many variants which have lost the ability to synthesize either H or L chains (Table 3) (12, 23). Those P3 clones that have lost the ability to synthesize H chains continued to produce approximately the same amount of L chains as the parent. When initially isolated, the H chain producing variants also continued to synthesize the same amount of H chain as the parental cells. However, within weeks synthesis decreased from approximately 5% of the cell protein to 0.5% and then was maintained at that level (23). The H chains synthesized in the absence of L chains were assembled into H chain dimers but were neither degraded nor secreted (23). We have been unable to obtain H chain producing variants from the MPC 11 cell line but the L chain producing variants also continue to synthesize the same amount of L chains as the parental cell lines (Table 3) (21). In fact, variants which synthesize complete H chains but no L chains have not been observed in human myelomas and have so far been reported only in the P3 (21) and MOPC-460 mouse myelomas (24). It is possible that such variants occur frequently but that in most cells the synthesis and intracellular accumulation of large amounts of relatively insoluble H chains is lethal. In the P3 cells, the intracellular accumulation of free H chains appears to result in decreased H chain synthesis, perhaps through a translational mechanism such as that suggested by Stevens and Williamson (25) or more likely through selection. Those human cells which synthesize only H chains always produce fragments (26) which are presumably more soluble than the intact H chain.

It is of interest that the C1 cell line, which synthesizes exactly equimolar amounts of H and L chains, does not appear to convert to either H or L chain producers but rather simultaneously loses the ability to produce both chains (12). It is possible that in this cell line there is either a linkage of the genes or a very tight coordination of H and L chain synthesis (27).

Those variants that have lost the ability to produce one or both chains provide an additional insight. In the H plus L chain producing parent the percentage of membrane associated ribosomes corresponds to the percentage of immunoglobulin produced. In those few variants studied so far, the loss of immunoglobulin production is not associated with a corresponding loss of membrane associated ribosomes. This suggests that the continued synthesis of secreted protein is not necessary for the maintenance of an extensive rough endoplasmic reticulum (28).

Our preliminary conclusion from these studies is that the synthesis of either immunoglobulin chain is not dependent on the continued synthesis of the other chain. In the case of H chains, L chain synthesis may be required if H chain synthesis is not reduced by some translational or transcriptional control, but L chain synthesis is probably a secondary requirement to maintain cell viability. The regulation of the amount of membrane associate ribosomes may be separable from the synthesis of secreted proteins.

ASSEMBLY, GLYCOSYLATION AND SECRETION

By comparing a number of mouse myeloma tumors synthesizing the different subclasses of IgG, we were able to show that different subclasses had different predominant covalent and non-covalent pathways of assembly (29,30). Since the L chains of all of these tumors were of the kappa subclass but the H chains differed in their constant regions, it was concluded that the amino acid sequence of the H chains determined the pathway of assembly (29,30). Within each subclass, different tumors showed different kinetics of assembly. These variations could have been due to different variable regions producing differences in the complementarity of the H and L chains or to some property of the cell. Through careful examination of the primary sequence variants we have isolated, it should ultimately be possible to obtain a clearer understanding of the structural features that determine the pathway and kinetics of assembly. The potential of this approach is illustrated in part by Figure 3.

Here we have incubated cells from the parent (P), a short H chain mutant (M3.11) and a 2a positive mutant (M2.24) with radioactive amino acids for 10 min. and then examined the labelled intracellular immunoglobulins by specifically precipitating them from the cytoplasmic lysate of the cell and analyzing them on SDS containing acrylamide gels. Since the SDS does not disrupt the disulfide bonds and the molecules separate based on their size, we can examine the intermediates in the assembly process and estimate the kinetics of their polymerization (31). Following the 10 min. labelling period, the incorporation of radioactive precursors was stopped by "chasing" with a large excess of unlabelled amino acids and the medium was examined for secreted material 3 hrs later. Since its H chains are smaller than those of the parent (middle panel Figure 3), all of the molecules of M3.11 are also smaller.

Figure 3

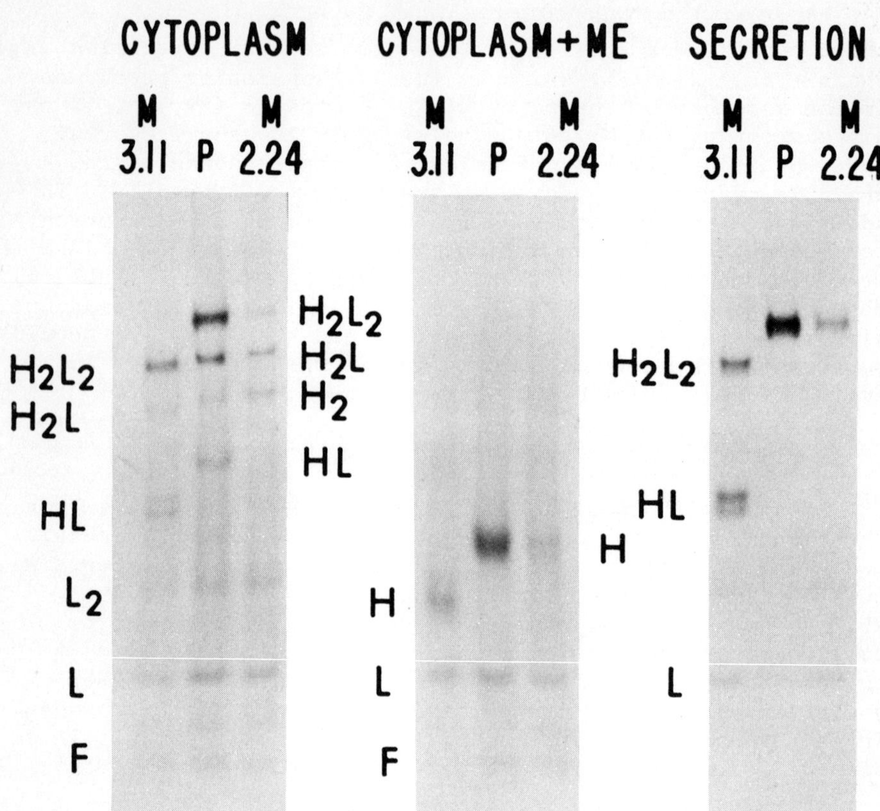

The other major differences are: 1) M3.11 does not form H_2, i.e. inter-H chain disulfide bonds are not formed prior to the inter H-L chain disulfide bonds; 2) large amounts of HL are secreted providing additional evidence for a block in the formation of the inter-H chain disulfide bonds; and 3) there is a double band for both HL and H chains. This double band is due to the non-glycosylation of a significant percentage of the M3.11 H chains (32). Since H_2L_2 and HL both contain non-glycosylated H chains, the carbohydrate moiety on the H chains does not seem necessary for the assembly of this mutant H chain. Furthermore, since the non-glycosylated HL molecules are secreted with the same kinetics as the glycosylated ones, carbohydrate is not necessary for secretion of H chain containing molecules (32).

M2.24, the 2a positive variant, has a normal sized H chain but differs greatly in sequence from the parental H chain (Table 2). HL, which is the distinguishing precursor in the assembly of the parental IgG_{2b} protein (29,30), is not a precursor of the M2.24 molecule. This is true of normal IgG_{2a} proteins (29,30)confirming that the sequence of the H chain is crucial in specifying the pathway of assembly. In addition, after 10 minutes of labelling, less H_2L_2 has been formed in the M2.24 variant than in the parent (17). Since we now have a number of short chain and 2a variants (Table 4) each of which differs from the others in its pattern and kinetics of assembly, glycosylation, and secretion, it should be possible to study the subtleties of these processes in great detail.

GENETIC CONTROL OF IMMUNOGLOBULIN PRODUCTION

As already noted, the most provocative finding in all of these studies is the unusually high rate at which variants occur and the increase in this frequency produced by certain mutagenizing agents. Those variants which have lost the ability to synthesize one or the other polypeptide chains could have arisen through chromosome loss, through some epigenetic change similar to those responsible for differentiation, or through true mutation resulting in the changes in the DNA sequence of structural or regulatory genes. These possibilities are being investigated by analysis of somatic cell hybrids in an attempt to complement these defects. In contrast the H chain primary sequence variants have the characteristics of true mutants: they arise through mutagenesis, are stable, and produce a gene product with a change in its amino acid sequence.

A detailed consideration of these primary sequence mutants should provide some insight into the structure and control of the immunoglobulin genes. Since the short chain mutations may be C-terminal and are produced with frame-shift agents (33), the most likely explanation is that a frame shift mutation has occurred in the Fc region with the production of a nonsense mutation and the resulting premature termination of the polypeptide chain. Needless to say, other possibilities such as a deletion in the C-terminal portion of molecule will have to be ruled out by detailed structural analysis.

The mutants that have switched to producing a 2a positive H chain are most easily explained by considering a shematic presentation of the part of the genome containing the H chain constant region genes (Figure 4).

Figure 4

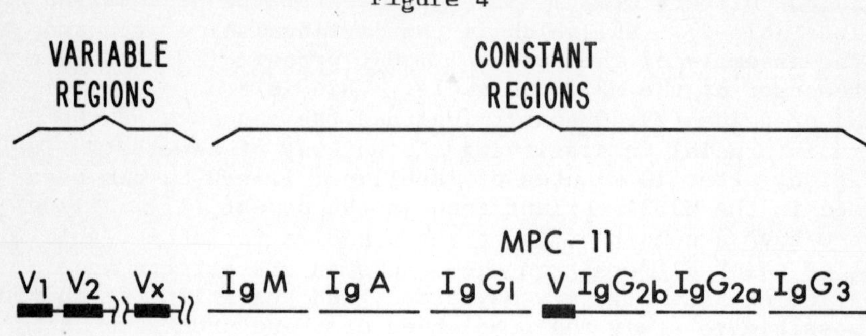

This drawing is based on Gally and Edelman's conception of the genome (34). Of course the order of the constant region genes is not known nor is it clear whether other genes or spacer sequences are interposed. Gally and Edelman (34) have suggested that one of the many available variable region genes is translocated from a neighboring region of the genome onto a constant region gene which in the case of MPC 11 codes for the IgG_{2b} subclass. Assuming the correctness of this thesis and using precedents from microbial genetics, there are three mechanisms which could explain the 2a positive mutants. First, the MPC 11 variable region gene could be "translocated" from the 2b to the 2a constant region gene. This would predict that all of the 2a positive mutants would have identical sequences since they would all reflect the same MPC 11 variable and IgG_{2a} constant region. Since no two of these variants are the same by peptide analysis, this mechanism is unlikely.

The second possibility is that a deletion has occurred between the 2b and 2a constant region genes with the loss of termination and a read-through into the adjoining 2a gene (35). The size of the deletion might vary yielding different size mutant gene products (i.e. the 75,000 dalton protein, Table 2). This mechanism predicts polarity. For example, if the scheme presented above were correct, a 2b myeloma could acquire part of a 2a gene, or less frequently part of a IgG_3 gene but should never acquire parts of any of the genes to its left in Figure 4. If one starts with a IgG_{2a} myeloma such as LPC-1, where the LPC-1 variable region is associated with the 2a constant region gene, it should never convert to the 2b subclass but only to the IgG_3 subclass etc. The polarity of such subclass switches can be tested and if deletions and read-throughs are occurring they would allow us to map the constant region genome.

The third and probably the most likely mechanism would require mismatching of DNA and crossing over between homologous tandem genes. This crossing over could be equal or unequal resulting in different size recombinant genes and gene products. This sort of mechanism is thought to give rise to Lepore type hemoglobins (36). Expression of such recombinant gene products would not show polarity but would reflect either the distance between genes or the degree of base homology between the different constant regions. In fact Kunkel and Natvig (37,38,39) and their colleagues have reported a series of "hybrid" human immunoglobulin molecules and suggested that they arose through crossing over. This recombinational mechanism raises other interesting possibilities. Since only one of two possible alleles is expressed (40), crossing over between allelic chromosomes could lead to non-expression and explain the high incidence of variants which have lost the ability to synthesize H chains. Crossing over between sister chromatids could lead to the 2a type variants described.

There are of course other possible mechanisms to explain the 2b to 2a switch including the turning on of normally unexpressed constant region genes (41). These and other possibilities can only be resolved by the isolation and detailed characterization of a large number of mutants.

CONCLUSION

A method for isolating mouse myeloma cells which have undergone mutations in immunoglobulin production has been developed. A variety of mutants have been isolated, their frequency determined, and some of their biochemical properties described. The detailed characterization of such mutants should provide a deeper understanding of the synthesis, assembly, and secretion of immunoglobulin. Examples of the preliminary steps toward such insights are presented here and will also be described by Milstein in the following chapter. Further studies should also allow us to determine whether the high mutation rates observed are due to one of the unusual aspects of the genetic control of immunoglobulin and provide information on the organization of the immunoglobulin genes.

ACKNOWLEDGMENTS

This work was supported by funds from the National Institutes of Health (AI 5231, AI 10702), the National Science Foundation (GB 29560X), and the American Cancer Society. B. Birshtein was a fellow of the New York Heart Association. W.M. Kuehl was supported by a Helen Hay Whitney Fellowship. D. Margulies was supported by NIH training grant 5T5 GM 1674 from the National Institute of General Medical Sciences. J.-P. Preud'Homme was supported by the French National Institutes of Health (Medical Research (INSERM) and a National Institute of Health John E. Fogarty International Fellowship (I FO 5TW-1862).

Dr. W.M. Kuehl's present address is in the Department of Microbiology at the University of Virginia Medical School. Dr. S.L. Morrison's present address is in the Department of Microbiology at Columbia Presbyterian Medical School. Dr. J.-L. Preud'homme's present address is at the Universite De Paris, Faculte de Medecine in France.

REFERENCES

(1) M.D. Scharff and R. Laskov. Progr. Allergy 14 (1970) 37.

(2) M.J. Bevan, R.M.E. Parkhouse, A.R. Williamson and B.A. Askonas. Progr. Biophysics 25 (1972) 133.

(3) J. Buxbaum. Seminars in Hematology 10 (1973) 33.

(4) R. Baumal and M.D. Scharff. J. Immunol. 108 (1972) 126.

(5) D. Zagury, J.W. Uhr, J.D. Jamieson and G.E. Palade. J. Cell. Biol. 46 (1970) 52.

(6) Y.S. Choi, P.M. Knopf and E.S. Lennox. Biochemistry 10 (1971) 668.

(7) E.W. Sutherland, III, D.H. Zimmerman and M. Kern. Proc. Natl. Acad. Sci. 69 (1972) 167.

(8) J.W. Uhr. Cell Immunol. 1 (1970) 228.

(9) L.Z. Herzenberg, H.D. McDevitt and L.H. Herzenberg. Annu. Rev. Genet. 2 (1968) 209.

(10) P. Coffino, R. Baumal, R. Laskov and M.D. Scharff. J. Cell. Physiol. 79 (1972) 429.

(11) P. Coffino and M.D. Scharff. Proc. Natl. Acad. Sci. 68 (1971) 219.

(12) R. Baumal, B.K. Birshtein, P. Coffino and M.D. Scharff. Science 182 (1973) 164.

(13) W.M. Kuehl and M.D. Scharff. J. Mol. Biol. 89 (1974) 409.

(14) W.M. Kuehl, P. Leder, M. Pace and M.D. Scharff. In preparation.

(15) J.-L. Preud'homme, J. Buxbaum and M.D. Scharff. Nature 245 (1974) 320.

(16) B.K. Birshtein, J.-L. Preud'homme and M.D. Scharff. Proc. Natl. Acad. Sci. 71 (1974) 3478.

(17) J.-L. Preud'homme, B.K. Birshtein and M.D. Scharff. In press.

(18) R. Lieberman and M. Potter. Personal communication

(19) B.K. Birshtein, J.-L. Preud'homme and M.D. Scharff. In Immune System, Genes, Receptors and Signals. Ed. Sercarz (Academic Press 1974) p.339.

(20) D.S. Secher, R.G.H. Cotton and C. Milstein. FEBS Lett. 37 (1973) 311.

(21) R. Laskov and M.D. Scharff. J. Exp. Med. 140 (1974) 1112.

(22) M.D. Scharff. Harvey Lecture, in press.

(23) S.L. Morrison and M.D. Scharff. Fed. Proc. 32 (1973) 1013.

(24) L.K. Bailey, K. Hammersted and H.N. Eisen. Fed. Proc. 32 (1973) 1013.

(25) R.H. Stevens and A.R. Williamson. J. Mol. Biol. 78 (1973) 505.

(26) B. Frangione and E.C. Franklin. Seminars in Hematology 10 (1973) 53.

(27) W.M. Kuehl. Personal communication.

(28) W.M. Kuehl and M.D. Scharff. Unpublished results.

(29) R. Baumal, M. Potter and M.D. Scharff. J. Exp. Med. 134 (1971) 1316.

(30) R. Baumal and M.D. Scharff. Transpl. Rev. 14 (1973) 163.

(31) R. Laskov, R. Lanzerotti and M.D. Scharff. J. Mol. Biol. 56 (1971) 327.

(32) S. Weitzman and M.D. Scharff. In preparation.

(33) J.R. Roth. Annu. Rev. Gen. 8 (1974) 319.

(34) J.A. Gally and G.M. Edelman. Nature 227 (1970) 340.

(35) B. Müller-Hill and J. Kania. Nature 249 (1974) 561.

(36) C. Baglioni. Proc. Natl. Acad. Sci. 48 (1962) 1880.

(37) H.G. Kunkel, J.B. Natvig and F.G. Joslin. Proc. Natl. Acad. Sci. 62 (1969) 144.

(38) J.B. Natvig and H.G. Kunkel. J. Immunol. 112 (1974) 1277.

(39) J.B. Natvig, T.E. Michaelson, J. Geddle-Pahl Jr. and S. Fisher. Immunogenetics 1 (1974) 33.

(40) J.J. Cebra. Bact. Rev. 33 (1969) 159.

(41) M. Bosma. J. Exp. Med. 130 (1974) 512.

DISCUSSION

G. KOCH: You mentioned transcriptional control and processing as a means of synthesizing immunoglobins up to a level of 20% of the total protein synthesis. I want to propose an additional way involving control at the translation level. Dr. Nuss in our laboratory, has shown that modification of the growth medium increases the amount of immune protein synthesized up to 90% of the total protein and significantly changes the ratio of L-chains and H-chains produced. This indicates that the mRNA for immunoglobins is translated under conditions which block translation of host mRNA.

M.D. SCHARFF: That is what I was alluding to when I referred to the papers by Stevens and Williamson. They never reported 90% of the protein was immunoglobin, but they showed you could change the ratio of heavy and light chains being made, that you could selectively decrease heavy chains synthesis and that you could get changes in immunoglobin synthesis and they ascribed this to a translational control. However, to say that there is a translational control is not to specify the mechanism by which the immunoglobin synthesis is amplified. My reading of the amount of messenger present is that in a myeloma tumor or cell line there is enough messenger to code for the amount of immunoglobin that is being made. I think that what you say is very interesting, that one can exert translational modulation superimposed on other controls, but the initial amplification still must result in the synthesis of enough messenger to make the immunoglobin and I guess that has to be either transcription or some sort of processing.

G. KOCH: Of course, I agree with that. I don't want to say that you don't have transcriptional control. I would suggest, however, that the mRNAs for immunoglobin have a higher affinity for ribosomes than do other mRNAs and that this also provides amplification for the synthesis of immunoglobins.

S. RAAM: You mentioned that you have worked with IgM secreting murine tumor cells. Did you come across any mutants with regard to J-chain biosynthesis and assembly?

M.D. SCHARFF: The answer is that we have not looked, because we have not been able to make antiserum against J-chain. However, it has been reported by Kaji and Parkhouse that IgG producing cells, as well as IgM and IgA producing myelomas, synthesise the J-chain found in the polymers of IgA and IgM.

R. SCHULMAN: Have you looked for reversion of short chain mutants by base analogs?

M.D. SCHARFF: I should have said something about that. We have not found a revertant anywhere. We tried to revert the original mutants with the mutagenizing agent that we used to produce them, and also with other agents, but in no case did we obtain reversion. There is a problem as to what one calls a revertant. We have found phenotypic changes. For instance, a variant that does not secrete and makes heavy chain of 50×10^3 can begin to secrete spontaneously. After it starts secreting, however, it makes heavy chains of 39×10^3, which for some reason or other, the cell is able to secrete. We have not found a legitimate structural revertant that has achieved a normal size chain.

C. BELL: Do you know whether the different synthesising capacities of the parental type myeloma cell synthesising H_2L_2 and the subsequent variants synthesising or secreting HL or H_2 are due to different mRNA's or to some other control mechanism preventing translation of mRNA in these variants?

M. D. SCHARFF: The only thing that we know is that in the cells that have lost the ability to make heavy and light chains Kuehl and Leder have failed to detect light chain messenger that has the same size as the parent. It could not be detected by either hybridization or translation. We know nothing about heavy chain messages.

E.A. KABAT: Have you found any evidence of V-region mutants?

M.D. SCHARFF: When we saw the high mutation rates we hoped that we were going to prove the somatic generation of antibody diversity. However, all the variants that I have described to you are in the constant region. By using antigens in the overlay to look at antigen binding myelomas, we have found some myelomas which secrete immunoglobins normally but no longer bind the antigen. One would guess that these have defects in the variable region. If we are finding variable region mutants they are not arising at much higher rates than constant region ones. I have one qualification. I have told you mainly about deletion mutations. We have not found any single amino acids substitutions so far. Although we have looked with the correct mutagenizing agents, our assay for finding them might well miss them. I think that is an important qualification because it could be that there are variable region changes occurring which we are not picking up either by isoelectric focusing or by defects in the assembly or secretion.

IMMUNOGLOBULIN GENES IN A MOUSE MYELOMA AND IN MUTANT CLONES

C. Milstein, K. Adetugbo, G.G. Brownlee, N.J. Cowan, N.J. Proudfoot, T.H. Rabbitts and D.S. Secher

MRC Laboratory of Molecular Biology, Hills Road, Cambridge, England

The requirements of multiple V-genes for the generation of antibody diversity was an inescapable corollary of the description of the three basic sequences of human kappa chains (1,2). Since the C-regions of the same chains were coded by single Mendelian genes (3,4) an integration involving V- and C-genes had to be postulated by both germ line and somatic mutation theories. A two genes-one polypeptide hypothesis had been previously proposed as an *ad hoc* solution to the paradox posed by the germ line theory of antibody diversity (5).

It soon became obvious that the pattern of diversity was different in different species. An expansion-contraction evolutionary model was proposed to explain the emergence of such differences (6). But an expansion-contraction evolutionary process could also be applied to explain the presence of well defined sub-groups in a germ line model of antibody diversity (7). Increasingly elaborate arguments almost exclusively based on protein sequence data become somewhat repetitive. Like Gally (8), we also became "weary of theoretical arguments, which are beginning to become a bit stale by now" and in recent years we attempted new approaches which could give a further insight into the genetic control of antibody diversity. The first line of attack was the isolation and chemical characterisation of mRNA suitable for studies of gene dosage by molecular hybridisation procedures. The second was a study of the clonal diversification of a myeloma cell line in tissue culture. This paper describes the progress made so far in our studies on a permanent tissue culture line (9) of the mouse myeloma MOPC 21.

Immunoglobulin mRNA

We consider that our structural studies on the light chain mRNA are sufficiently advanced to permit the unambig-

4 10 19 21 38

--- Met - Thr - Gln - Ser - Pro - Lys - Ser - Met ---- Val - Thr - Leu ---- Tyr - Gln - Gln -

(G)A-C-C-C-A-A-U-C-U-C-C-C-A-A-A-U-C-C-A-U-G (G)U-C-A-C-C-U-U-G U-A-U-C-A-A-C-A-G

t3 t15 t17

70 73 85 88 105 108

------ Asp - Phe - Thr - Leu ---- Asp - Tyr - His - Cys ---- Glu - Ile - Lys - Arg ---------

(G)A-U-U-U-C-A-C(U-C)U-G (G)A-U-U-U-A-U-C-A-C-U-G (G)A-A-A-U-A-A-A-A-C-G

t9 t10 t11b

115 120 137 140

- Val - Ser - Ile - Phe - Pro - Pro - Ser - Ser ---- Asn - Asn - Phe - Tyr - Pro - Lys -

(G)U-A-U-C-C-A-U-C-U-U-C-C-C-A-C-C-A-U-C-C-A-G A-A-C-A-A-C-U-U-C-U-A-C-C-C-C-A-A-A-G

t2 t5

145 171 174 177 180 188

Asp - Ile - Asn - Val ---- Ser - Thr - Tyr - Ser ---- Ser - Thr - Leu - Thr ---- Arg - His -

-A-C-A-U-C-A-A-U-G (G)C-A-C-C-U-A-C-A-G (G)C-A-C-C-C-U-C-A-C-G (G)A-C-A-U-

t16 t22 t20 t13

190 195 200

Asn - Ser - Tyr - Thr - Cys - Glu - Ala - Thr - His - Lys - Thr - Ser - Thr - Ser - Pro -

A-A-C-A-G-C-U-A-U-A-C-C-U-G (G)C-C-A-C-U-C-A-C-A-A-G-A-C-A-U-C-A-A-C-U-U-C-A-C-C-C-

t14 t19 t4

205 210

Ile - Val - Lys - Ser - Phe - Asn - Arg

A-U-U-G (G)C-U-U-C-A-A-C-A-G

t18

Fig. 1. Proposed alignment of the larger T_1 oligonucleotides of the mRNA and the amino acid sequence of MOPC 21 light chain

uous statement that there is one continuous mRNA molecule which codes for both the V- and C-regions of the light chain (10). The possibility of the V- and C-regions being translated from two separate mRNA molecules had been a matter of considerable speculation and we would like to summarise the structural evidence for the presence of a single mRNA.

The light chain mRNA can be chemically identified by the presence of nucleotide sequences (11) which correspond to sequences predicted by the genetic code and the known amino acid sequence (12) of the protein. Our original analysis has been extended to 25 T1 oligonucleotides ranging from 8 to about 45 bases (10). These account for about 345 nucleotide residues which represent one third of the length of the molecule (excluding the 200 residues of A at the 3' end). Of these, 194 bases have been assigned to the coding region accounting for 65 amino acids out of a total of 214 of the light chain. Sequences from both V- and C-regions are included, as shown in Fig. 1. The other 150 nucleotides were present in nine oligonucleotides larger than eight residues which could not be fitted in the amino acid sequence. If the preparation is pure, these oligonucleotides should be part of the non-coding region of the light chain mRNA, presumably located at the 5' or the 3' end. Those which are located at the 3' end should be nearer to the poly(A) sequence than any of the oligonucleotides which have been assigned to the coding region. This linear arrangement was investigated by introducing random breaks in the ^{32}P-mRNA by means of alkali digestion. The population of fragments was fractionated by sucrose gradient centrifugation and oligo(dT) chromatography. The fraction of about 6S which contained poly(A) was then studied by fingerprint analysis (Fig. 2). This showed the presence of almost all the oligonucleotides assigned to the untranslated region, in variable yields. Since all the fragments in the population start at poly(A) but differ in total length, the yields of oligonucleotides will be inversely proportional to their distance from the poly(A). Most of the nucleotides assigned to the coding region were totally absent. Trace amounts of oligonucleotides t18, t19 and t4 were, however, detectable. As expected, these are the coding oligonucleotides nearest to the poly(A) region (see Fig. 1).

A different approach to define the 3' end of the mRNA involved the sequence analysis of complementary ^{32}P-labelled DNA (^{32}P-cDNA). This was prepared by reverse transcription of mRNA by DNA polymerase I from Escherichia coli (13) primed by oligo(dT)$_{12}$. By this procedure, a unique sequence of 52 bases adjacent to poly(A) could be established and is shown

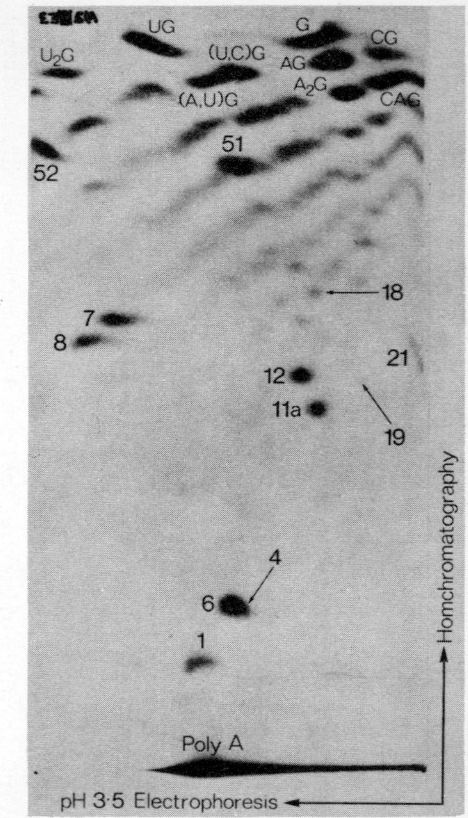

Fig. 2. Two-dimensional fraction of the T1 RNase digest of the poly(A)-containing 6S fraction prepared by partial alkaline hydrolysis. Prominent spots were analysed by further degradation. Some of them are complementary to the cDNA transcript described in Fig. 3. Spots 1,6,7,8, 11a, 12a and 21 could not be correlated with the amino acid sequence of the light chain. Most of the oligonucleotides described in Fig. 1 could not be detected, but trace amounts of t18, t19 and t4 are just visible. They must derive from the longest fragments in the population. This permits an estimation of a distance of 250 bases between the end of the coding region and the poly(A) (10). An alternative estimation of this distance can be made by adding the lengths of all the numbered oligonucleotides (except 18, 19 and 4) and assuming a minimum contribution of about 40 residues for the smaller un-numbered ones (13 of them have been located - see Fig. 3). This gives a minimum distance of 150 residues. The average of 200 between these two independent estimations has been used in Fig. 4.

cDNA (HO)G-A-T-T-A-T-A-A-A-C-T-A-C-A-G-C-G-T-C-T-T-T-T-A-T-A-

mRNA C-U-A-A-U-A-U-U-U-G-A-U-G-U-C-G-C-A-G-A-A-A-A-U-A-U-

←— 8 —→ ←→ ←→ ←→ ←— 6 —

A-G-T-T-A-T-T-T-C-A-C-T-C-A-G-A-A-A-C-G-T-G-A-A-C-G T_n T_{12}

U-C-A-A-U-A-A-A-G-U-G-A-G-U-C-U-U-U-G-C-A-C-U-U-G-C A_n(OH)

— 6 —→ ←→ ←— ←— 52 —→ ←— 51 —→

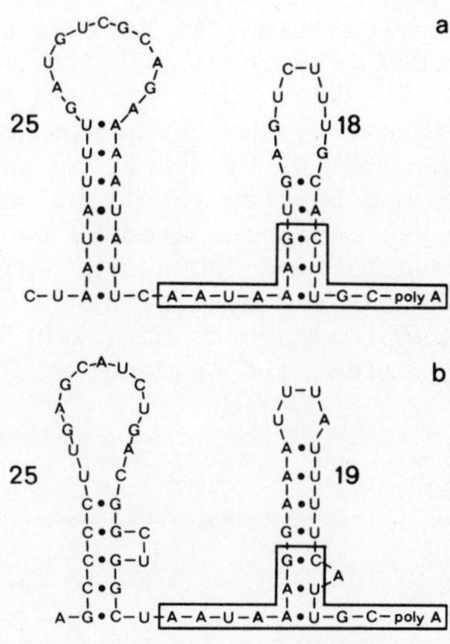

Fig. 3. Sequence of cDNA transcript of MOPC 21 light chain mRNA. The complementary mRNA sequence is shown to contain T1 oligonucleotides which correspond to previously identified products of the ^{32}P-mRNA fingerprint. A possible secondary structure of this section of the mRNA is shown below (a) and is compared with the homologous section from β-globin mRNA isolated from rabbits (b).

in Fig. 3. The sequence derived contains the complement of four T1 oligonucleotides which had been previously assigned to the 3' end of the mRNA. These oligonucleotides occurred in good yields (Fig. 2). The linear arrangement indicated by the fingerprint analysis of the mRNA fragments obtained by partial alkali degradation and the sequence analysis of the ^{32}P-cDNA were in complete agreement.

It could still be argued that there are two molecules with identical sequences at the 3' end. If so, the oligonucleotides assigned to the 3' untranslated region should occur in twice the molar yield to those oligonucleotides derived from either the V- or the C-region. Molar yields have been measured and gave no such indication (14). This, together with the fact that a unique sequence at the 3' end of the mRNA was deduced shows that there is only one major molecular component. Since both V- and C-region oligonucleotides are present in the same preparation, it follows that they occur in a single, integrated, mRNA.

The results obtained by these experiments permitted a linear diagram of the mRNA to be drawn, as shown in Fig. 4. The length of the 3' end between the light chain coding sequence and the poly(A) was estimated by two procedures (Fig. 2) to be between 150 and 250 bases, while the 5' untranslated region was derived by difference (10). The diagram shows 642 bases coding for the light chain and about 400 extra bases (the amino acid sequence of P is not known).

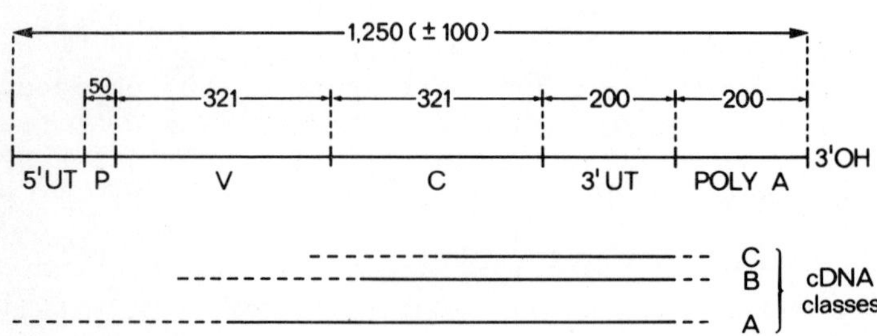

Fig. 4. Diagrammatic representation of the mRNA for the L-chain of MOPC 21. The figure also shows the size classes of cDNA used for hybridisation studies. The heterogeneity of the poly(T) tract was experimentally shown to span from 14 to 70 bases.

If, on the other hand, the V- and C-regions occurred on two different mRNA molecules, each containing 1,250 bases and 200 residues in a poly(A) sequence at the 3' end, the number of bases coding for V- and C-regions in each would be 321 and the rest (730 bases in each) would occur as extra bases. In the mixture the total number of bases coding for light chain would be 642 while the extra bases would be about 1460. One would therefore expect on average to find more bases in oligonucleotides which do not fit the amino acid sequence than oligonucleotides which do. Clearly this is not so, since in T1 oligonucleotides larger than eight residues we account for 195 bases in the translated region (Fig. 1) and so far only 150 which are not translated as light chain.

Number of Genes

One of the main reasons for the studies above was to provide a firm basis for RNA(or cDNA)-DNA hybridisation studies to determine the reiteration frequency of immunoglobulin genes. We (15), and others (16,17), have shown that the hybridisation of L-chain mRNA from several sources to cellular DNA is biphasic. Such biphasic profiles could result from single species of mRNA containing segments which hybridise with repetitive and non-repetitive genes respectively. The unique genes could represent the C-region while the repetitive could represent parts of the V-region or untranslated sections. Such profiles could also result from mixtures of molecules, some of which hybridise to repetitive, and others to non-repetitive genes. That the first interpretation was correct was suggested by the fact that cDNA copies prepared with reverse transcriptase fail to show the repetitive component (18,19,20,21). The implication that the repetitive component was a segment located beyond the transcribed 3' end of the mRNA was indicative of the existence of very few or unique genes for the C-region. The cDNA transcripts were, however, too short to permit speculations about the participation of the V-region in the profiles.

In the previous section it was shown that transcription of mRNA primed by oligo$(dT)_{12}$ starts in the poly(A) region. The longer transcripts will therefore include increasing sections of the mRNA towards the V-region and the 5' untranslated end. By suitable fractionation procedures (described in detail in ref. 21) three size classes were prepared as shown schematically in Fig. 4. A number of detailed studies were made to describe the cDNA populations accurately. These included size determination on denaturing gels, using restriction fragments from ØX 174 as markers and determination of the length of oligo(dT) tracts (by depurination and gel electrophoresis) to estimate the extent of poly(A) transcription.

The cDNA populations were used to measure the rate of hybridisation with nuclear DNA. Figs. 5 and 6 show the results when hybrid formation was measured by hydroxyapatite fractionation and by S1 nuclease digestion respectively. What emerges clearly from these profiles is that the biphasic kinetics characteristic of the intact mRNA can only be obtained when the largest of the cDNA populations is tested by hydroxyapatite. To interpret the results, it is important

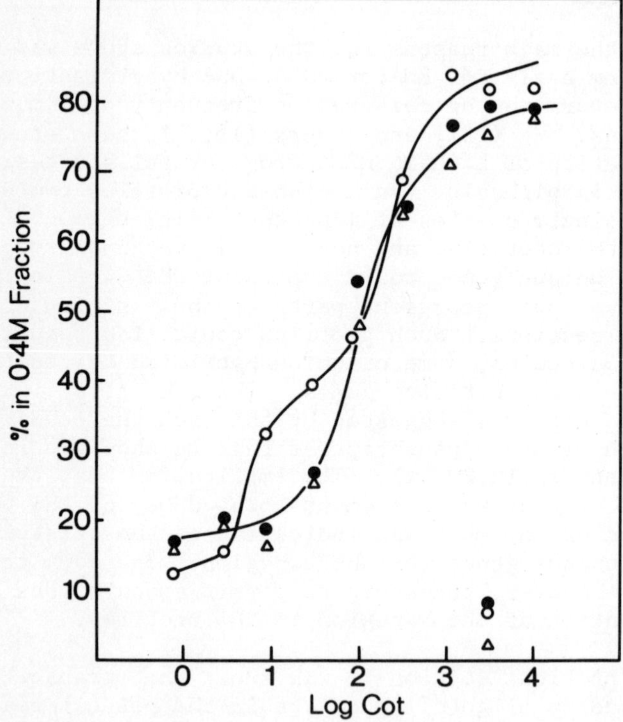

Fig. 5. Hybridisation of the three size classes of cDNA to excess myeloma nuclear DNA measured by hydroxyapatite fractionation. cDNA fractions A —○— , B —●— and C —△— as shown in Fig. 4. Zero points shown at bottom right hand corner. For experimental details see (19).

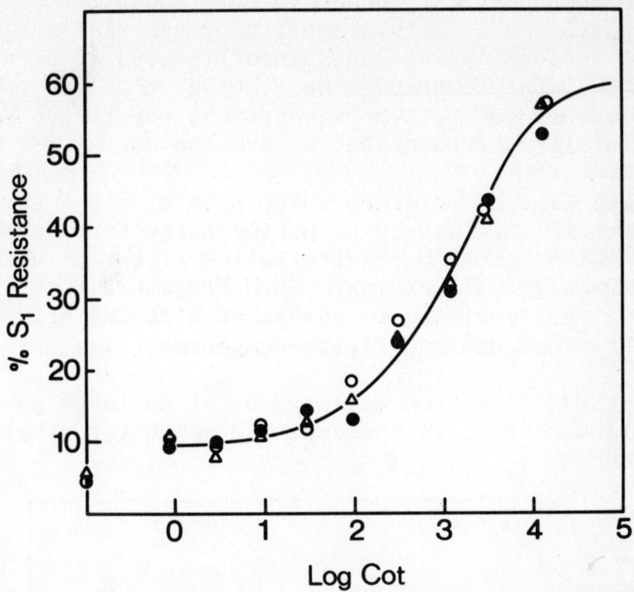

Fig. 6. Hybridisation of cDNA to excess myeloma DNA as measured by S1 nuclease digestion. Other details as Fig. 5.

to remember that S1 nuclease digests single stranded regions while hydroxyapatite retains partly hybridised molecules. The single stranded tails are therefore computed as hybrids by hydroxapatite analysis but not by S1 nuclease resistance.

Fraction B does not show the repetitive component and contains a considerable proportion of the V-region. About 70% of the molecules of fraction B are of sufficient length to include enough V-region to form stable hybrids. As we estimate that the purity of the cDNA is 50% or better, the percentage of cDNA retained by hydroxyapatite through hybridisation to V-genes will be at least 35% (70% x 50%). Even assuming that our preparation is only 30% pure (instead of 50%) and only 50% (rather than the 70% value given above) contains hybridisable V-region, the putative repetitive component should have been 15% of the hydroxyapatite pattern and hence easily detectable. The conclusion that the V-region gene for MOPC 21 light chain is not repetitive seems inescapable. The fact that the rapidly hybridising component was detected in fraction A and then, only when analysed by hydroxyapatite, was reassuring. It indicates that the repetitive component is present in only about 25% of the longest copies and is only a small fragment (and for that reason not detected by S1 resistance) located at or near the 5' end of the mRNA template. We conclude that the repetitive component is not due to hybridisation to repetitive V-genes which are similar or identical to the one coding for MOPC 21.

Another line of evidence which points to the same conclusions was obtained by preparing large fragments (about 12S) of ^{32}P-mRNA after partial alkaline digestion which were retained by oligo(dT) columns. Such fragments lack, therefore, the 5' end region. In agreement with the previous results they lose the repetitive component (Fig. 7).

The hybrid formation measured by S1 nuclease gave a $Cot^{d}_{\frac{1}{2}}$ of about 1,000. This is the expected value for single copy

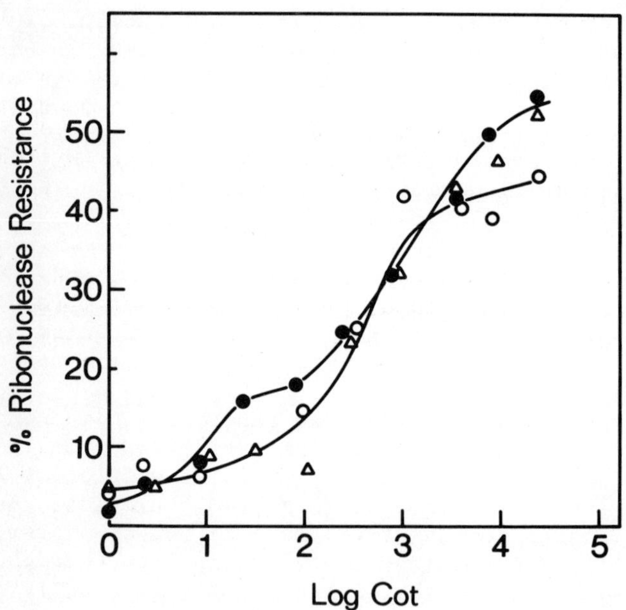

Fig. 7. DNA excess hybridisation of ^{32}P-L-chain mRNA fragments. Partial alkaline digested ^{32}P-mRNA was fractionated by size and by oligo(dT) chromatography. —△— 12S and —○— 6S poly(A)-containing fragments; —●—6S non-poly(A)-containing fragment.

genes under our experimental conditions. The reasons for the higher values obtained with hydroxyapatite have been investigated and fully discussed elsewhere (21). We have concluded, therefore, that within experimental error there is a single gene which codes for both V- and C-regions of MOPC 21 light chain. A similar conclusion, based on competition experiments, has been indicated for the light chain of the MOPC 70E myeloma (22). If we generalise, we could conclude that each basic sequence will be coded by few genes. We are, however, fully aware that this is a generalisation and that the possibility that some basic sequences may be coded by a larger number of genes is still possible. On the other hand, the possibility that different basic sequences are coded by a single gene has not been disproved either. The nature and selection of somatic mutants and their possible role in the generation and maintenance of antibody diversity remain as exciting puzzles.

Somatic Mutants

A better understanding of spontaneous somatic mutation at the molecular level is of general importance in biology and may be critical in understanding the generation of antibody diversity. In the past few years we have been isolating and characterising spontaneously arising clonal variants of the MOPC 21 cells kept in tissue culture. The choice of myeloma cells has a number of advantages but unfortunately certain limitations. In particular we are well aware of the possibility that, by studying the end cell of the differentiation pathway, we may diminish or totally eliminate our probability of finding specific mutational mechanisms. Our primary interest (23) was to obtain information on frequency and nature of spontaneous mutations unaffected by antigen selection and for that reason we have avoided selective pressures and the use of mutagens as a means of concentrating variants.

Two classes of variants have been isolated - variants which do not secrete immunoglobulin and variants which secrete an altered immunoglobulin. We will call them mutants when the variation has been reasonably established to be the result of a change in the sequence of the DNA.

The non-secreting variants have been classified (24) into three types (Table 1). NS I type variants are by far the most common and only one example of type NS II has been observed. The latter is particularly interesting in that it reveals the presence of a heavy chain (H*) of reduced

TABLE 1

Three types of non-secreting (NS) variants of MOPC 21 myeloma cells

Type	Intracellular chains present		
	H	H*	L
NS I	-	±	+++
NS II	-	++	-
NS III	-	±	-
P3K (wild type)	+++	-	+++

molecular weight (24). The nature of the heavy chain abnormality is not yet known. A major difficulty in its chemical analysis is the low amounts of available material due to its intracellular destruction. A puzzling observation is the presence of trace amounts of H* in other non-secreting variants. It must be emphasised, however, that so far we have not been able to obtain positive evidence on the chemical identity between the H* component of different variants. Whether the emergence of this component is the result of a mutation or another change in the expression of the cell remains uncertain. The fact that H* could be synthesised in a reticulocyte cell-free system directed by polysomes from the variant cells (24) suggests that the alteration is the result of a mutation.

Two of the variant clones (IF1 and IF2) secrete Ig of altered electrophoretic properties which have been shown to be the result of a deletion in the heavy chain (25,26). We would like now to report the characterisation of a third mutant, IF3. This mutant was detected by the screening procedure which detects alterations in the isoelectric point of the secreted immunoglobulin, as described previously (23). The alteration was the result of a shorter heavy chain as revealed by SDS-acrylamide gel electrophoresis. Gross differences were also detected by amino acid composition. Analysis of the cyanogen bromide fragmentation pattern revealed the absence of the two fragments which constitute the last (CH3) domain.

A more detailed study of the other fragments did not reveal any other abnormality except for the fragment that extends from residue 304 to 352 (Fig. 8). This latter fragment gave an abnormal amino acid analysis, and preliminary

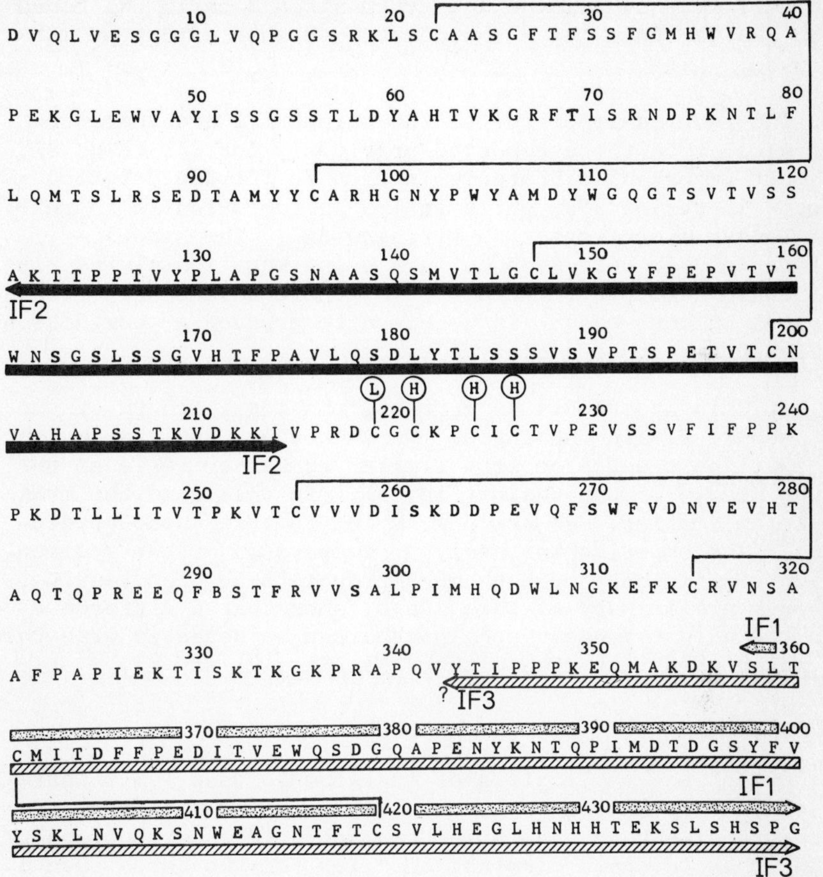

Fig. 8. Tentative sequence of the H-chain of MOPC 21 and of three deletion mutants. The horizontal arrows indicate the extent of the deletion in each mutant. IF1 and IF2 are taken from ref. 26. The mutant IF3 is discussed in the text (Adetugbo and Milstein, unpublished). The question mark indicates that the results are only based on the amino acid composition of the cyanogen bromide fragments. A discrepancy between mobility in SDS gels (Fig. 9) and the molecular weight as calculated from the sequence of IF1 is being investigated.

results show that the abnormality is the result of a deletion starting with the tyrosine-343 (Fig. 8). This deletion of the C-terminal domain does not seem to be the result of a post-translational modification. The isolated heavy chain mRNA from the IF3 cells has been used in a rabbit reticulocyte cell-free system and the synthesised H-chain was found to be smaller than the H-chain obtained when wild type mRNA was used.

The results reported for the mutant IF3 are therefore very similar to those reported previously for IF1 (Fig. 8). The most important difference is that in IF1 the deletion started in serine 358, while in IF3 the deletion is 15 residues longer and starts with tyrosine-343. The simple explanation for both mutants is a point mutation giving rise to a chain termination triplet. A single base change (transversions in both cases) is required to produce a termination triplet from either serine or tyrosine.

If this hypothesis is correct, the total length of the mRNA should remain unchanged. On the other hand, the mutant IF2 involves a deletion of a similar number of residues but in the middle of the chain (Fig. 8). In this case the mRNA should be smaller. We are now trying to test these predictions. The experiments involve a comparison of the sedimentation coefficients of each mRNA preparation. The results, although preliminary at this stage, show that a difference with the wild type heavy chain mRNA can be detected with the IF2 mutants but not with either IF1 (Fig. 9) or IF3.

Final Remarks

Out of the 64 triplets of the genetic code, only three are chain termination triplets. Random point mutations are therefore likely to give rise to amino acid substitutions rather than to chain termination. Yet, of the three spontaneous mutants fully characterised so far, the two explained by point mutations involve a chain termination.

This may partly reflect our inability to detect neutral amino acid exchanges. In any case, the number of characterised mutants is still too low to allow confident conclusions about the non-random nature of spontaneous mutations. But it is possible that we are detecting certain preferred mutational patterns resulting from mutational events which are not randomly distributed along the DNA. In addition, the proportion of amino acid substitutions, which may be quite

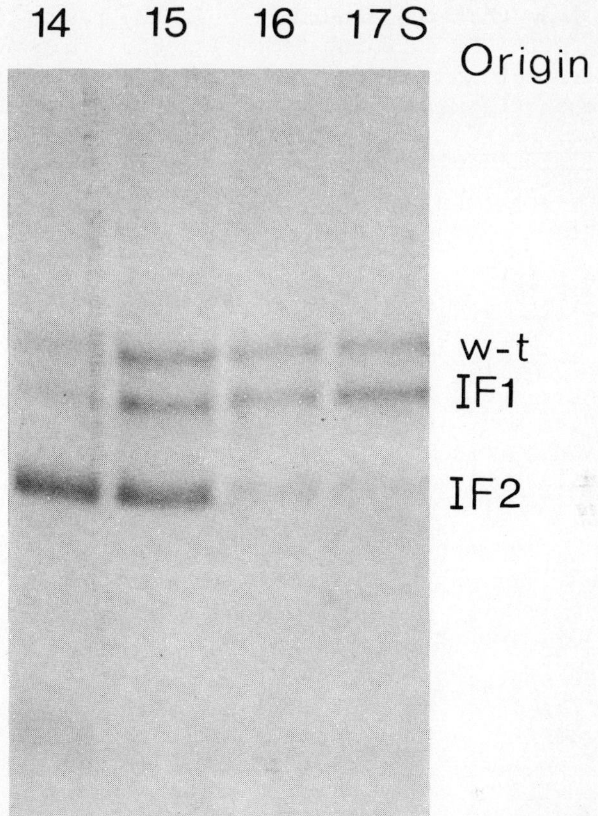

Fig. 9. The translation of a mixture of wild type P3K (w-t), IF1 and IF2 H-chain mRNAs in a rabbit reticulocyte cell-free system. The figure shows that the IF2 H-chain is translated from the fractions containing mRNA of about 14S 15S, whereas both IF1 and wild type H-chains are translated from fractions containing higher molecular weight mRNA.

Polysomes were prepared separately from each of the three cell cultures and then mixed. The RNA dissociated from the mixed polysomes was fractionated on a sucrose density gradient and RNA from fractions in the region 14-22S were assayed in the cell-free system. Ig chains were precipitated with sheep antiserum to mouse Ig (24). The figure shows the analysis of the ^{35}S-Met labelled products by SDS gel electrophoresis and autoradiography. w-t, IF1 and IF2 indicate the positions of the primary translation products of the corresponding H-chain mRNAs. The number above each channel refers to the approximate S-value of the RNA assayed in that incubation.

considerable, introduce distortions in the protein structure. Such distortions could affect properties such as solubility which, in turn, could affect the proliferation of the mutant clones. In this context it is interesting to note that all the deletions involve complete domains. The four residues which define the deletions in the three mutants are located between the S-S loops and yet in MOPC 21 heavy chain there are fewer residues between the loops (192 residues) than within loops (247 residues).

These mutations (and a few others uncharacterised) have been observed in a survey of about 7,000 clones. Of course, this frequency of almost 10^{-3} includes also an accumulation factor due to the proliferation of mutant clones. If the growth characteristics of the mutant clones are the same as in the wild type, the frequency of mutants is about n x f where n is the number of generations in a culture and f the mutation frequency/cell/generation. Taking into consideration the age of our cultures, the point mutations described occur at a frequency of about 2×10^{-6}/cell/generation. This must represent an underestimate of the overall mutation frequency because due to our screening procedure we only detect electrophoretic changes. In addition we have argued above that many of the mutants may be deleterious and for those the n x f argument would not apply.

A model for the immune system in which germ line genes serve the dual purpose of providing for protection against common pathogens as well as the raw material for the development of suitable somatic variants (27,28) seems in harmony with the results discussed in this paper.

References

(1) C. Milstein. Nature (London), 216 (1967) 330.

(2) C. Milstein, FEBS Lett. 2 (1969) 301.

(3) H. Ritter, C. Ropartz, P.Y. Rousseau, L. Rivat and H. Walter. Blut, 13 (1966) 373.

(4) H. Hunger and P. Herzog. Vox. Sang. 10 (1965) 635.

(5) W.J. Dreyer and J.C. Bennett. Proc. Natl. Acad. Sci. U.S.A. 54 (1965) 864.

(6) C. Milstein and J.R.L. Pink, in: Progress in Biophysics and Molecular Biology, Vol. 21, ed. J.A.V.Butler and D. Noble (Pergamon Press, Oxford and New York, 1970) p. 209.

(7) L. Hood and J. Prahl. Adv. Immunol. 14 (1971) 291.

(8) J.A. Gally, in: The Antigens, Vol. 1, ed. M. Sela (Academic Press, New York and London, 1973) p. 283.

(9) K. Horibata and A.W. Harris. Exp. Cell Res. 60 (1970) 61.

(10) C. Milstein, G.G. Brownlee, E.M. Cartwright, J.M. Jarvis and N.J. Proudfoot. Nature (London), 252 (1974) 354.

(11) G.G. Brownlee, E.M. Cartwright, N.J. Cowan, J.M. Jarvis and C. Milstein. Nature (London), New Biol. 244 (1973) 236.

(12) J. Svasti and C. Milstein. Biochem. J. 128 (1972) 427.

(13) N.J. Proudfoot and G.G. Brownlee. FEBS Lett. 38 (1974) 179.

(14) T.M. Harrison, G.G. Brownlee and C. Milstein. Eur. J. Biochem. 47 (1974) 621.

(15) T.H. Rabbitts, J.O. Bishop, C. Milstein and G.G. Brownlee. FEBS Lett. 40 (1974) 157.

(16) T. Delovitch and C. Baglioni. Cold Spring Harbor Symp. Quant. Biol. 38 (1973) 739.

(17) S. Tonegawa, A. Bernardini, B.J. Weimann and C. Steinberg. FEBS Lett. 40 (1974) 92.

(18) T.H. Rabbitts. FEBS Lett. 42 (1974) 323.

(19) C.H. Faust, H. Diggelman and B. Mach. Proc. Natl. Acad. Sci. U.S.A. 71 (1974) 2491.

(20) J. Stavnezer, R.-C.C. Huang, E. Stavnezer and J.M. Bishop. J. Mol. Biol. 88 (1974) 43.

(21) T.H. Rabbitts and C. Milstein. Eur. J. Biochem. (1975) in press.

(22) S. Tonegawa, C. Steinberg, S. Dube and A. Bernardini. Proc. Natl. Acad. Sci. U.S.A. 71 (1974) 4027.

(23) R.G.H. Cotton, D.S. Secher and C. Milstein. Eur. J. Immunol. 3 (1973) 135.

(24) N.J. Cowan, D.S. Secher and C. Milstein. J. Mol. Biol. (1974) in press.

(25) D.S. Secher, R.G.H. Cotton and C. Milstein. FEBS Lett. 37 (1973) 311.

(26) C. Milstein, K. Adetugbo, N.J. Cowan and D.S. Secher, in: Progress in Immunology, Vol. 2 (1974) in press.

(27) C. Milstein and J. Svasti, in: Progress in Immunology, Vol. 1 (1971) 33.

(28) M. Cohn, B. Blomberg, W. Geckeler, W. Raschke, R. Riblet and M. Weigert, in: The Immune System, ed. E.E. Sercarz, A.R. Williamson and F.C. Fox (Academic Press, New York and London, 1974) p. 89.

DISCUSSION

M.D. SCHARFF: About the last point you made concerning the frequency of mutations and the possibility of selection, I think it is worthwhile to reemphasize the difference between the way we find our variants and to report our experience with variants that do not secrete and may be missing part of a domain. These variants are very unstable and we first select them, carry out a rapid serological screening and then find ones that are making defective heavy chains. Then we reclone a number of times. Each time the majority of the sub-clones of the unstable variants lose the ability to make heavy chains, as if there was a selective disadvantage in growth rate or in viability. Ultimately the non-secreting variants stabilize so I think we have confirmatory evidence that some variants have a hard time surviving. Only by immediate characterization, recovery and recloning are we able to identify them.

C. MILSTEIN: How do you know that it is not the whole of a domain (domains) that is missing?

M.D.SCHARFF: I'm guessing from the molecular weight.

C. MILSTEIN: I do not think that the molecular weight is sufficiently accurate to tell that you are not splitting or missing in between domains.

H.H. FUDENBERG: Why are there no mutations, neither substitutions nor deletions, in the variable region? Some would be expected if mutation were purely random.

C. MILSTEIN: The chain termination mutants, as far as I can see, are point mutations leading to chain termination rather than to substitution. Statistically, this is something that beats me. We are not getting what we expected. However, you must remember that the mutation rates that we are finding are still high and that mutants of the V-region may occur at lower frequency.

G. KOCH: It becomes more and more important to look for the structure of the 5' end of the mRNA. Have you, or anyone else, looked to see if the 5' end of the myeloma mRNA is methylated or blocked?

C. MILSTEIN: We are looking into this but I am not yet able to answer that question.

L.A. HERTZENBERG: This is addressed to both Dr. Scharff and Dr. Milstein if they care to comment. I was struck by Mattie Scharff pointing out the 5 variants he now has which have gamma 2a and gamma 2b chains. As he knows, such variants also occur in mice. Noel Warner and I found one of these in a myeloma some years ago and recently Noel Warner has found several more. They might, therefore, occur not only in myelomas but also in the germ line, or at least be present in normal immunoglobulins. A number of the kinds of variants of which both of you have spoken are found in patients, and do not seem to be a random assortment of the possible mutations which one might expect. Milstein did not really answer Dr. Fudenberg's question as to why one does not find any mutants or variants in the variable region. The answer may be that the kinds of variants which are seen are a non-random set of the possibilities one might expect a priori because, in fact, none of them is truly a variant but rather an expression of something which is there in a latent form and not being translated. It is a far out possibility, but would either of you care to comment in a positive or negative way?

M.D. SCHARFF: I think that is a real possibility in that there are an increasing number of rumors and published papers concerning unexpressed genes in immunoglobulin. These occur either spontaneously or under pressure, for example idiotypic suppression. In addition to your comments which are correct on the mouse, Kunkel and Natuig have reported a number of what they call "hybrid" immunoglobulin molecules, but in the context of this discussion what we would call "recombinant immunoglobulin molecules" between two constant regions. Interestingly, as you suggested, one of them was in an abnormal protein, and was also found elsewhere as a representative of a germ line gene My answer to the question is that it is possible that a "2a variant" is an unexpressed gene but that there would have to be a lot of such unexpressed genes because each "2a variant" is different from the other. As one reads the bacterial genetic literature, which I try to do more and more these days, one realizes that there are hot spots in all bacterial systems. There is a beautiful review by Roth on frame shifts, both spontaneous and mutagenized, in the Annual Review of Genetics in which he discussed these hot spots in various systems. Reemphasizing what Milstein said, I don't think we should be surprised to see these, rather we should be surprised to see anything else. I don't believe that we've looked properly for the variable region mutants, but I think that they are there and that their frequency may be a function of hit size; the size of the variable region as opposed to the size of the constant region.

C. MILSTEIN: I would like to emphasize the point you are making by raising another point. I think it is also your experience, that most of the mutations so far found are on the heavy chain, few on the light chain. Now the size of the light chain is half of the heavy chain, and therefore one would expect an average of one light chain mutant for every two heavy chain mutants. There is obviously a lack of balance, and either the light chain is much more stable or the mutant more unstable.

M. COHN: There have been reports of B-cells in humans that carry both IgD and IgM on the surface and secrete IgG. Pernis told me recently that there is some evidence that they carry the same idiotype. Now this would imply a single V region that is associated with several heavy chains and from this you would say that when you translocated a V region you would have to gene duplicate it in order to have simultaneous transcription of the VC cistrons. As you might imagine such a situation is embarrassing for a somatic mutation theory for when you switch classes you would switch to a different specificity if you had independent mutations in each one of these genes. So the question I want to ask is, do we have a very strong argument that V and C are not joined at the mRNA level?

C. MILSTEIN: You have indeed raised a critical point. What I presented is a very strong argument that the final product is a single messenger RNA from which you translate. I think that's clear enough. Now how do you make a single integrated mRNA? I do not think you make it out of two different RNA pieces. I say this based on an experiment which we did about two years ago. (Nature, 244, 42 (1973). We fused a rat myeloma cell which secretes kappa chain with a mouse cell which also secretes a kappa chain. The hybrid cell made the two light chains, that is, you destroy allelic exclusion. We did not detect molecules of the types, V mouse-C rat or V rat-C mouse. This indicates that there are no "half messenger" molecules formed, which are then linked together.

E. BRILES: About the V region not showing any mutations whereas the constant region does; I just want to suggest the possibility that this might be a reflection of the polarity of translation. If you have a frame shift mutation early on in the variable region, the protein molecule that is generated may look so unlike an antibody that it would not be picked up and would therefore be scored as an absent antibody rather than as a mutant. However, if a frame shift mutation, a deletion or a terminating nonsence codon occurred in the constant region, there may be enough protein sequence synthesised for the molecule to be recognized as an antibody molecule.

C. MILSTEIN: We have not found any frameshift mutant yet. Are you suggesting that all mutants are going to be chain terminations?

E BRILES: Not necessarily but some, or even many, of them may be.

C. MILSTEIN: Well some of them may be and as you suggest, we may miss them, but they should be in the minority on a statistical basis.

P. LEDER: Actually, my comment was similar to the one made by Dr. Briles. To just reiterate what you've said, the testing techniques have intrinsic limitations which would not be expected to pick up point mutations which result in neutral amino acid substitutions, but they will pick up changes of charge. Perhaps that was what you were referring to when you said you have no such amino acid substitutions that you are ready to talk about. Perhaps there are such known. The possibili that a termination occurring in the variable region results in a strong polarity effect is a very real one and this would have several consequences. First, it might result in a short peptide that is simply not recognized by your assay or is degraded very quickly. Second, it might result in a mRNA which would be subject to immediate degradation and would not survive in the cell. Combination of these possibilities would account for the fact that you see only constant region deletion or termination mutants.

C. MILSTEIN: What surprises me is that we get so much chain termination. I have described three randomly picked mutants. IF1, IF2, and IF3, and two of them are chain terminations which are presumably single base changes. Not one is an amino acid substitution involving a change in charge which we would be able to pick up. Until we have characterized more mutants all these arguments are weak because they may not be representative of the average events.

A. R. WILLIAMSON: May I switch the discussion to your elegant cDNA experiment? Your cDNA experiment appears to say that the reiterated sequences code for the untranslated portion, although I don't know how precise you would need to be in your numerology to say that it did not include the N terminal end of the V region, which after all might show more cross hybridisation between different kappa genes. Let me ask you whether the untranslated part, which you can partially define from the sequence of the precursor molecule, is identical from one kappa chain to another? If that is the reiterated portion, you might expect to find sequence identity.

C. MILSTEIN: First of all let me say that the numerology is not sufficiently accurate for me to say whether the N terminal is included or not. It is possible that one could put 10 residues of the amino acid into fragment A, but I am dubious about it being much bigger. Concerning the second point, I have no sequence data on the precursor part of this myeloma.

F.W. PUTNAM: If there are no further questions let me just summarize our dilemma for a moment before we close the session. In immunoglobulins there are as many light chains as there are heavy chains and the V region of the light chain is as variable if not more so that the V region of the heavy chain. However, so far only one or two mutants of light chains have been picked up in contrast to all the mutations described today that appeared in the C region of the heavy chains.

GENES CODING FOR ANTIBODIES

A.R. WILLIAMSON and A.J. McMICHAEL
Department of Biochemistry
University of Glasgow
and National Institute for Medical Research
Mill Hill, London

Abstract: The nature and extent of antibody diversity are discussed. The genotypic basis of this diversity appears to be multiple V genes and single C genes. A system is described showing coinheritance of the antibody combining site and the V region containing that site. Somatic processes leading to V gene amplification and VC joining are proposed.

INTRODUCTION

Two fascinating questions are posed by the problem of antibody diversity: 1. What is the germ line basis of antibody diversity? 2. What somatic processes are needed for the expression of the phenotype?

This article discusses the nature and extent of diversity in the antibody phenotype and the possible genetic basis for this diversity. Data are presented showing the inheritance of a complete V gene (or family of V genes). A separate marker shows stable co-inheritance of the fine specificity of the antibody combining site. At least one somatic process required for antibody synthesis is the formation of a VC gene pair. A model is discussed in which multiple copies of a V_H gene are involved in the joining process.

PHENOTYPE

Antibody diversity can be considered as being made up of three elements. 1. The different functional classes of antibody, IgG, IgM, IgA, IgD, IgE, etc. The number of antibody classes is already well defined with the largest number being known in the best studied species - man. It is unlikely that there are many more classes of antibody to be discovered. 2. Combining site diversity. This occurs within and between classes of antibody and it would appear that any combining site can be expressed in any class of antibody. 3. Non-combining site diversity. Diversity of this type extends the number of antibody molecules of a given specificity and class.

The separate basis for the three types of diversity has been revealed by amino acid sequence studies of individual antibody molecules, largely obtained as myeloma immunoglobulins. Each immunoglobulin polypeptide chain, L or H, consists of a C-terminal constant region which is common to all chains of the same isotype and an N-terminal variable region which has a different sequence in every chain. This paradox was pointed out ten years ago (1). As more sequences became available a pattern of variability emerged. This was pointed out by Wu and Kabat (2), who showed that when many V_K region sequences are compared there are a limited number of positions at which many different amino acids are found and these were termed hyper-variable regions.

The naming of constant, variable and hyper-variable regions has been emotively misleading since the names are often taken to imply active processes maintaining constancy or creating variability. Current knowledge of the evolution of variable regions tends to deny this. Comparison of the amino acid sequences of constant regions of comparable chains from a variety of species shows that these constant regions are evolving in a similar manner to most other proteins. The variable regions of immunoglobulin chains also fit within this pattern and are at least as conserved between species as the constant regions.

It was initially tempting to implicate the hyper-variable regions as being the most important parts of the V region in determining antibody specificity and therefore to invoke special mechanisms for deriving hyper-variability (2). The combining sites of two hapten binding myeloma proteins have now been described in three dimensions by X-ray crystallographic analysis (3,4). These studies finally confirmed that both V_H and V_L contribute to the antibody combining site and showed that five of the seven hyper-variable regions are proximal to the hapten binding site; the other two hyper-variable regions are however remote. One of the more striking features of the three dimensional structure is the highly conserved folding of each variable region in order to form an antibody combining site. The detailed specificity of that site could be controlled by changing only a few amino acids, presumably in the hyper-variable regions, but there must be a strong conservation of V region sequence outwith the hyper-variable regions in order to obtain a viable combining site. The presence of the hyper-variable regions within the conserved combining site appears to contribute diversity to combining sites. The problem now is how does the diversity arise such that in combination with the overall constancy of V region structure it results in a specific binding site. The original problem of diversity and constancy appeared to have been solved by the evidence for the separation of V and C genes in the germ line. However the new problem arises from the mosaic nature of V regions themselves. This problem can be tackled by studying separate markers for the combining site and for the rest of the V gene. Such studies will be discussed in a later section but first a brief discussion of the problem of the extent of antibody diversity.

EXTENT OF ANTIBODY DIVERSITY

One of the most striking things about the repertoire of antibodies which all vertebrates are able to make is our apparent failure to find any gaps in the armoury. The extent of antibody diversity can not be mapped by plotting a range of chemical determinants to which antibodies can not bind. Moreover, for every antibody there is another antibody (or set of antibodies) which will specifically recognise the binding site of the first antibody. Each antibody therefore leads to a progression of anti-combining-site antibodies and I have referred elsewhere to this as being an uncertainty principle governing the number of antibody combining sites (5). The limit must be set by the level of discrimination which an antibody can show in recognition of different determinants. Each antibody combining site will bind many antigenic determinants, though there will be quantitative discrimination in the binding; a much larger number of antigenic determinants will fail to be bound in a measurable way to a given combining site. Unpredictable cross-reactions at enzyme combining sites have been reported by Glazer (6) and recently Varga *et al* (7) have shown that each individual combining site can bind a range haptenic determinants. That multiple shared specificities of individual antibody molecules are consistent with the specificity of antisera was pointed out by Talmage in 1959 (8). In essence his argument was that an antiserum consisted of a population of antibody molecules having the common property of binding the eliciting antigen. This would make the antiserum more specific for the eliciting antigen than any of the individual antibody molecules present in the antiserum. The converse of this argument is that the fewer the number of antibody molecules contributing to an antiserum the greater the number of shared specificities the antiserum will show. Each antibody combining site can be defined by its set of shared specificities.

Direct attempts to measure the number of antibodies capable of binding particular haptens have yielded large numbers. Kreth and Williamson (9) found that CBA/H mice could produce about 5,000 V_LV_H pairs which are capable of binding NIP. This is a most probable value calculated from the number of repeat spectrotypes found in an analysis of CBA/H anti NIP antibodies by isoelectric focusing. It is important to note that the spectrotype reflects heterogeneity of the entire V regions and not just the combining site. The same combining sites might be repeated any number of times in different V region settings. In a similar study using CBA/H and C3H/HE mice, Pink and Askonas (10) compared only the subset of spectrotypes of DNP binding antibody which was able to strongly bind TNP. They found that about 500 different VLVH combinations showed this particular cross-reaction. Again we can not decide whether the diversity lies in the antibody combining site or outwith that site. I now wish to turn to the description, in a little more detail, of a system in which the combining site and the V region in which it is contained can both be followed.

INHERITANCE OF V GENES AND COMBINING SITES

Mäkelä has elegantly developed the use of cross reactions to map the fine specificity of an antibody and has shown that this can be used as a genetic marker. Imanishi and Mäkelä (11) showed that when C57BL/6 mice are immunized with the hapten NP conjugated to a protein the antibody produced in either a primary or a secondary response shows a higher affinity for the related haptens NIP, NBrP and NNP than for NP. An antibody showing a higher affinity for a hapten other than the eliciting hapten has been termed heteroclitic. The reasoning outlined in the previous section leads one to the conclusion that an antiserum exhibiting very defined fine specificity properties such as a heteroclitic property must contain relatively few different combining sites. The heterogeneity of C57BL/6 anti NP antibodies was analysed by analytical isoelectric focusing to see whether the number of antibody molecules present in each antiserum was also limited. This study (12) has allowed us to follow simultaneously, with separate markers, a combining site and the complete V gene(s) in which it is contained.

Isoelectric focusing of C_{57}BL/6 serum collected 14 to 28 days after priming with NP protein revealed that each antiserum contained a restricted $NI^{131}P$-cap binding antibody spectrum. The spectra showed no additional heterogeneity when development was carried out with NP-SRC. Most strikingly, one spectrotype, designated N1, was present in 38 out of 42 spectra. N1 antibody comprised the major part of each response and when this antibody was isolated by preparative isoelectric focusing it was shown to contain the heteroclitic combining site. Where non N1 antibody was present in a primary response this too was isolated and also proved to have a heteroclitic combining site. Both N1 and non N1 spectrotypes were shown to be due to $IgG_1\kappa$ antibodies by by developing them with NP-SRC and specific anti-IgG_1 or anti-κ and complement. This finding implies that very similar binding sites can be formed by the use of different V_LV_H combinations. The secondary response of C_{57}BL/6 mice to NP further supports this notion, for the antibody obtained is much more heterogeneous than in the primary response and N1 antibody is only a minor constituent but the serum retains its heteroclitic property.

Imanishi and Mäkelä (13) studied the inheritance of the heteroclitic combining site in crosses of C_{57}BL/6 mice against CBA mice which produced conventional (i.e. non heteroclitic) antibodies against NP. They found that (CBA x C_{57}BL/6)F_1 mice made heteroclitic anti NP antibodies as frequently and as well as the C_{57}BL/6 parents. In backcrosses against the recessive CBA parent the heteroclitic combining site was inherited as a single Mendelian marker closely linked to the Ig-1b allotype marker of the H-chain constant region. This allotype linked inheritance is only clearly seen in their studies of primary sera, now known to be of restricted heterogeneity. The same studies conducted using antibody from secondary responses (now known to be more heterogeneous) led Imanishi and Mäkelä (14) to propose multiple gene inheritance of the heteroclitic property with the involvement of a gene or genes unlinked to the H-chain allotype.

The inheritance of the N1 spectrotype was investigated by isoelectric focusing analysis of the F_1 and backcross anti NP antisera. The anti NP spectrum of primary response sera from F1 mice resembled a mixture of the two parental type primary responses. The dominant N1 spectrotype of the C57BL/6 parent was present in about the same percentage of F1 sera as of parental sera but in addition the F1 primary responses were more heterogeneous than those of either parent. In the F1 x CBA backcross generation 70% of the progeny heterozygous at the H-chain allotype locus showed the N1 spectrotype in their primary anti NP response. The N1 spectrotype thus behaves as though it is controlled by a single gene, which we will call V_HN1, linked to the H-chain constant region gene. This poses a problem, for the spectrotype must depend on both the light and the heavy chains contributing to the antibody. The genes coding for L-chains have not previously been shown to be linked to the H-chain loci so the high rate of appearance of the N1 spectrotype in backcross mice suggests that both the CBA and the C57BL/6 L-chain repertoires contain an L-chain capable of constituting the N1 spectrotype when the appropriate H-chain is supplied. CBA mice can by the same token also supply a V_L region capable of making, in combination with the V_HN1 region, a heteroclitic combining site. One interpretation of the secondary response data of Imanishi and Mäkelä would be that other C57BL/6 V_H regions are capable of making heteroclitic combining sites only in combination with L-regions present in the C57BL/6 repertoire and not present in the CBA repertoire.

The linkage between V_HN1 and Ig-1b was further tested by studying two congenic strains of mice. The first strain was Potter's CB20 congenic, homozygous for the Ig-1b allotype of C57BL/KA on a BALB/c background. Imanishi and Mäkelä found that both the b-allotype parent and the CB20 congenic mice made heteroclitic anti-NP antibody. By isoelectric focusing we found the N1 spectrotype present in primary CB20 anti-NP sera. Linkage between the V_HN1 gene and the C_H locus has thus been preserved through 20 backcrosses. Moreover we can add that the BALB/c repertoire of V_L genes contains a gene capable of complementing the V_HN1 gene for the production of heteroclitic combining site and the N1 spectrotype. The second congenic strain of mice used in this study was Dresser's CBA b/b line which is homozygous for the Ig-1b allotype on a CBA background. Only four mice at the twelfth backcross generation were available for study. None of these mice produced the N1 spectrotype upon primary immunization with NP-chicken gammaglobulin. The potential of these cogenic mice to produce the N1 spectrotype was further tested by taking the spleens three months after priming and using each one to reconstitute ten irradiated (660r) conventional CBA mice. An adoptive secondary response to NP was elicited and examined for the Nl spectrotype but this could not be found in any of the 40 recipients. This result suggests that the linkage between V_HNl and the CH locus has been broken by a crossover event at some point during the twelve backcrosses used to make the cogenic strain. Table 1 summarises the linked inheritance of fine specificity and V_HNl.

TABLE 1

	Positive	Negative	
C_H allotype	b	a	b
NP/NIP	C57BL/6	BALB/C	SJL/J
	LP/J	C3H	
	CB20	CBA	
Nl	C57BL/6	CBA	SJL/J
	CB20	BALB/C	LP/J*
			CBAbb12

*In LP/J mice a repeat spectrotype differing from Nl has been seen.

It should be added to this story that when C_{57}BL/6 mice are immunized with NIP protein the Nl spectrotype can be detected in both the primary response (all of 6 mice) and in the secondary response (9 of 14 mice). Thus the Nl antibody which binds the two related haptens is not only elicited by both haptens but also forms a dominant part of the response to either hapten. This property of dominance remains to be explained.

Two striking examples of the conservation of combining sites have recently been reported. The first example provides direct evidence for the relationship between combining site, hypervariable regions and idiotype.

Capra et al (15) have sequenced the complete variable regions of the heavy chains of two human IgM cold agglutinins. The two proteins (LAY and POM) have similar combining specificities and similar idiotypic determinants. The two V_H regions were found to differ at only eight positions, three of these being in hypervariable regions and five elsewhere in the V region. Two complete hypervariable regions had an identical sequence in each of the two H chains. These striking findings for two V_H regions obtained from outbred members of the same species are hard to reconcile with any rapid or special accumulation of mutations in the hypervariable regions. Each entire V region appears to have evolved from the same precursor V region with the combining site (hypervariable region or idiotypic determinant) evolving at the same rate as the rest of the V region.

Further strong evidence for the evolutionary stability of the antibody combining site comes from the studies of Claflin and Davie (16) on anti-phosphorylcholine antibodies in the mouse. These workers produced, in a rabbit, a site directed anti-idiotypic antibody. This anti-idiotypic antibody could not distinguish between anti-phosphorylcholine antibodies raised in any of a large number of different mouse strains. Even where the anti-phosphorylcholine antibody of two strains had previously been distinguished using other anti-idiotype sera (17) the site directed reagent revealed no differences. The idiotypic determinants which distinguish anti-phosphorylcholine antibodies from different strains are thus behaving as very restricted V region allotype markers. The combining site for anti-phosphorylcholine antibodies appears to have been conserved in all mice although other mutations in the variable region have accumulated. Another example of inter-strain idiotypic cross reactions has been reported for the group A streptococcal antibody responses in mice (18).

GENOTYPE

The antibody phenotype points to an unusual pattern of genes. All of the evidence points to only a single gene carried in the germ line for each constant region. On the other hand there appear to be three multiple V gene sets also carried in the germ line, one linked to all of the C_H loci, one linked to the C_κ locus and one to the C_λ locus. This pattern can be tested by using mRNA or complementary DNA in hybridisation assays with nuclear DNA. The rate of hybridisation of the probe mRNA or cDNA measures the number of copies of that sequence in the nuclear DNA. The result using H chain mRNA (mRNA - H) as a probe is that a substantial part of the mRNA hybridises to unique DNA sequences (19,

20). This is consistent with the predicted single C_H gene coding for the C region of H chain. A minor part of the mRNA-H hybridises to reiterated DNA sequences. It was initially plausible to assume that the reiterated sequences might represent multiple V_H genes. While this remains neither proven nor disproven the more thorough study that has been made of the rapidly hybridising portion of mRNA-L has shown that the reiterated sequences mainly code for the untranslated part of the mRNA located at the 5' end of the V region sequence (21,22). The presence in DNA of reiterated sequences coding for an untranslated V region proximal sequence may provide a measure of the number of V genes in the DNA without the complication of cross hybridisation between different V gene sequences. The accuracy of the estimate will depend on the amount and nature of impurity in the mRNA probe used for the hybridisation: this is all too clearly seen in the two disparate estimates of 300 and 5,000 genes coding for the reiterated portion of mRNA-H (19,20). The data for the light chain, which are described in the following paper by Leder, provide a clearer picture.

All of the studies whether of the antibody phenotype or of the genotype by molecular hybridisation agree on the fact that only a single gene for each constant region is carried in the germ line but that the basis of V gene diversity is a multiple gene set. It has been suggested that this multiple gene set might code for only the hypervariable regions or combining sites of antibody molecules (2,23). The evidence described in the previous section and an analysis of available V region sequence point to the inheritance and evolution of V region sequences as entire units. The total number of V genes in each multiple gene set will no doubt be more clearly defined by further molecular hybridisation studies and eventually by isolation of the genes coding for the V regions. Whatever the final number it is necessary to consider how much of the phenotypic diversity arises at the somatic level. If a limited number of V genes are available then somatic processes will be necessary to amplify diversity. On the other hand the larger the pool of V genes which is available the greater the rate of accumulation of mutations in V regions. The joining of V and C region information is one somatic process which appears to be mandatory for the synthesis of an antibody. This process is discussed in the next section.

GENOME REARRANGEMENT

Joining of V and C gene information to give a complete heavy or light chain could occur at either the DNA, the RNA or the protein level. No evidence favouring joining at the RNA or protein levels has stood the test of time. The mRNA-H or mRNA-L molecules that have been isolated code for both V and C regions. Milstein and co-workers (24) have sequenced an overlap region between V and C in mRNA-L. Stevens and Williamson (25) have isolated a nuclear pre mRNA-H 2½ times the length of the cytoplasmic mRNA-H. This nuclear pre mRNA-H contains poly A and codes for the entire H chain. The evidence thus points to the transcription of a VC gene pair so it would appear that we are looking for a VC joining process at the DNA level.

For the synthesis of any complete immunoglobulin molecule by a given cell two VC gene pairs must be formed in that cell, one coding for heavy chain and one for a light chain. If a single V_H gene is joined, by a translocation of the appropriate piece of DNA, to one of the possible C_H genes on the same chromosome then this would lead to a restriction for this cell and its progeny to the synthesis of a single class of antibody of the specificity coded for by the chosen V_H gene. The sequential synthesis of different classes of antibody of the same specificity during clonal expansion requires either that the chosen V_H gene be re-translocated or that multiple copies of that V_H gene are made and joined to other C_H loci (26). A test of these two models might be provided by a study of single cells simultaneously producing two different classes of antibody. The continuous human lymphocyte cell lines provide a well documented source of cells simultaneously producing more than one class of antibody. Recently Steel <u>et al</u> (27) have described a fascinating human lymphocyte cell line, which is producing two different classes of antibody, IgM and IgA, each having the ability to agglutinate glutaraldehyde-fixed sheep red cells. Clearly a detailed study of the V regions of these antibodies is called for but to a first approximation it seems reasonable to assume that similar antibody specificity of two products of the same cell reflects V regions derived from the same original V gene. Pernis <u>et al</u> (28) have recently described a case of Waldenström's macroglobulinemia in which were found lymphocytes producing both IgD and IgM with a similar specificity, the antigen in this case being human IgG. It is unlikely that in each of these cases two different V genes chosen at random code for similar specificities or different specificities present on the same antigen. The evidence therefore favours a copy-choice-multiple-entry programming system for the C_H loci (26). In this system the selected V_H gene will be copied several times to give an episomal set of replica V_H genes, each of of which can then be joined to a different C_H gene without any translocation of the original germ line copy of the chosen V_H gene. It is possible that the duplication of a given V_H gene occurs within the multiple V gene set long before the joining of V and C takes place. In this case the V regions of different classes in the same cell might not be identical. If the V_H gene duplication is a somatic process then differences in the sequence of V_H regions of different classes in the same cell will give a measure of the rate and pattern of accumulation of somatic mutations.

SOMATIC MUTATION AND SELECTION

Much has been written about the possible roles of these processes in antibody diversity. A few comments are added here on the occurrence of these processes in a multiple V-gene system. The rate of accumulation of V region mutations will be proportional to the number of V genes. For a mutant to be acted upon by selective forces it needs to be expressed as a receptor antibody on a lymphocyte. This implies a programming event, as described in the previous section, that will allow selection to act only on one V gene product. The finding that in double-producing cells one class of antibody behaves like a surface receptor molecule while the other is secreted (29) limits the usefulness of any mutations which might occur in somatically duplicated V_H genes. Reprogramming events in which the integrated V genes are exchanged for new V genes from the multiple set are a less plausible way of allowing variants to occur within a selected clone. Subtle changes of specificity in the antibody produced by a single clone (30, 31) should be due to changes in a single V gene. The variants of mouse λ chain (32) should be a model for this process but the mechanism remains unknown. Any variation mechanism has to account for the remarkable stability of clonal products whether the clone is expanded by a neoplastic event as in a myeloma tumour or by antigen (33,34).

GENES CONTROLLING IMMUNE RESPONSIVENESS (Ir)

Since it has been suggested that Ir genes code for a set of antibodies expressed on T cells (35,36) the role of

Ir genes should be briefly mentioned here although they will be more extensively discussed by Katz in a later chapter. Control of immune responsiveness by Ir gene products can be explained without postulating that Ir genes code for T cell receptor antibodies. The fact that Ir products are present on B cells (See Katz) argues against the T-cell receptor hypothesis. Katz data strongly support the idea that Ir products are involved in cell interactions. The Ir gene system may have evolved from a primative self recognition system, such as that operating in the colonial ascidions(37).

Colony formation in the ascidions is controlled by a single genetic locus with multiple alleles. Fusion occurs only between colonies whose cells have one allele in common. Rejection occurs when cells have two different pairs of alleles. These rules are remarkably similar to those governing cooperation between T and B cells in the immune response. A model for the control of responsiveness to non-self antigens by a self recognition system on B and T lymphocytes has been described elsewhere (38).

REFERENCES

(1) W.J. Dreyer and J.C. Bennett, Proc. Nat Acad. Sci. U.S.A., 54 (1965) 864.

(2) T.T. Wu and E. Kabat, J. Exp. Med., 132 (1970) 211.

(3) E.A. Padlan, D.M. Segal, G.H. Cohen, D.R. Davies, S. Rudikoff and M. Potter, in: The Immune System. Genes, Receptors, Signals, eds. E.E. Sercarz, A.R. Williamson and C.F. Fox (Academic Press, New York, 1974) p.7.

(4) L.M. Amzel, R.J. Poljak, F. Saul, J.M. Varga and F.F. Richards, Proc. Nat. Acad. Sci. U.S.A., 71 (1974) 1427.

(5) A.R. Williamson, E. Premkumar and M. Shoyab, Fed. Proc., in press (1974).

(6) A.N. Glazer, Proc. Nat. Acad. Sci. U.S.A., 65 (1970) 1057.

(7) J.M. Varga, W.H. Koningsberg and F.F. Richards, Proc. Nat. Acad. Sci. U.S.A., 70 (1973) 3269.

(8) D.W. Talmage, Science, 129 (1959) 1643.

(9) H.W. Kreth and A.R. Williamson, Eur. J. Immunol., 3 (1973) 141.

(10) J.R.L. Pink and B.A. Askonas, Eur. J. Immunol., 4 (1974)

(11) T. Imanishi and O. Mäkelä, Eur. J. Immunol., 3 (1973) 323.

(12) A.J. McMichael, J.M. Phillips, A.R. Williamson, T. Imanishi and O. Mäkelä, Immunogenetics (1975) in press.

(13) T. Imanishi and O. Mäkelä, J. Exp. Med., (1975) in press.

(14) T. Imanishi and O. Mäkelä, Ann. Immunol. Inst. Pasteur, 125C (1974) 199.

(15) J.D. Capra, R.L. Wasserman, P. Querinjean and J.M.Kehoe, Proc. 9th FEBS Meeting, Budapest (1974) in press.

(16) J.L. Claflin and J.M. Davie, J. Exp.Med. 140 (1974) 673.

(17) M. Potter and R. Lieberman, J. Exp. Med., 132 (1970) 737.

(18) D.E. Briles and R.M. Krause, J. Immunol., (1974) in press.

(19) A. Bernardini and S. Tonegawa, FEBS Letters, 41 (1974) 73.

(20) E. Premkumar, M. Shoyab and A.R. Williamson, Proc. Nat. Acad. Sci. U.S.A., 71 (1974) 99.

(21) S. Tonegawa, C. Steinberg, S. Duke and A. Bernardini, Proc. Nat. Acad. Sci., (1974) in press.

(22) T.H. Rabbits, C. Milstein and G.G. Brownlee, Proc. 9th FEBS Meeting, Budapest (1974) in press.

(23) J.D. Capra and T.J. Kindt, Immunogenetics (1974) in press.

(24) C. Milstein, G.G. Brownlee, E.M. Cartwright, J.M.Jarvis and N.J. Proudfoot, Nature 252 (1974) 354.

(25) R.H. Stevens and A.R. Williamson, Nature, New Biol., 245 (1973) 101.

(26) A.R. Williamson, Nature, 231 (1971) 359.

(27) C.M. Steel, J. Evans, A.W.L. Joss and E. Arthur, Nature 252 (1974) 604.

(28) B. Pernis, J.C. Bronet and M. Seligmann, Eur. J. Immunol., 4 (1974) 776.

(29) A.R. Williamson, R.H. Stevens, E. Premkumar and P.A. Singer, Proc. 9th FEBS Meeting, Budapest, (1974) in press.

(30) A.J. Cunningham and L.M. Pilarski, Eur. J. Immunol., 4 (1974) 757.

(31) L.M. Pilarski and A.J. Cunningham, Eur. J. Immunol., 4 (1974) 762.

(32) M. Weigert, I. Cesari, S. Yonkovitch and M. Cohn, Nature, 228 (1970) 1045.

(33) N.R. Klinman, J. Immunol., 106 (1971) 1345.

(34) B.A. Askonas and A.R. Williamson, Nature, 238 (1972) 339.

(35) B. Benaceraff and H.O. McDevitt, Science, 175 (1972) 273.

(36) M. Cohn, in: Genetic Control of Immune Responsiveness, eds. H.O. McDevitt and M. Landy (Academic Press, New York, 1972) p.367.

(37) M. Oka, in: Profiles of Japanese Science and Scientists (1970) p.196.

(38) A.R. Williamson, Transpl. Revs., 23 (1975) in press.

We wish to acknowledge close and friendly collaboration with Dr. O. Mäkelä, Dr. T. Imanishi and Dr. J. M. Phillips.

Abbreviations:

NP: (4-hydroxy-3-nitrophenyl)acetyl
NBrP: (4-hydroxy-5-bromo-3-nitrophenyl)acetyl
NIP: (4-hydroxy-5-iodo-3-nitrophenyl)acetyl
NNP: (4-hydroxy-3,5-dinitrophenyl)acetyl
NIPcap: NIP-amino-caproate
SRC: sheep red cells

DISCUSSION

H. FUDENBERG: Two comments and a question: first, although not the case for cell lines, fresh cells from human chronic lymphocytic leukemia obtained from peripheral blood almost invariably have two immunoglobulins on their surface with monoclonal light chains usually with IgM heavy chains, but sometimes IgG, and almost always IgD in association. I think any theory of antibody formation and evolution must account for this. Secondly, in terms of the use of continuous cell lines, I wonder if it is releveant to extrapolate the data obtained therein to what goes on *in vivo*. It is conceivable, since all genes are present in all cells but perhaps not expressed because of *in vivo* repression mechanisms, that once the cells are outside the body the regulatory mechanisms are lost. It then would not be surprising to find multiple V and C regions made by the same cell. Lastly, as I remember, you had data that the messenger for heavy chains was considerably longer than was needed for continuous synthesis of a VC joined heavy chain. I forget the controls you used to ensure that, when you added the messenger to the appropriate system, only IgG was being made and not something else. Was the size of the messenger, considering the size of the heavy chain, not longer then need be? I just want to make sure that the protein produced is IgG and solely IgG. Those are the three points that I would like you to comment on.

A. R. WILLIAMSON: Well, let me comment on the last one first. The messenger is only about 450 nucleotides longer than is needed to code for a heavy chain and the evidence on the translation of that message was based on fingerprint analysis of the product, not complete sequence. Fingerprint analysis showed that the peptides were as one would expect for the particular myeloma protein for which the message should code. We have looked in the oocyte products to see whether other classes of immunoglobulin are made because of the possibility that the messages are there in abnormal cells even though they are not normally being translated in those cells. We haven't found such products; that does not mean that they are not there. They could be there at a level below our discrimination. On the second point, which is related to the last one concerning the products of the continuous cell lines. I think you are making a very good point. I think that it is very likely that the instances of double production in these abnormal cell lines is high because there is a loss of some normal control. However, I think that this is an accident of nature that might be very useful because it is probably a way of finding out what the total programming is in that cell; that is whether all of the C regions have V regions attached to them. The fact that we get expression of more than one C region (and cell lines have now been described making several classes) leads us to ask whether the V regions can be shown to be very similar or identical in those cases. Such a finding would say that there is a multiple programming of different C genes occurring in the cell. The cell somehow regulates, even after multiple programming, which gene is expressed, thus leading to an ontogenic switching mechanism. To summarize, yes I think multiple antibody class expression may well be an accident of the transformation with EB virus.

R. K. GERSHON: In your analysis of the spectrotypes in clones did you look at any different carriers, or was your carrier always the same?

A. R. WILLIAMSON: The carrier in the first experiment was usually CGG, because it is a very good carrier. We have also used BGG and we have not seen a spectrotype difference. We also put a spacer molecule between hapten and protein; using NIP-amino-caproate BGG we also saw exactly the N-1 spectrotype in the primary responses, in fact they were some of the least heterogeneous responses we saw.

R. K. GERSHON: Differences between mouse strains in the fine specificity of antibodies have been shown to be thymus-dependent in a number of cases. Suppose you take your F1 cells and put the F1 T-cells into either of the parents.

Is it possible that this would show whether the genetic material or the genetic information for the antibody specificities is operationally carried in the T-cell rather than in the B-cell?

A. R. WILLIAMSON: It is a possibility. Would you accept an allogeneic T-cell stimulation which revealed the same clone?

R. K. GERSHON: Not really, because these are primed animals and the F1 T-cells would have already acted if they do determine any of the fine specificity. The allogeneic effect would just be boosting those cells which had already been T-cell influenced.

A. R. WILLIAMSON: Yes it is a secondary response in that situation.

P. LEDER: I think that you would agree that it is important to realize that no direct evidence rules out a joining mechanism taking place at the level of the message. It is quite clear from a variety of studies, in particularly those presented yesterday by C. Milstein, that the message occurs as a single polynucleotide chain coding for both the constant and variable regions. I certainly favor the joining mechanism having occurred at the level of DNA, but we can not rule out the possibility that it also occurs at the level of RNA fragments.

A. R. WILLIAMSON: No, thank you for adding that. I tried to say that, although there is no absolute proof, the data favors joining at the DNA level, but maybe I didn't place the right emphasis on the lack of absolute proof. I do think the evidence as you say points towards a DNA integration step.

P.LEDER: My point is that there isn't any evidence favoring either model, its only a teleological argument. We know that the message ends up as a single continuous polynucleotide chain. I don't feel that there is any experimental or observational evidence to favor either hypothesis, one just seems a lot more reasonable teleologically.

A.R. WILLIAMSON: But I think one would have to say that there is absolutely no evidence favoring joining at the mRNA or protein level. The finding of an intact precursor molecule in the nucleus, even though it is probably not the original transcript, and our failure to find anything smaller, does suggest that the VC gene pair is transcribed as a single entity. I agree it is not proof but taken together with the H chain deletion mutants spanning V and C regions the evidence is highly suggestive.

C. BELL: I have a question concerning the intrinsic capabilities of a cell to express more than one specificity. Was this done with cells kept in culture or with cells drawn continuously from peripheral blood? In a similar situation Pat Jones has shown in heterozygous rabbits a high incidence of PNBC expressing two IgM on their surface. The incidence of double producers within the same cell was from 20 to 63%, which would clearl show that there is no allelic exclusion. However, when she did a fluorescence study and differentiated the cells and stripped them with pronase, then the amount of the double producer went down to 3%, which clearly showed that there was some kind of adherence on the surface. Were the same studies done in cells drawn from the peripheral blood or were they kept in culture so that the IgD or IgM might have adhered to them?

A.R. WILLIAMSON: Well, the answer to your question is that the studies on the human lymphocytes by Steel _et al_ (Ref. 27) were performed using continuous lines in culture. But I think Len Herzenberg ought to answer the point about Pat Jones studies since he knows that data.

L. HERZENBERG: This is to straighten the record, as an author on the paper. The interpretation that we made was clearly that there was cytophilic antibody found on the B-cells when they were taken out of the rabbit. It wasn't a matter of it being synthesized by those cells at all and there is extensive evidence for that; it is published in the Journal of Experimental Medicine in August 1974 by Jones _et al_.

A. R. WILLIAMSON: Whereas the two cases of double producing cells that I quoted have been shown to be due to synthesis.

L. HERZENBERG: Yes

C. MILSTEIN: You said that the binding of the heavy chain by the messenger is at the 5' end. What is the evidence?

A. R. WILLIAMSON: The evidence is published in the European Journal of Biochemistry (42 (1974) 553) by Ron Stevens, and, as I said, is not conclusive evidence. The evidence is based on the translational control effect, in which there appears to be an inhibition of initiation of translation and so we interpret that as being due to binding of immunoglobulin at a site near the initiation site.

E.A.KABAT: If I may assume the prerogative of the Chairman, I just want to ask you if there is evidence that your untranslated portion at the 5' end really might be involved in synthesis of many other proteins which are not immunoglobulin and that it really does not give you an estimate of the number of immunoglobulin V genes.

A. R. WILLIAMSON: There is no firm evidence, one way or the other.

THE ORGANIZATION AND DIVERSITY OF IMMUNOGLOBULIN κ AND λ GENES

P. LEDER, T. HONJO, D. SWAN, S. PACKMAN, M. NAU and B. NORMAN

Laboratory of Molecular Genetics
National Institute of Child Health and Human Development
National Institutes of Health
Bethesda, Maryland 20014

Abstract: Our studies have focused on several hypotheses put forward to account for the diversity of immunoglobulin genes. These studies have shown that the constant regions of the mouse κ and λ chains are represented as relatively unique sequences in the genome of the mouse. Experiments which have attempted to focus on the genetic representation of the variable region of the κ chain are not as readily interpreted. They do, however, rule out thousands of closely related germ line sequences. As a result of ambiguities in the κ system, we have turned our attention to a simpler model, the mouse λ light chain. Since detailed analyses have shown that there are at least seven very closely related λ light chains, this class provides a very useful model for studies involving molecular hybridization. Utilizing mouse λ chain ^{3}H-cDNA, hybridization kinetic analyses indicate that these sequences are represented among the relatively unique genetic sequences in the mouse genome. This result tends to rule out a germ line model for antibody diversity. The reservations with respect to reaching such a conclusion are also discussed.

INTRODUCTION

The unique features of immunoglobulin light and heavy chains obviously require a unique genetic explanation, which involves accounting for the constant and variable portions of these molecules in genetic terms. A variety of structural and serologic studies carried out over the past decade have provided a remarkable insight into the nature of the genetic problem. These provide the basis for several contending hypotheses which, until recently, could not be subject to direct experimental test (see Ref. 1 for detailed references). Recent advances in the isolation of a variety of immunoglobulin mRNAs and our ability to use them in molecular hybridization experiments have altered this situation dramatically (1-15). Such studies are the subject of this report.

THE HYPOTHESES

Three major types of hypotheses have been advanced to account for the organization and diversity of the immunoglobulin genes (Fig. 1). The simplest of these, the stringent germ line hypothesis, requires a single continuous genetic sequence encompassing variable and constant region for each light and heavy chain in the organism's immunologic repertoire. Thus, 1,000 light chains would require 1,000 variable region genetic sequences immediately adjacent 1,000 constant region genetic sequences (assuming an antibody repertoire of approximately 10^6 different molecules) (16).

In contrast to this straightforward model, the recombinational germ line hypothesis incorporates a critical feature originally suggested by Dreyer and Bennet (17), namely, that variable and constant regions are encoded by two separate genes which are (or whose products are) ultimately joined to form an intact immunoglobulin sequence. This model requires one or very few copies of the constant region sequence which combine with one of the thousand or so variable region gene sequences encoded in the germ line genome. Obviously the major difference between this hypothesis and the stringent germ line hypothesis is the former's requirement for very few constant region genes.

The above two models hold that the diversity of the variable region sequences have arisen during evolution of

Figure 1.

PREDICTED FREQUENCIES OF LIGHT CHAIN CONSTANT AND VARIABLE GENE SEQUENCES IN CLONED IMMUNOCYTE DNA

		Theoretical Gene Frequency		Expected Frequency as Determined by Hybridization with MOPC-41 Light Chain mRNA	
		Variable	Constant	Variable	Constant
Stringent Germ Line Hypothesis					
DNA Source					
MOPC-41	V_{41} C_k V_2 C_k V_3 C_k	~ 1000	~ 1000	<50	~ 1000
Other	V_{41} C_k V_2 C_k V_3 C_k	~ 1000	~ 1000	<50	~ 1000
Recombinational Germ Line Hypothesis					
DNA Source					
MOPC-41	V_{41} V_2 V_3 V_4 ... $V_{10^2-10^3}$ C_k	~ 1000	<10	<50	<10
Other	V_{41} V_2 V_3 V_4 ... $V_{10^2-10^3}$ C_k	~ 1000	<10	<50	<10
Somatic Mutation Hypothesis					
DNA Source					
MOPC-41	V_{41} V_2 V_3 V_4 ... V_{10-10^2} C_k	<100	<10	<<50	<10
Other	V_1 V_2 V_3 V_4 ... V_{10-10^2} C_k	<100	<10	<<50*	<10

*According to the somatic mutation hypothesis, the gene sequence corresponding to the variable region of the MOPC-41 subgroup in a MOPC-41 immunocyte should differ from the comparable sequence in other clones. Therefore, hybrids of the MOPC-41 variable region mRNA and the comparable DNA regions derived from other clones should be mismatched and incomplete were this hypothesis correct.

the species. A rather different view, in its most modern form, holds that while much diversity between variable region sequences has arisen through evolution, critical diversity continues to be generated in the genome during the somatic differentiation of the immunocyte. According to this hypothesis, the somatic mutation hypothesis, the number of germ line genes corresponding to variable regions is very few, possibly corresponding to the variable region subgroups, and these undergo changes during somatic differentiation which result in the final production of the immunologic repertoire.

The three models clearly differ from one another in the number of constant and variable gene sequences they require. As shown in figure 1, the stringent germ line hypothesis requires many copies of the constant region sequence, the remaining hypotheses require very few. The recombinational germ line hypothesis requires many variable region gene sequences, the somatic mutation hypothesis requires few. In addition, the last hypothesis holds that the genetic make up of one immunocyte clone will differ from that of another, inasmuch as both have undergone somatic mutation. In view of these differences each model has predictive value in terms of the number of variable and constant region sequences it requires.

THE EXPERIMENTAL APPROACH

The approach we have taken has relied very heavily on advances which we have been able to make in the study of the organization and regulated expression of the globin genes (18, 19). These studies led to techniques for the assay, purification and, most importantly, the ability to reverse transcribe purified mRNA into stable, highly radioactive DNA sequences corresponding to specific mammalian genes. These techniques have been applied by ourselves and others to the purification and reverse transcription of several immunoglobulin light chain mRNAs.

Synthesis of DNA complementary to purified light chain mRNA. Quantitation of the immunoglobulin genes has depended upon our having suitably radioactive probes for molecular hybridization studies. Early studies showed that the purified immunoglobulin mRNA would serve as an efficient template for the synthesis of complementary MOPC-41 cDNA (7, 20, 21). As we have pointed out previously (1), by annealing an oligo(dT) primer to the 3' poly(A) end of the message we were able to phase RNA-dependent DNA polymerase and assure that the light chain mRNA is copied from the 3' to the 5' end. Careful chain length determinations showed that the MOPC-41 cDNA had a chain length of approximately 630 nucleotides (1). Since reverse transcription occurs from the 3' end of the mRNA, the cDNA probe corresponds to the C terminal (or constant region) portion of the immunoglobulin light chain mRNA. A number of control studies indicated that the MOPC-41 cDNA indeed contained such a sequence (1).

Early studies also addressed the very important question of the purity of the mRNA preparation used and the purity of the probe itself (1). In addition to directing the synthesis of the immunoglobulin light chain and to migrating as a single, homogeneous band on formamide polyacrylamide gel electrophoresis, the technique of hybridization kinetic analysis was used to assess the purity of message and probe. According to these studies, the rate of hybridization of the MOPC-41 message and probe was such that its purity was comparable to that of rabbit and mouse globin mRNAs.

GENETIC REPRESENTATION OF THE κ CONSTANT REGION GENE SEQUENCE

As noted above, the stringent germ line hypothesis requires hundreds if not thousands of copies of the constant region sequence. A number of genetic analyses (22-29) which have examined the linkage, allotype and cross-over of heavy and light chain C regions have buttressed the arguments of Dreyer and Bennet (17) suggesting that only few copies of the C region gene are required. Implicit in their argument was the notion that at least two genes encode one polypeptide chain.

This hypothesis can be tested directly using the MOPC-41 cDNA as a hybridization probe to assess the reiteration frequency of the constant region gene sequence. The relevant experiment is shown in figure 2 wherein ^{3}H-cDNA MOPC-41 was hybridized to a vast excess of unlabeled total DNA derived from MOPC-41 tumor. A similar analysis using globin cDNA is shown for comparison. A $Cot_{1/2}$ value for MOPC-41 cDNA of 1130 was obtained as compared to a $Cot_{1/2}$ value of 3000 for "unique" mouse DNA. This corresponds to a reiteration frequency of 2.7 copies per haploid genome. The sharp thermal elution profile (Fig. 2 inset) indicates the closely

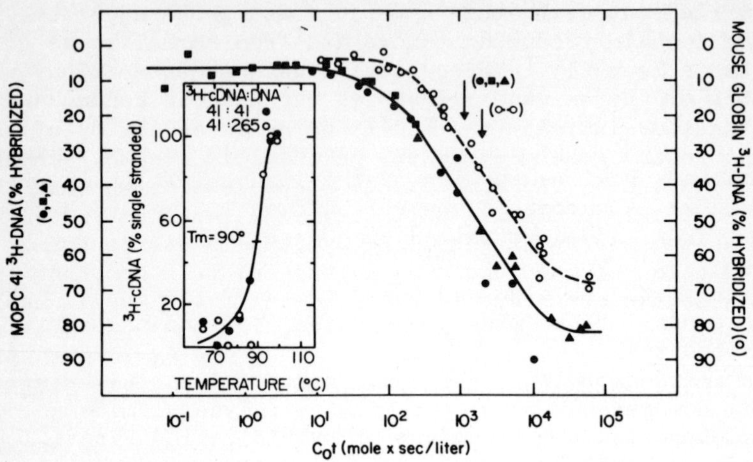

Fig. 2. Kinetics of annealing of MOPC-41 cDNA to a vast excess total cellular MOPC-41 DNA. Hybridization kinetics of MOPC-41 ^{3}H-cDNA were carried out in the presence of up to a 1.2 x 10^7-fold excess of unlabeled, sheared MOPC-41 cellular DNA. [For comparison, the kinetics of hybridization, under similar conditions, of mouse globin ^{3}H-cDNA with MOPC-41 cellular DNA are shown.] The cDNA and cellular DNA were prepared as described (1), with the former having a specific activity of 4.6 x 10^7 dpm/μg, and a base length of 630 by alkaline sucrose gradient centrifugation. The hybridization procedure and S_1 nuclease assays were as described (1), and were performed at DNA concentrations and salt concentrations appropriate for each portion of the kinetic curve (see below). The Cot values on the abscissa are those that would obtain at 0.18 M Na^+ (34). $Cot_{1/2}$ for MOPC-41 DNA x MOPC-41 DNA equals 1130. $Cot_{1/2}$ for globin cDNA x MOPC-41 DNA equals 2100. The filled symbols represent MOPC-41 cDNA x MOPC-41 DNA: (■) 0.99 mg/ml DNA, 0.18 M Na^+; (●) 9.9 mg/ml DNA, 0.54 M Na^+; (▲) 9.9 mg/ml DNA, 1.06 M Na^+. The open symbols (O) represent globin cDNA x MOPC-41 DNA. Thermal elution profiles (inset) were determined by diluting the hybrid to 0.24 M Na^+, heating at each temperature for 8-10 minutes and determining resistance to S_1 nuclease (1). In the inset, the closed symbols (●) represent MOPC-41 cDNA vs. MOPC-41 DNA; the open symbols (O) represent MOPC-41 cDNA vs. MOPC-265 DNA.

matched nature of the hybrid formed. Similar analyses have been carried out using this hybridization probe and total DNA from λ chain producing tumors and from normal mouse liver and spleen (1). These results gave a reiteration frequency of approximately 3 copies per haploid genome and taken together indicate that only two or three copies of the constant region gene are present per haploid genome. These are represented to the same extent regardless of whether the cell is actively producing κ chains. The result obviously rules out the stringent germ line hypothesis and conforms to the prediction of the remaining hypotheses that constant region gene sequences are represented but few times in the genome.

SOMATIC MUTATION OR EVOLUTION AS A SOURCE OF κ CHAIN DIVERSITY?

The recombinational germ line hypothesis and the somatic mutation hypothesis address the question of how the diversity of the variable region arises. The former hypothesis requires many, possibly thousands, of variable region gene sequences whereas the latter requires few. While these requirements are quite clear, there are consequences in terms of the hybridization experiment which require qualification.

Referring to Fig. 1 we may ask what results might be expected from hybridization analyses were either model correct? It is clear that the differences in amino acid sequences between variable regions from different κ subgroups are so great that stable hybrids would not form between sequences derived from different subgroups (11, 21). At best, variable sequences derived from the same subgroup which agree in over 80% of their amino acid sequences would be expected to form stable cross-hybrids. Therefore, if each subgroup contained approximately 50 different variable sequences, and were the germ line hypothesis correct, we would only observe a reiteration frequency of about 50, corresponding to about 50 or fewer closely related copies for the variable region. Were the somatic mutation hypothesis correct and each subgroup represented by a single germ line gene, the expected $Cot_{1/2}$ value would be consistent with a unique representation of this gene.

In contrast to the previously described experiments which focused on the reiteration frequency of the constant region sequence, the intact immunoglobulin light chain mRNA was iodinated with ^{125}I in order to assess the reiteration frequency of constant and variable portions of the κ light chain message. A very detailed hybridization kinetic analysis is shown in figure 3. There is no very highly reiterated material. In addition, the Crt curve is not obviously biphasic. At best, a small proportion, approximately 25%, of the ^{125}I mRNA does hybridize over a Crt range between 5 and 800. This material can be assigned a reiteration frequency of 30 to 50 copies per haploid genome, though it is difficult to feel secure about this number. The remaining and major portion of the hybridization reaction occurs over a range of Crt that is clearly unique. Similar experiments have been carried out using this iodinated MOPC-41 mRNA preparation and DNA derived from other myeloma tumors as well as normal spleen and liver tissue (12).

The results of this experiment are, unfortunately, subject to several interpretations. It is possible that the variable as well as constant region sequences are represented in the RNA that hybridizes as a unique sequence. The moderately reiterated material may be a contaminant or a portion of RNA beyond the variable region sequence. We have carried out a number of hybridization experiments of the type originally described by Tonegawa and his coworkers (30, 31) and have not been able to resolve this problem to our satisfaction. Clearly our experiments fail to reveal a major proportion of highly reiterated material. It is possible that the 30 to 50 times reiterated material does correspond to the variable region, a result which would be entirely consistent with the recombinational germ line hypothesis and the number of germ line variable genes expected in the MOPC-41 subgroup. However, since we cannot estimate the size of such a subgroup, such an interpretation leaves a great deal to be desired. Realizing that these difficulties could only be settled by a more focused use of hybridization probe, we turned our attention to the λ class of mouse immunoglobulin light chains.

THE ORIGIN OF DIVERSITY OF λ VARIABLE SEQUENCES: A SIMPLER CLASS

While λ light chains represent a minor proportion of light chains in circulating mouse antibody, Cohn and his associates (32) have pointed out that λ light chains derived from myeloma tumors fall into what seems to be a single

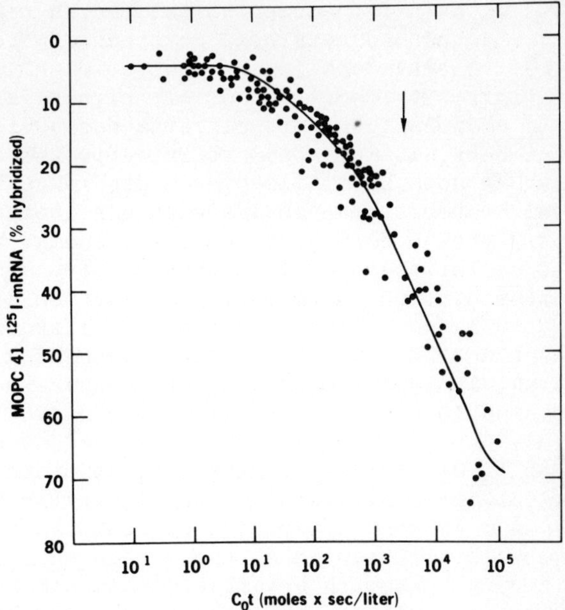

Fig. 3. Kinetics of annealing of MOPC-41 ^{125}I-mRNA to a vast excess of total, cellular MOPC-41 DNA. Hybridization kinetics of MOPC-41 ^{125}I-mRNA in the presence of up to a 2.94×10^6-fold excess of unlabeled, sheared MOPC-41 cellular DNA. Cellular DNA was prepared as described (1). MOPC-41 mRNA was prepared as described (1). Iodination was performed according to the procedure of Prensky et al. (35); specific activity of the MOPC-41 ^{125}I-mRNA is 3.2×10^6 cpm/μg. Hybridization was performed at 65°-67°C in 1.04 M Na^+ - 0.02 M Tris-Cl, pH 7.0, with 0.18 M Na^+ used at the lower Crt values. DNA concentration was 10 mg/ml, with 0.94 mg/ml used at the lower Crt values. Crt values on the abcissa are those that would be obtained at 0.18 M Na^+ (34) in a DNA-DNA reannealing reaction. At each time point, aliquots were diluted 100-fold into 0.3 M NaCl - 30 mM Na-citrate, and assayed (37° x 40 min.) for resistance to 60 μg/ml RNase A, according to the procedure of Melli et al. (36). Reaction mixtures were acid-precipitated and collected on GFC glass fiber filters. Filters were eluted with NCS, and counted in solution in a standard toluene-fluor mixture in a Beckman LS-250 β-scintillation spectrometer. The symbols represent: (●) MOPC-41 ^{125}I-mRNA x MOPC-41 DNA, $Crt_{1/2}$ equals 3200.

subgroup. Of the eighteen mouse λ light chains thus far analyzed, seven sequences have been determined which differ from one another at the most in one, two or four amino acids located in the hypervariable portion of the variable region. Such small differences in amino acid sequences which could be accounted for by not more than four or five base changes suggest genetic sequences so closely related that they would certainly form stable cross-hybrids with one another. Thus the λ myeloma proteins form a very well-defined subgroup which contain a minimum of seven members. If the recombinational germ line hypothesis were correct, we would expect, as a minimum, seven germ line λ variable gene sequences to be present in the mouse genome. These sequences would be virtually identical to one another so that the hybridization should correspond to this reiteration frequency. We have emphasized that seven separate λ chains represent the minimum value. It is possible, even likely, that this subgroup has many more closely related members. The major difference, then, between the λ and κ subgroups are that in λ, we have a defined amino acid sequence which assures us the formation of a stable hybrid. Thus, hybridization kinetic analysis for the variable region sequence should be unique for the constant region and reiterated at least 7-fold for the variable region if the recombinational germ line hypothesis is correct. If it is not correct, hybridization kinetics should reveal a unique sequence.

Experiments using RPC-20 cDNA: A λ constant and variable region probe. Somewhat in contrast to results obtained using the κ chain mRNA template, RPC-20 mRNA directs the synthesis of a relatively long cDNA reverse transcript (33). Relatively detailed studies of sized cDNA yielded a family of probes with an average chain length of 830 nucleotides. Taking into account the fact that the RPC-20 mRNA was approximately 1150 bases long and assuming that the poly(A) sequence was approximately 200 bases long, this probe should clearly cover a 150-200 base long untranslated sequence, the 325 base long constant region sequence and a major portion, if not all, of the variable region sequence as well. The probe, therefore, in contrast to the κ light chain probe, should represent both constant and variable regions. The behavior of this λ cDNA in hybridization kinetic analyses using total DNA derived from RPC-20 tumor and mouse spleen is shown in figure 4. The $Crt_{1/2}$ values of 1200 are consistent with about two copies of this sequence per haploid genome.

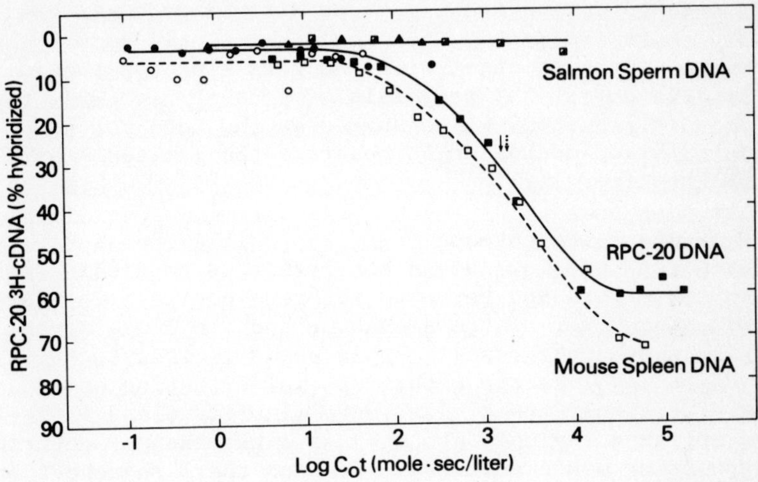

Fig. 4. Kinetics of annealing of RPC-20 ^{3}H-cDNA to total RPC-20, mouse spleen and salmon sperm DNA. The hybridization reaction was carried out under conditions described in the legend to figure 2. The curves are appropriately labeled in the figure. The $Cot_{1/2}$ values obtained are 1200 and 13^^ for mouse spleen and RPC-20 DNA respectively.

CON SIONS AND CAVEATS

While the matter of genetic representation of the κ constant region sequence seems settled and is relatively unique, the genetic representation of the variable region sequence remains a problem. Our results viewing the hybridization of the κ light chain mRNA have produced somewhat ambiguous results, but nevertheless, rule out a variable sequence corresponding to thousands of closely related genetic sequences. To overcome the difficulties intrinsic in interpreting the results from studies of the κ sequence, we have turned to the simpler λ system in the mouse. Here we are assured of at least seven sequences of a single subgroup which are so closely related that they would produce stable hybrids in our kinetic experiments. Studies using ^{3}H-cDNA give results relevant to both constant and variable regions. Constant and variable λ sequences seem to be represented one or two times per diploid genome, certainly no more frequently than the mouse globin genes. Such a result is not consistent with the germ line hypothesis. The results support the proposals of Cohn et al. (32), based on the mouse λ system, which suggested the need for a somatic mutation mechanism to generate the limited λ variable region diversity.

What about the caveats? It is possible that the hybridization technique would not permit us to distinguish between one or two and seven to ten gene copies. In view of the resolving power of the technique and the close agreement with globin sequence results, this seems unlikely. Further reservation involves the rather special situation of mouse λ chains. Certainly the λ class is a minority class in the mouse, representing only about 5% of light chains occurring in circulating mouse antibody. Perhaps the λ sequences have undergone a massive deletion in this species and their unique or relatively unique representation is a consequence of this and is, therefore, not representative of the mouse variable region genome. This point, of course, will be clarified when we are able to focus in greater detail upon the hybridization kinetics of several different κ chain subgroups.

ACKNOWLEDGEMENT

We are most grateful to Ms. Catherine Kunkle for coordinating the editorial efforts necessary to write this paper.

REFERENCES

(1) T. Honjo, S. Packman, D. Swan, M. Nau and P. Leder. Proc. Nat. Acad. Sci. USA 71 (1974) 3659.

(2) J. Stavnezer and R.C. Huang. Nature New Biol. 230 (1971) 172.

(3) G.G. Brownlee, T.M. Harrison, M.B. Mathews and C. Milstein. FEBS Lett. 23 (1972) 249.

(4) C. Milstein, G.G. Brownlee, T.M. Harrison, and M.B. Mathews. Nature New Biol. 239 (1972) 117.

(5) R.H. Stevens and A.R. Williamson. Nature 239 (1972) 143.

(6) D. Swan, H. Aviv and P. Leder. Proc. Nat. Acad. Sci. USA 69 (1972) 1967.

(7) B. Mach, C. Faust and P. Vassalli. Proc. Nat. Acad. Sci. USA 70 (1973) 451.

(8) I. Schechter. Proc. Nat. Acad. Sci. USA 70 (1973) 2256.

(9) M. Smith, J. Stavnezer, R.C. Huang, J.B. Burdon and C.D. Lane. J. Mol. Biol. 80 (1973) 553.

(10) T.M. Harrison, G.G. Brownlee, and C. Milstein. Eur. J. Biochem. 47 (1974) 621.

(11) P. Leder, T. Honjo, S. Packman, D. Swan, M. Nau and B. Norman. in: Proceedings of the ICN-UCLA Symposium on Molecular Biology, ed. C.F. Fox (Academic Press, Inc., New York, 1974) p. 299.

(12) P. Leder, T. Honjo, S. Packman, D. Swan, M. Nau and B. Norman. Proc. Nat. Acad. Sci. USA 71 (1974) 5109.

(13) T.H. Rabbitts. FEBS Lett. 42 (1974) 323.

(14) T.H. Rabbitts, C. Milstein and G.G. Brownlee. Symposium of the 9th Meeting of the Federation of European Bio-Chemical Societies, September, 1974.

(15) J. Stavnezer, R.C.C. Huang, E. Stavnezer and J.M. Bishop. J. Mol. Biol. 88 (1974) 43.

(16) J.K. Inman. in: Proceedings of the ICN-UCLA Symposium on Molecular Biology, ed. C.F. Fox (Academic Press, Inc., New York, 1974) p. 37.

(17) W.J. Dreyer, and J.C. Bennett. Proc. Nat. Acad. Sci. USA 54 (1965) 864.

(18) H. Aviv and P. Leder. Proc. Nat. Acad. Sci. USA 69 (1972) 1408.

(19) J. Ross, H. Aviv, E. Scolnick and P. Leder. Proc. Nat. Acad. Sci. USA 69 (1972) 264.

(20) H. Aviv, S. Packman, D. Swan, J. Ross and P. Leder. Nature New Biol. 241 (1973) 174.

(21) P. Leder, J. Ross, J. Gielen, S. Packman, Y. Ikawa, H. Aviv and D. Swan. Cold Spring Harbor Symp. Quant. Biol. 38 (1973) 753.

(22) R. Liberman and M. Potter. J. Mol. Biol. 18 (1966) 516.

(23) R. Hamers and C. Hamers-Casterman. Cold Spring Harbor Symp. Quant. Biol. 32 (1967) 129.

(24) M. Koshland. Cold Spring Harbor Symp. Quant. Biol. 32 (1967) 119.

(25) J.B. Natvig, H.G. Kunkel and S.D. Litwin. Cold Spring Harbor Symp. Quant. Biol. 32 (1967) 173.

(26) L.A. Herzenberg, and H.O. McDevitt. Annu. Rev. Genet. 2 (1968) 209.

(27) H.G. Kunkel, J.B. Natvig and F.G. Joslin. Proc. Nat. Acad. Sci. USA 62 (1969) 145.

(28) S.L. Tosi, R.G. Mage and S. Dubiski. J. Immunol. 104 (1970) 145.

(29) R.G. Mage, G.O. Young-Cooper and C. Alexander. Nature New Biol. 230 (1971) 63.

(30) S. Tonegawa and I. Baldi. Biochem. Biophys. Res. Commun. 51 (1973) 81.

(31) S. Tonegawa, C. Steinberg, S. Dube and A. Bernardini. Proc. Nat. Acad. Sci. USA 71 (1974) 4027.

(32) M. Cohn, B. Blomberg, W. Geckeler, W. Raschke, R. Riblet and M. Weigert. in: Proceedings of the ICN-UCLA Symposium on Molecular Biology, ed. C.F. Fox (Academic Press, Inc., New York, 1974) p. 89.

(33) T. Honjo, S. Packman, D. Swan and P. Leder. J. Mol. Biol., submitted.

(34) R.J. Britten and J. Smith. Carnegie Inst. Washington Yearb. 68 (1970) 378.

(35) W. Prensky, D.M. Steffensen and W.L. Huges. Proc. Nat. Acad. Sci. USA 70 (1973) 1860.

(36) M. Melli, C. Whitfield, K.V. Rao, M. Richardson and J.O. Bishop. Nature New Biol. 231 (1971) 8.

DISCUSSION

T WU: In the mRNA-DNA hybridizing experiment should the poly A give a diphasic curve?

P. LEDER: I'd like to emphasize that the last experiment that I showed you was done with DNA not mRNA. There is no problem because the hybridizations are carried out under such conditions and the assays are done in such a way, that the poly dT interactions play no role. In the iodinated RNA experiments, the chemistry is such that the iodine is on the cytidine.

F. W. PUTNAM: If you can't be sure that you don't have at least 7 to 10 V region genes for the lambda chain then in the kappa chain, where there are many more variable sequences the number of V kappa genes could be 20 to 50 times greater. You could easily have several hundred V kappa genes, couldn't you?

P. LEDER: I don't think that our results can be interpreted to determine the reiteration frequency of the kappa variable region. I made no interpretation of the results I showed in terms of the reiteration frequency of the variable region.

S. B. GREER: My question refers to the problem of joining. I know that you are using the RNA dependent DNA polymerase as a probe, but it might be interesting, concerning the mechanism of joining that I have in mind, if you took two different populations of messenger RNA molecules, and utilized the reverse transcriptase to see if you obtained a DNA product that is a combination of the two templates.

P. LEDER: As a pencil and paper experiment that might be alright.

S.B. GREER: On the subject of pencil and paper joining mechanisms, one might consider the findings of So, Downey, and Byrnes at the University of Miami on the existence of an RNA replicase in mammalian cells. Instead of being joined by a ligase one could imagine two templates being copied to result in a combination of parts of two molecules.

P. LEDER: Right, I'm familiar with the enzymatic activity and I have given it some thought. About joining constant and variable regions, in the case of lambda where you have only one sequence, you don't have to postulate any joining mechanism yet. So keep this in mind, it doesn't speak to the Dryer and Bennet model. Lambda gets around that problem completely.

CELL SURFACE ANTIGENS AND CELL SURFACE PROTEINS

Problems and Approaches for Protein Chemistry

BRUCE A. CUNNINGHAM
The Rockefeller University

Abstract: Cell-cell interactions and cell-ligand interactions depend upon the physico-chemical interactions of receptors, the specificity of these receptors, and their linkage to metabolic events within the cell. Analyses of these phenomena at the molecular level are providing challenges for the protein chemist that require a greatly expanded view and closer interaction with the cell biologist than in previous structural studies in immunology and enzymology. This paper reviews studies in our laboratory that provide the biological framework for our characterization of cell surface receptors at the molecular level. These studies include: 1) experiments on the mobility and redistribution of cell surface receptors and the modulation of receptor and cell movements by lectins such as concanavalin A and various drugs which suggest that these receptors may have a common anchorage system under the plasma membrane; 2) analysis of the initial events in the mitogenic stimulation of lymphocytes by Con A which suggests that the same colchicine-binding protein system may be involved in mediating the modulation of receptor mobility and mitogenic activation; and 3) direct analysis of the chemical structure of surface molecules such as β_2-microglobulin which suggests that it may be possible to classify receptors into groups of molecules with common evolutionary origins.

Introduction

Interactions and events taking place at the cell surface are of major importance in cell development, for cell function, and in the control of cell growth. Analysis of these events at the molecular level is defining a new role for the protein chemist in cell biology. Because of the large scope encompassed by the biological questions, the complex assemblies of proteins, the interactions between these components, and the complex assays of activity, a larger view is required for structural studies in these systems than for previous studies in immunology and enzymology.

Consideration of the composition of cell membranes and their associated molecules shows that a variety of different interactions must occur in the membrane complex. The sum of these interactions should eventually be reflected in the behavior of particular receptor molecules. A variety of antigenically distinct moieties have been identified on the surfaces of lymphocytes, but little is known about the chemical structure or function of these molecules (1,2). Furthermore, the total number of different receptors present on a single cell and the number of different kinds of molecules they represent have not been established. A single receptor may be exposed to a number of different environments simultaneously as shown in Figure 1 (3). Molecules on the cell surface function in the predominantly hydrophilic region outside the cell and can interact with ligands and metabolites in the media, be associated with proteins, glycoproteins, carbohydrates, and glycolipids on the cell surface, and may be anchored to components at or just under the membrane. Receptors that penetrate through the membrane may be involved in hydrophobic interactions with the lipid bilayer or be imbedded in a matrix of other molecules in intramembranous particles. In addition these receptors may extend through the membrane and be involved in functions associated with the hydrophilic interior of the cell where contacts with intracellular enzymes and molecular assemblies are possible. Any one receptor might serve a variety of cellular functions and could interact with a number of molecules both on the surface and beneath it. These numerous arrangements and potential interactions raise key questions about the polarity and detailed structural features of the proteins, the relationships between the various receptors and the phases they encounter, and the coupling between the various phases. It is equally important to define the anchorage systems and the molecules that regulate receptor dynam-

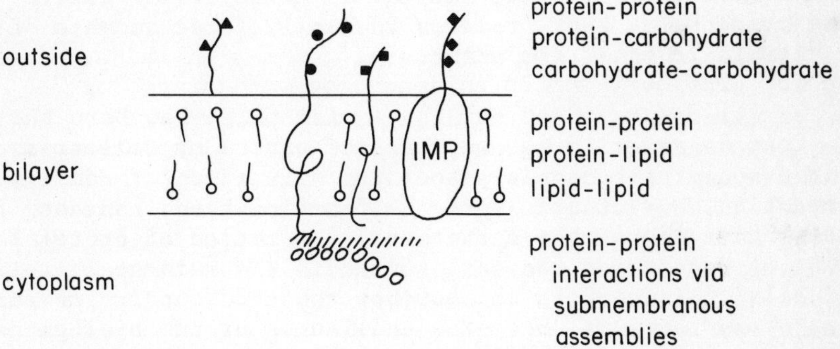

Fig. 1. Environments in which cell surface receptors can interact with external ligands, each other, membrane components and cytoplasmic constituents. Proteins or glycoproteins on the cell surface can function in two distinct hydrophilic regions, the cell periphery and the cytoplasm, as well as in the hydrophobic lipid bilayer (adapted from references 3 and 10).

ics. In such complex systems, the approach for the structural chemist is intimately directed by the biological framework in which hypotheses can be formulated and tested.

In addition to the complexity of the biological activities and the molecular interactions mediating such activities, another challenge is provided by the fact that most of the proteins on the cell surface can be obtained in only minute amounts. To solve this problem microchemical methods must be developed and purification procedures adapted for the isolation of small amounts of proteins from large amounts of tissues or large volumes of cultured cells. In addition, many cell surface proteins are deeply embedded in the cell membrane, interact strongly with each other or with carbohydrates or lipids, and are insoluble in simple aqueous solvents. New detergents and other dissociating solvents are therefore required. Many of these solvents will result in a loss of biological activity or will prevent the use of certain classical methods for protein characterization. One hope for decreasing such technical demands lies in the identification of the appropriate "accidents of nature" such as cells that display an enlightening genetic defect or a tumor that produces unusually large amounts of a particular surface component.

To illustrate these points, I wish to review here the work, not necessarily my own, carried out by my colleagues on some dynamic processes associated with receptors on lymphocytes. These studies form the functional environment for our analyses of the structure and function of proteins and glycoproteins on the cell surface. The main goal in presenting this work is to show how the structural approach must be reoriented to meet the challenges of the biological questions. Three types of systems will be considered: 1) the modulation of receptor mobility in which the biological phenomena are well described, but the molecules and molecular assemblies involved are unknown; 2) the stimulation of mitosis in lymphocytes in which the initial interactions at the cell surface are known but the receptors involved and the events that lead to the transmission of a stimulatory signal into the interior of the cell are not defined; and 3) the analysis of specific cell surface components for which detailed structural information is being obtained, but the biological functions of these molecules are unknown.

Modulation of Lymphocyte Receptor Mobility by Con A

An experimental system for testing the factors that may regulate receptor anchorage, distribution, and mobility was provided by examining the effects of the lectin concanavalin A (Con A) on the mobility of lymphocyte receptors (4). Lymphocyte receptors appear to be distributed randomly on the cell surface (Figure 2). In the presence of multivalent ligands such as antibodies to immunoglobulins, however, the receptors to which these ligands bind can undergo patch formation and subsequent cap formation (5). Patch formation depends upon the local diffusion of the receptors in the plane of the membrane. Cap formation results from the movement of these cross-linked receptor complexes toward one pole of the cell and depends upon cellular metabolism.

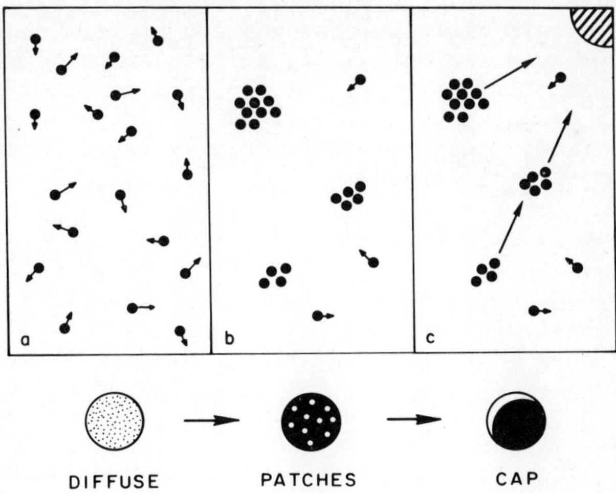

Fig. 2. A schematic diagram (10) of the redistribution of surface immunoglobulin molecules on lymphocytes after binding with anti-immunoglobulin antibodies. The initial random distribution of receptors results in a diffuse labelling pattern. Cross-linking of receptors by the bound ligand leads to cluster or patch formation and coalescence of patches at one pole of the cell results in cap formation (4,5).

Global cell movement or translocation is not required for cap formation (6) but microfilaments may be involved (7).

It was shown by Yahara and Edelman (4) that Con A inhibits the ability of cell receptors to form patches and caps. If Con A is added at concentrations of 100 μg/ml to lymphocytes at 21° C before treatment with anti-Ig both patch formation and cap formation are inhibited (Table 1). This effect depends on the dose of Con A and is reversed by addition of a competitive inhibitor of Con A such as α-methyl-mannoside (αMM). In addition to inhibiting the movement of Ig molecules on B lymphocytes, Con A inhibits cap formation by a variety of other receptors including the Θ antigen of thymocytes, the Con A glycoprotein receptors, and H-2 molecules on lymphocytes and fibroblasts.

The ability of the lectin to influence receptor mobility appears to depend upon its ability to cross-link receptors because of its multivalence. Succinyl-Con A (8), a dimeric derivative of the tetravalent native lectin, competes with Con A for the cell surface receptors. Unlike native Con A, however, the modified lectin does not modulate the mobility of other receptors. Treatment of cell-bound dimeric succinyl-Con A with divalent antibodies directed against Con A, however, results in the inhibition of patch formation (Table 1). Monovalent F_{ab}' fragments of the antibodies to Con A show little or no effect. Thus, the effective valence and possibly the charge of the lectin may be critical in inducing the inhibition of cell receptor mobility. While we know the structure of the lectin in considerable detail (9) and can define to some extent the properties that might influence its effects on cell surface receptor mobility, we know very little about the receptors and other molecules of the cell involved in these processes.

Model for Modulation of Receptor Mobility

Analysis of the effect of temperature and various drugs on the ability of Con A to inhibit receptor mobility has provided clues to the possible nature of the cellular structures involved in the modulation of cell surface receptors (10). When fluorescein-labelled Con A is added to cells at 37°, the cells are diffusely stained and remain so. If, however, cells are treated with fluorescein-Con A applied at 4°, washed, and returned to 37°, the Con A receptors themselves patch and cap (11). In addition, Con A, under these conditions, does not inhibit the movement of any of the other receptors of the cell. These results suggested that proteins capable of dissociation at low temperature such as cytoplasmic microtubules may be involved in controlling receptor distribution. Further evidence was provided by showing that colchicine, vinblastine, vincristine, and podophyllotoxin, reagents known to affect microtubules, partially reverse the inhibition of receptor mobility by Con A at 37° and allow formation of both Con A and anti-Ig caps (Table 1) (10,12). Neither lumicolchicine, a photo-inactivated derivative of colchicine (13) nor strychnine, which affects erythrocyte membranes (14), showed any effect in the system. The effects of colchicine and related drugs on receptor mobility do not appear to be due to non-specific interactions of

Table 1

Modulation of receptor mobility by Con A and anti-mitotic drugs[a]

Treatment	% Cap-forming cells
Control	87
Con A	4
Succinyl-Con A[b]	86
Succinyl-Con A + anti-Con A[c]	53
Succinyl-Con A + F_{ab}' anti-Con A	80
Con A + colchicine[d]	30
Con A + vinblastine	51
Con A + vincristine	15
Con A + podophyllotoxin	10

[a]To test for the inhibition by Con A of immunoglobulin receptor cap formation, the percent of cap-forming cells obtained with fl-anti-Ig (100 μg/ml) was measured in the presence of Con A (100 μg/ml).

[b]Succinyl-Con A, 50 μg/ ml.

[c]Succinyl-Con A, 50 μg/ml; antibody reagents, 100 μg/ml.

[d]Colchicine, vinblastine and vincristine, 10^{-4}M; podophyllotoxin, 10^{-3}M.

these drugs with the lymphocyte membrane and are not due to the interactions of the drugs with Con A. Colchicine does not bind to Con A nor does it cause changes in the aggregation of its subunits. In addition, colchicine does not inhibit the binding of Con A to saccharides or to the cell surface.

Based on these results and a variety of additional data (4-8,15,16) Edelman *et al*. have formulated a model (10,15) for the modulation of the mobility of cell surface proteins. The model (Figure 3) assumes that some receptors penetrate the lipid bilayer and interact with submembranous proteins. These receptors can exist in either a free or anchored state. The effects of cytochalasin B and colchicine on cap formation and its inhibition (15,16) suggest that the central elements in this system of anchorage are the microfilaments and microtubule-like proteins. Cross-linkage of lectin receptors is assumed to influence the association-dissociation equilibrium of these macromolecular assemblies, shifting their interaction with other receptors or the inner lamella of the bilayer. This provides a system for communicating receptor states through the membrane as well as for altering receptor states via intracellular events. This model suggests that at least four sets of equilibria may be involved: 1) cross-linkage of glycoproteins or other receptors with various ligands; 2) interaction of receptors with microfilaments; 3) interaction of microfilaments with formed microtubules; and 4) interaction of tubulin subunits to form the microtubules.

In the analysis of such an intricate system at the level of protein structure an essential first step is to establish that a colchicine-binding protein exists near the cell surface and show that it can interact directly or indirectly with surface receptors. The biological studies suggest that the next most valuable step would be to establish the number of components in the assembly, their distribution, and the order of their interactions. This could proceed by the isolation of microtubular-like and microfilament-like proteins using approaches and assays described for other systems such as the isolation of the actin-like protein from red cells (17) and the isolation and characterization of brain tubulin (18). Such an approach, however, could be lengthy and may result in the loss of biological functions because of components lost during the isolation or because the molecules may function only as complexes. A more fruitful approach may be to devise chemical means for cross-linking the assembly so that it can be isolated as a unit. Gel electrophoresis and immunological methods could then be used to catalog the contents of the assembly and each component could then be isolated by other methods from various cell extracts or from the cross-linked assembly.

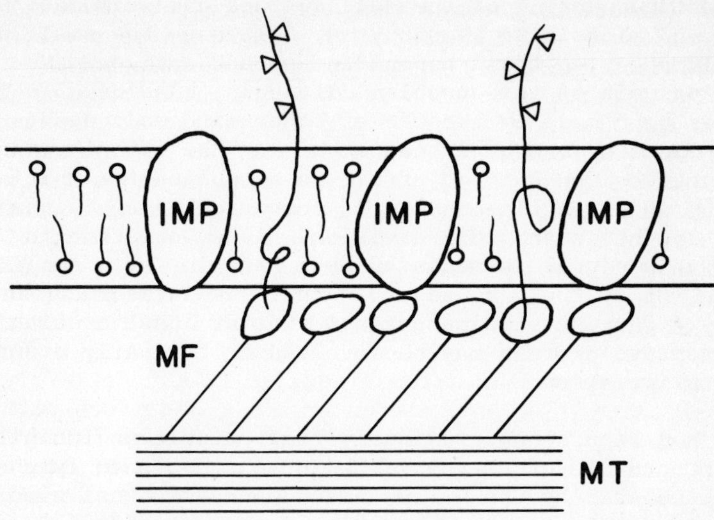

Fig. 3. A hypothetical model (10,15) for modulation of cell surface receptors by submembranous structures. The model assumes that microfilaments (MF) interact with receptors, possibly via a myosin- or spectrin-like structure and that the microfilaments interact in turn with microtubules (MT). The interactions among the various components are assumed to involve reversible association-dissociation reactions. Intramembranous particles (IMP) are not involved in these equilibria.

An alternative approach would be to search for other cellular functions mediated by this hypothesized receptor anchorage system. These new activities may provide other clues for the identification and characterization of the structural components of the anchorage system. The hypothesis that such a cytoplasmic assembly is linked to the exterior of the cell suggests that the same system might be involved in the transmission of signals from the cell surface to the interior of the cell, as in mitogenic stimulation.

Mitogenic Stimulation of Lymphocytes by Con A

One of the key problems in immunology is to understand how an antigen acting at the cell surface can stimulate maturation and mitosis in lymphocytes. Although the small number of lymphocytes that respond to any one antigen makes a direct analysis of this problem difficult, considerable progress has been made by the use of other mitogenic agents such as lectins. We have been examining the stimulation of lymphocytes by Con A in an effort to establish the initial events by which lectin-binding is converted into a signal for DNA synthesis and cell division. A key question is whether this signal is mediated by a protein, by a small molecule, or by the same assembly that regulates receptor mobility. Current studies suggest that at least a colchicine-sensitive protein may be involved in the early events of cell stimulation.

It had been shown previously that colchicine inhibits the incorporation of ^{3}H-thymidine in mouse splenic lymphocytes stimulated by Con A (10) and human peripheral blood lymphocytes activated by PHA (19). Recent studies (20) in our laboratory have shown that at concentrations of 10^{-7} M or above, colchicine reduced the response of human lymphocytes to Con A by 70 to 90% as measured by the incorporation of ^{3}H-thymidine between 48-50 hours after the start of the culture. The number of blast cells was also significantly lower in cultures containing Con A and colchicine. The effects of the drug could be due to killing of the cells, the selective killing of blast cells, interference with DNA synthesis, or the blocking of first generation cells at metaphase.

Analysis of the activation of human lymphocytes by Con A suggests that the inhibitory activity of colchicine could not be accounted for by diminution in cell viability. In addition, studies were performed on Con A stimulated cells collected at the G_1/S boundary by blocking with hydroxyurea. Addition of colchicine to these cultures containing preformed blast cells did not result in the selective killing of blast cells. Furthermore, these studies also showed that the inhibition of ^{3}H-thymidine incorporation was not due to blockage of thymidine transport or DNA synthesis inasmuch as colchicine had no effect on cells in the S phase of the cell cycle. At the times when appreciable inhibition is observed (36-40 hours after stimulation), only a small percentage of the lymphocytes present are daughter cells (21,22), so the inhibition by colchicine of the mitogenic response is not due to a simple blockage of the first generation cells at their metaphases. These results suggest that the depressed level of ^{3}H-thymidine incorporation seen in cultures containing colchicine represents an inhibitory effect of the drug on lymphocytes prior to their transformation into blast cells.

Kinetic data have now been obtained to indicate that colchicine blocks stimulation early in the sequence of events following addition of the mitogen and that the time of inhibition may be correlated with the kinetics of cellular commitment to lectin activation. The kinetics of colchicine inhibition were analyzed by introducing the drug into cultures at various times after Con A stimulation (Figure 4b). When colchicine is added at the start of the culture, the incorporation of ^{3}H-thymidine as measured at 48 hours is inhibited by about 90% compared to controls. The extent of inhibition decreases the later colchicine is added, and no inhibition is observed if the drug is added 30 hours after the addition of Con A.

This is strikingly similar to the curve obtained using the inhibitor αMM which removes Con A from the cell surface (Figure 4a). The later the saccharide inhibitor is added, the less inhibition is observed. No inhibition was found if αMM was added 30 hours after the start of the culture. Other experiments have shown that the rising level of ^{3}H-thymidine incorporation with later additions of both αMM and colchicine is proportional to the number of cells committed to lectin stimulation. The fact that the kinetics of inhibition of stimulation by αMM and by colchicine are similar suggests that the inhibitory effect of the drug might be temporally correlated with cellular commitment.

The effects of colchicine on the modulation of receptor mobility and on the stimulation of lymphoid cells suggests that a colchicine-binding protein system such as the cellular microtubules may be involved in both processes. Inasmuch as microtubules have only been identified in the cytoplasm, this system may represent an example of receptor-cytoplasmic interaction and could be a key component in the control of cell growth.

The series of cellular events following lectin binding that lead to mitogenic stimulation remains obscure. One possibility is that the lectin cross-links receptors which

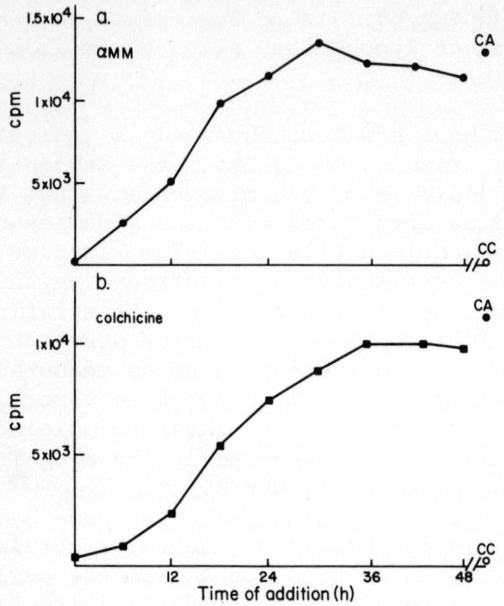

Fig. 4. Effect of αMM (a) and colchicine (b) added at different times after the start of the cultures, on the incorporation of ^{3}H-thymidine in human lymphocytes stimulated by Con A (20). Inhibitors were added to cultures containing Con A at the indicated time points, and the cultures were continued until 48 hours at which time they were pulsed with ^{3}H-thymidine and harvested for analysis.

in turn alters the hypothesized microtubular assembly. The alteration in the assembly could then result in the stimulation of a specific enzymatic activity, the release of a small molecule, alterations in the levels of cyclic nucleotides, or the generation of additional changes in the structure of the cell membrane so as to alter the transport of a critical metabolite. All of these possibilities present major challenges for the protein chemist in identifying the assemblies and macromolecules involved.

Furthermore, recent analysis (21) of the kinetics of cellular commitment in the stimulation of lymphocytes by Con A suggests that resting lymphocytes are dispersed in different states with regard to their ability to respond to the lectin. These cells may be distributed in a loop within G_1 and such temporal heterogeneity may be reflected by differences in the number, the distribution, or the types of specific receptors on the cell surface presenting a major challenge for the chemist to devise methods for looking in detail at specific receptors on single cells.

Structure of Cell Surface Proteins

Important generalizations may also come from direct analysis of cell surface proteins. Although the structure and function of most cell surface receptors remains unknown, we do know a considerable amount about one cell surface protein, namely immunoglobulin (23). The mode of attachment of this protein to the cell surface is unknown, however, and no detailed mechanism has been provided for how the interaction of immunoglobulins with specific antigens triggers a specific immune response. Our knowledge of immunoglobulin structure, however, may provide an important basis for comparison with other receptors.

β_2-microglobulin (24) is a low molecular weight human protein found on the surfaces of a variety of cell types (25). We have determined the amino acid sequence of this protein (26,27) and shown that it is homologous to the C_L, C_H1, C_H2, and C_H3 homology regions of IgG (Figure 5). β_2-microglobulins also exist in other species and the protein appears to be highly conserved in evolution (28,29). Recent studies have indicated that β_2-microglobulin is closely associated with the HL-A antigens and may represent the smaller polypeptide chain of these antigens (30,31). If β_2-microglobulin is an integral chain of the histocompatibility antigens, these antigens may show a common evolutionary origin with immunoglobulins (32). The histocompatibility antigens and β_2-microglobulin are general cell surface proteins found on nearly all cells. The striking homology between β_2-microglobulin and immunoglobulin, which is restricted to lymphocytes, suggests that while there may be a large number of different cell surface proteins, they may have only a few evolutionary origins and, therefore, can

	1									10	
β_2-MICROGLOBULIN	ILE	GLN	ARG	THR	PRO	LYS	ILE	GLN	VAL	TYR	SER
EU C_L (RESIDUES 109-214)	THR	VAL	ALA	ALA	PRO	-	-	SER	VAL	PHE	ILE
EU C_H1 (RESIDUES 119-220)	SER	THR	LYS	GLY	PRO	-	-	SER	VAL	PHE	PRO
EU C_H2 (RESIDUES 234-341)	LEU	LEU	GLY	GLY	PRO	-	-	SER	VAL	PHE	LEU
EU C_H3 (RESIDUES 342-446)	GLN	PRO	ARG	GLU	PRO	-	-	GLN	VAL	TYR	THR

													20							
ARG	HIS	PRO	ALA	-	GLU	-	-	-	-	ASN	GLY	LYS	SER	ASN	PHE	LEU	ASN	CYS	TYR	VAL
PHE	PRO	PRO	SER	ASP	GLU	GLN	-	-	LEU	LYS	SER	GLY	THR	ALA	SER	VAL	VAL	CYS	LEU	LEU
LEU	ALA	PRO	SER	SER	LYS	SER	-	-	THR	SER	GLY	GLY	THR	ALA	ALA	LEU	GLY	CYS	LEU	VAL
PHE	PRO	PRO	LYS	PRO	LYS	ASP	THR	LEU	MET	ILE	SER	ARG	THR	PRO	GLU	VAL	THR	CYS	VAL	VAL
LEU	PRO	PRO	SER	ARG	GLU	GLU	-	-	MET	THR	LYS	ASN	GLN	VAL	SER	LEU	THR	CYS	LEU	VAL

		30												40						
SER	GLY	PHE	HIS	PRO	SER	ASP	ILE	GLU	VAL	-	-	ASP	LEU	LEU	LYS	ASP	GLY	GLU	ARG	ILE
ASN	ASN	PHE	TYR	PRO	ARG	GLU	ALA	LYS	VAL	-	-	GLN	TRP	LYS	VAL	ASP	ASN	-	ALA	LEU
LYS	ASP	TYR	PHE	PRO	GLU	PRO	VAL	THR	VAL	-	-	SER	TRP	ASN	SER	-	GLY	-	ALA	LEU
VAL	ASP	VAL	SER	HIS	GLU	ASP	PRO	GLN	VAL	LYS	PHE	ASN	TRP	TYR	VAL	ASP	GLY	-	-	VAL
LYS	GLY	PHE	TYR	PRO	SER	ASP	ILE	ALA	VAL	-	-	GLU	TRP	GLU	SER	ASN	ASP	-	-	GLY

					50										60					
GLU	LYS	VAL	-	GLU	HIS	SER	ASP	LEU	SER	PHE	SER	LYS	ASN	-	TRP	SER	PHE	TYR	LEU	LEU
GLN	SER	GLY	ASN	SER	GLN	GLU	SER	VAL	THR	GLU	GLN	ASP	SER	LYS	ASP	SER	THR	TYR	SER	LEU
THR	SER	GLY	-	VAL	HIS	THR	PHE	PRO	ALA	VAL	LEU	GLN	SER	-	SER	GLY	LEU	TYR	SER	LEU
GLN	VAL	HIS	ASN	ALA	LYS	THR	LYS	PRO	ARG	GLU	GLU	GLN	TYR	-	ASP	SER	THR	TYR	ARG	VAL
GLU	PRO	GLU	ASN	TYR	LYS	THR	THR	PRO	PRO	VAL	LEU	ASP	SER	-	ASP	GLY	SER	PHE	PHE	LEU

						70											80			
TYR	SER	TYR	-	THR	GLU	PHE	THR	PRO	THR	-	GLU	LYS	-	ASP	GLU	TYR	ALA	CYS	ARG	VAL
SER	SER	THR	LEU	THR	LEU	SER	LYS	ALA	ASP	TYR	GLU	LYS	HIS	LYS	VAL	TYR	ALA	CYS	GLU	VAL
SER	SER	VAL	VAL	THR	VAL	PRO	SER	SER	SER	LEU	GLY	THR	GLN	-	THR	TYR	ILE	CYS	ASN	VAL
VAL	SER	VAL	LEU	THR	VAL	LEU	HIS	GLN	ASN	TRP	LEU	ASP	GLY	LYS	GLU	TYR	LYS	CYS	LYS	VAL
TYR	SER	LYS	LEU	THR	VAL	ASP	LYS	SER	ARG	TRP	GLN	GLN	GLY	ASN	VAL	PHE	SER	CYS	SER	VAL

						90														100
ASN	HIS	VAL	THR	LEU	SER	GLN	PRO	-	-	-	LYS	ILE	VAL	-	LYS	TRP	ASP	ARG	ASP	MET
THR	HIS	GLN	GLY	LEU	SER	SER	PRO	VAL	THR	-	LYS	SER	PHE	-	-	ASN	ARG	GLY	GLU	CYS
ASN	HIS	LYS	PRO	SER	ASN	THR	LYS	VAL	-	ASP	LYS	ARG	VAL	-	-	GLU	PRO	LYS	SER	CYS
SER	ASN	LYS	ALA	LEU	PRO	ALA	PRO	ILE	-	GLU	LYS	THR	ILE	SER	LYS	ALA	LYS	GLY		
MET	HIS	GLU	ALA	LEU	HIS	ASN	HIS	TYR	THR	GLN	LYS	SER	LEU	SER	LEU	SER	PRO	GLY		

Fig. 5. Comparison of the amino acid sequence of β_2-microglobulin with the various homology regions of the immunoglobulin Eu (26,27). Positions where residues identical to those in β_2-microglobulin appear are in boxes.

be classified into groups of proteins with similar structures and functions. Many of these may also have homologues among the soluble proteins, which would greatly simplify such analyses. More importantly, such similarities between a surface molecule and a soluble protein may provide some clues to the biological functions of membrane proteins, which for the most part remain unknown. The task of deducing function from structure is enormously difficult and probably requires even closer interaction with biological studies for the design of assays and functional tests. Even if it can be demonstrated in every way that the histocompatibility antigens are homologous to immunoglobulins in chain structure and in the organization of the heavy chain into immunoglobulin-like domains, the designing of a meaningful assay for the biological function of these antigens remains as the most important step.

References

(1) G.M. Edelman, ed., Cellular Selection and Regulation in the Immune Response (Raven Press, New York, 1974).

(2) M.F. Greaves, J.T., Owen and M.C. Raff, T and B Lymphocytes (North-Holland, Amsterdam, 1973).

(3) G.M. Edelman, in: The Cell Surface, Immunological and Chemical Approaches, eds. B.D. Kahan and R.A. Reisfeld (Plenum Press, New York, 1974) p. 245.

(4) I. Yahara and G.M. Edelman, Proc. Nat. Acad. Sci. U.S. 69 (1972) 608.

(5) R.B. Taylor, P.H. Duffus, M.C. Raff and S. de Petris, Nature (New Biol.) 233 (1971) 225.

(6) U. Rutishauser, I. Yahara and G.M. Edelman, Proc. Nat. Acad. Sci. U.S. 71 (1974) 1149.

(7) M.C. Raff and S. de Petris, Fed. Proc. 32 (1973) 48.

(8) G.R. Gunther, J.L. Wang, I. Yahara, B.A. Cunningham and G.M. Edelman, Proc. Nat. Acad. Sci. U.S. 70 (1973) 1012.

(9) G.M. Edelman, B.A. Cunningham, G.N. Reeke, Jr., J.W. Becker, M.J. Waxdal and J.L. Wang, Proc. Nat. Acad. Sci. U.S. 69 (1972) 2580.

(10) G.M. Edelman, I. Yahara and J.L. Wang, Proc. Nat. Acad. Sci. U.S. 70 (1973) 1442. G.M. Edelman and J.L. Wang, Proceedings of International Workshop on Cell Surfaces and Malignancy, Fogarty International Series (1974) in press.

(11) I. Yahara and G.M. Edelman, Exp. Cell Res. 81 (1973) 143.

(12) I. Yahara and G.M. Edelman, Nature, 246 (1973) 152.

(13) L. Wilson and M. Friedkin, Biochemistry 6 (1967) 3126.

(14) H. Jacob, T. Amsden and J. White, Proc. Nat. Acad. Sci. U.S., 69 (1972) 471.

(15) I. Yahara and G.M. Edelman, Exp. Cell Res., (1974) in press.

(16) S. de Petris and M.C. Raff, Ciba Foundation Symp., 14, (1973) 27.

(17) T.L. Steck, J. Cell Biol., 62 (1974) 1.

(18) J.B. Olmsted and G.G. Borisy, Ann. Rev. Biochem., 42 (1973) 507.

(19) E. Medrano, R. Piras and J. Mordoh, Exp. Cell Res., 86 (1974) 295.

(20) J.L. Wang, G.R. Gunther and G.M. Edelman, (1974) manuscript submitted.

(21) G.R. Gunther, J.L. Wang and G.M. Edelman, J. Cell Biol. 62 (1974) 366.

(22) M.S. Sasaki and A. Norman, Nature, 210 (1966) 913.

(23) G.M. Edelman, Science, 180 (1973) 830.

(24) I. Berggård and A.G. Bearn, J. Biol. Chem., 243 (1968) 4095

(25) K. Nilsson, P.-E. Evrin, I. Berggård and J. Pontēn, Nature (London), 244 (1973) 44.

(26) B.A. Cunningham, J.L. Wang, I. Berggård and P.A. Peterson, Biochemistry, 12 (1973) 4811.

(27) P.A. Peterson, B.A. Cunningham, I. Berggård and G.M. Edelman, Proc. Nat. Acad. Sci. U.S., 69 (1972) 1697.

(28) B.A. Cunningham and I. Berggård, Transplant Rev., vol. 21, ed. G. Möller (1974) 3.

(29) O. Smithies and M.D. Poulik, Proc. Nat. Acad. Sci. U.S. 69 (1972) 2914.

(30) K. Nakamuro, N. Tanigaki and D. Pressman, Proc. Nat. Acad. Sci. U.S., 70 (1973) 2863.

(31) P.A. Peterson, L. Rask and J.B. Lindblom, Proc. Nat. Acad. Sci. U.S., 71 (1974) 35.

(32) J.A. Gally and G.M. Edelman, Ann. Rev. Genet., 6 (1972) 1.

Acknowledgement

I am grateful to Professor G.M. Edelman for his advice and discussion, and to my other colleagues, particularly J.L. Wang, G.R. Gunther and I. Yahara, for allowing me to discuss their work. The studies described here were supported by grants from the U.S. Public Health Service and the National Science Foundation.

DISCUSSION

H. HEINGER: I have two questions: Rittenhouse and Fox have demonstrated a temperature-transition-dependent increase in Con A binding between 14° and 18°. This transition is quickly reversible and is not related to the microtubule system. Could you find this difference in Con A binding in your experiments? We recently found that, if lymphocytes are stimulated by phytohemagglutinin, a peak of cholesterol synthesis precedes the DNA synthesis phase in these cells. If the synthesis of cholesterol is specifically inhibited by blocking the HMG-CoA reductase activity with 25-hydroxycholesterol the later occurring DNA synthesis is also inhibited. What is the role of cholesterol in the process of Con A binding and the subsequent activation of lymphocytes?

B.A. CUNNINGHAM: With regard to the effects of temperature, our patching and capping experiments have been carried out primarily at 4° and 37°. We do not believe that the Con A effect is due to a phase transition in the lipid. A large number of early events are known to be associated with the stimulation of mitosis in lymphocytes and anyone of these may be critical for the subsequent activation. The problem is to establish which of these are on the direct pathway of the signal.

M.D. POULIK: I have isolated rabbit β_2-immunoglobulin in collaboration with Dr. Smithies, University of Wisconsin, and sequenced 42 amino acids. Our sequence differs from that of Drs. Cunningham and Berggård only at residue 20, but this difference may be because our β_2-immunoglobulin was obtained from a single rabbit whereas theirs was obtained from a pool of perhaps two rabbits. We recently isolated the β_2-microglobulin of rat and determined its partial amino acid sequence. Antibodies to this protein may help us to detect and isolate the enigmatic mouse β_2-microglobulin. With respect to the presence of β_2-microglobulin on the cell surface, Dr. Cunningham mentioned the absence of this protein in the membrane of the mature red cell. We have studied erythroblasts of patients in hemolytic crises and, using an immunofluorescence technique, we have demonstrated the presence of β_2-microglobulin on these cells. The β_2-microglobulin disappears when the nucleus is excluded. A similar observation was made with human platelets.

B. A. CUNNINGHAM: Would you comment on position 25 in your β_2-microglobulin sequences?

M.D. POULIK: We are sure that it is cysteine as in your sequence.

B. A. CUNNINGHAM: I should emphasize that the sequence of rabbit β_2-microglobulin was primarily determined in the automatic sequencer. Because half-cystine is usually difficult to identify, we used a radioactively labeled half-cystine derivative and measured the release of the radioactive label at position 25.

R.K. GERSHON: A cell-cell type interaction may explain the increased recruitment of cells by Con A rather than there being different stages in the cell cycle in which the cell can be stimulated. It may be that certain cells are dependent on factors released by other cells in order to respond to Con A in a number of immunological systems. Is there anything in your data that would rule out such an interpretation?

B. A. CUNNINGHAM: We cannot rule out cell-cell interaction. One of the important challenges in these studies is to design a method which will allow one to look at the entire process at the single-cell level. If stimulation is dependent upon the production of a factor from another cell, the problem is simply shifted to analysis of the kinetics of factor production. Data suggest that these cells may be heterogeneous with regard to their ability to make such a factor.

G. ROELANTS: If I am not mistaken, Con A binds and redistributes in patches and caps equally well on T-and B-lymphocytes, but triggers only the T-lymphocytes. Would you agree that there is no clear relationship between these surface phenomena and triggering of the cells?

B. A. CUNNINGHAM: We have a more convincing experiment that shows that capping is not directly involved in stimulation. Succinyl-Con A neither inhibits cap formation nor forms caps itself. However, it is as mitogenic as native Con A , giving an optimal response at the same concentration. This does not mean that the submembraneous system is not involved in stimulation , but I would agree that capping and patching are not involved.

A. WHITE: How homogeneous is the population of your lymphoid cells with respect to cell size and what is the time interval required to recover the Con A effect after washing the cells free of colchicine?

B. A. CUNNINGHAM: The cells we used are mostly small lymphocytes, either mouse spleenic lymphocytes or human peripheral lymphocytes. It takes 24 to 48 hours to wash out sufficient colchicine in order to see a response to con A.

M.M. SIGEL: In the experiment on Con A interference with the cap formation by anti-immunoglobulin, you are obviously dealing with B-cells. Have you used anything, for example anti-theta, to clarify this point regarding T-cells?

B. A. CUNNINGHAM: I probably went over this point too fast. Yes, we used anti-theta, and showed that Con A inhibits cap formation by anti-theta on T-cells.

E. KONDRACKI: In order to clarify the point on lymphocyte responses at the single cell level, I would like to mention some results obtained in our laboratory, using a lymphocyte culture in agarose gel in which most cells remain separated from each other. The response to PHA-P is at most 10% of that in liquid cultures, while the responses to Con A, pokeweed mitogen, $ZnCl_2$, $NaIO_4$, lipopolysacharide, fetal calf serum and PPD are totally abolished, as measured by liquid scintillation spectrometry. In the case of PHA-P, autoradiography of agarose gel cultures shows that only 1.5% of the total lymphocyte population is incorporating ^{3}H-thymidine at 48 hours. Therefore, I would caution against any interpretation of membrane phenomena occurring in single cells as necessarily being related to lymphocyte proliferation, and also caution against explanations of experimental results that are based on the assumption that most single cells can proliferate in response to all mitogenic stimuli under any conditions.

B. A. CUNNINGHAM: Can you show any kind of proliferation in your system?

E. KONDRACKI: Yes, because the incorporation of optimal amounts of 1) autologous erythrocytes 2) untreated stromata 3) sonicated stromata 4) supernatant fluid of sonicated stromata 5) carrageenan iota into the agarose gel results, in each case, in a marked increase of the proliferative response to PHA-P stimulation. The first three also potentiated proliferation with Con A stimulation but the supernatant fluid and carrageenan iota have not yet been tested in the system. We have also studied the kinetics of the proliferative response of two-fold decreasing numbers of lymphocytes to an optimal dose of several mitogens. When cell numbers versus ^{3}H-thymidine incorporation were plotted on a full logarithmic scale, the slope value varied from 1.7 to 3.3, depending on the mitogen used. The addition of autologous erythrocytes brought the slope value close to 1.0, thus showing by a different technical approach the existence of cell cooperation in the lymphocyte proliferative response.

THE ROLE OF PRODUCTS OF THE HISTOCOMPATIBILITY GENE COMPLEX IN IMMUNE RESPONSES

DAVID H. KATZ, MARTIN E. DORF, DIETER ARMERDING AND BARUJ BENACERRAF

Department of Pathology
Harvard Medical School

Abstract: The data of our most recent investigations have mapped the relevant gene or genes coding for *CI* molecules to the *I* region of the *H-2* complex of the mouse. Thus, T and B lymphocytes from donor mice which differ at genes in either the *K*, *S* or *D* regions of *H-2* (or combinations of the latter), but which are identical for genes in the *I* region, are capable of developing cooperative immune responses. Conversely, gene differences in the *I* region, more precisely in the *Ir-1A* and *Ir-1B* subregions, prevent the development of T-B cell interactions irrespective of the existence of gene identities elsewhere in the *H-2* complex (including the *I-C* subregion).

Those data demonstrating the existence of *CI* genes in the *I* region of *H-2* are supported by recent experimental evidence demonstrating that active products obtained in culture supernatants of appropriately stimulated T lymphocytes are themselves most likely *I* region gene products. Thus, purified fractions of a factor from alloantigen-stimulated T cells, termed allogeneic effect factor (AEF), which are known to stimulate B cell differentiation in the presence of antigen, manifest several biochemical and immunological properties which indicate that the active moiety is derived from or related to gene products of the *H-2* complex. The AEF derived from T cells of the $H\text{-}2^d$ haplotype is specifically removed by immunoadsorbents prepared from antibodies reactive with $H\text{-}2^d$. Moreover, immunoadsorbents prepared with anti-Ia sera reactive with *I* region specificities of the $H\text{-}2^d$ haplotype are effective in removing the biological activity of AEF. Finally, the active moiety in AEF appears to be a bimolecular complex comprised of a heavy molecule (around 35,000 daltons) and a lighter molecule (around 12,000 daltons) suggesting the participation of a β_2-microglobulin-like component in the active complex.

INTRODUCTION

Over the past two years, observations from our own laboratories, as well as those of others, have demonstrated the involvement of histocompatibility gene products in governing the cell-cell interactions concerned with development and regulation of immune responses in several species (1-5). These discoveries have placed histocompatibility gene products on a more complex level of biologic function than was heretofore generally considered (6). Thus, the hypothesis was made from these observations that genes in the *H-2* complex coded for products involved in the development of effective cell-cell interactions in the immune response (2,3,6).

In this paper, we shall review the data that have demonstrated genetic restrictions of T-B lymphocyte interactions and describe our recent studies on the isolation and characterization of an active T cell mediator which appears to be involved in such interactions and which bears determinants known to be associated with certain histocompatibility gene products. The conclusion we draw from these findings is that the regulatory role of T lymphocytes in immune responses, which appears to be related to control of differentiation processes of other lymphocytes of both T and B classes, is mediated via molecules that are comprised, at least in part, of gene products of the major histocompatibility gene complex which are phenotypically interrelated on the surface membranes of such cells.

EVIDENCE FOR GENETIC RESTRICTIONS IN COOPERATIVE CELL INTERACTIONS

The data that will be reviewed in this section demonstrate, we believe, that the participation of histocompatibility gene products in cell-cell interactions reflects a physiological control mechanism utilizing readily accessible structures that are dynamic constituents of the surface membranes of lymphoid cells. We wish to emphasize at the outset, however, that like other physiologic control mechanisms, it is not an absolute system in the sense of precluding alternate, albeit less efficient routes to the same end.

The evidence for the existence of genetic restrictions in T-B cell interactions can be succinctly summarized as follows: Under conditions in which isogeneic or syngeneic lymphoid cells interact together to develop humoral immune responses, cells lacking certain critical identities in histocompatibility genes fail to successfully interact (1-3, 5-11). The succinctness of the preceding statement must be elaborated upon to include the very important qualifications that: 1) demonstration of a "failure" to obtain a response in the system employed in our studies has been shown *not* to reflect a suppression phenomenon (8), and 2) the positive responses obtained are those which are elicited by interactions between antigen-specific T and B cells and not by allogeneic cell interactions. Initially, the central problem was to design an experimental scheme that specifically circumvented the possible contribution to the results of a complicating allogeneic effect. This was accomplished for *in vivo* cell transfer studies by using an F_1 hybrid as the recipient of T and B cells from the respective parental strains against which the semiallogeneic host would be genetically incapable of reacting. The intricacies of the experimental protocol employed have been described in detail elsewhere (2,3).

The protocol and data from a representative experiment using congenic-resistant mouse strains demonstrating the involvement of the *H-2* gene complex in physiologic lymphocyte interactions is shown in Fig. 1. The DNP-primed B cells were derived from congenic-resistant B10.A ($H\text{-}2^a$) donor mice and the relevant genetic similarities and/or differences are listed for each combination (3). Groups I and II demonstrate the intact cooperative functional capacities of the irradiated (*in situ*) bovine gamma globulin (BGG)-primed T cells and the anti-Θ-treated DNP-primed B cells of syngeneic B10.A origin within the environs of (A x B10)F_1 irradiated recipients (Group I). Similarly, BGG-primed T cells derived from A/J donors, which are identical with B10.A at the major $H\text{-}2^a$ locus but dissimilar with respect to background genotypes are capable of exerting a clear helper effect in cooperating with B cells of B10.A origin. In sharp contrast, T cells from A.By or B10 donors, which are both $H\text{-}2^b$, fail to cooperatively interact with B lymphocytes from B10.A mice. This is true irrespective of whether or not the genetic background other than *H-2* is identical such as in the case of

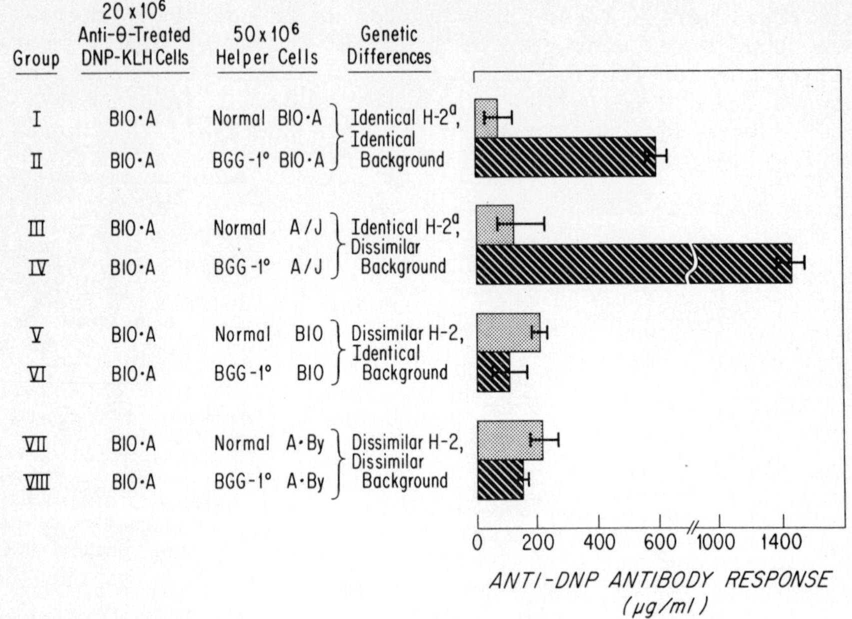

Figure 1. Failure of physiologic cooperative interactions to occur between T and B lymphocytes differing at the major histocompatibility locus. The scheme followed is described in the text. Recipients for all cell combinations were (A x B10)F_1 hybrids. Combinations and strain origins of T and B cells and the relevant genetic differences are indicated. Recipients in groups I-VIII were secondarily challenged with 50 μg of DNP-BGG. Mean serum anti-DNP antibody levels of groups of five mice on day 7 after secondary challenge are illustrated. Horizontal bars represent ranges of the standard errors (Ref. 3).

B10 donor cells.

Among the various possible explanations for the failure of physiologic T-B cell cooperation to occur across the major histocompatibility barrier certain possibilities which are trivial in terms of biological significance have been ruled out either by experimental design or by direct experimentation (2,3,8). These possibilities have been described and discussed in detail elsewhere (2,3,6,8) and will not be reiterated here. These findings led us to conclude, therefore, that a relevant gene or genes in the major histocompatibility complex control physiologic cooperative interactions between T and B cells in the immune response. Subsequent studies were designed to determine more precisely the intra-*H-2* localization of the postulated cell-interaction or *CI* genes.

In our initial studies (2), no cooperation occurred with mixtures of T and B cells from BALB/c (H-2^d) and A/J (H-2^a) donors, respectively. Since these particular strains are identical at *S* and the entire *D* end of the *H-2* complex, these results indicated that gene identities only at *S* and *D* are insufficient to permit optimal cooperative interactions. In subsequent experiments we asked the reciprocal question--i.e. whether identities at only *K* and *I* are sufficient to allow effective cooperation. One such experiment was carried out *in vitro* using lymphocytes from A/J and B10.BR mice which differ from one another at genes in the *S* and *D* regions of the *H-2* complex but are identical at *K* and *I* regions (9). As shown in Fig. 2, DNP-primed B cells from A/J donors developed effective cooperative responses with keyhole limpet hemocyanin (KLH)-primed T cells from both isogeneic A/J donors and from B10.BR donors. In the reciprocal mixed cell cultures, DNP-primed B cells from B10.BR mice interacted with KLH-primed T cells from A/J as well as isogeneic T cells in response to DNP-KLH. These data do not reflect non-specific allogeneic effects as an explanation for successful cooperation between A and B10.BR lymphocytes since, as shown here, reciprocal controls using irradiated normal rather than KLH-primed cells failed to develop secondary responses to DNP-KLH. The development of cooperative responses between A/J and B10.BR which differ for genes in *S* and *D* but are identical for *K* and *I* region genes indicate that the critical *CI* genes involved in T-B cell cooperation exist in the latter regions.

This observation has quite recently been corroborated in a totally *in vivo* double adoptive transfer scheme as well. The protocol and data from such a complementation experiment are illustrated in Fig. 3 (11). Before discussing the data shown in Fig. 3, it is pertinent to cite the following data from independent control experiments that are not shown in the figure: 1) All of the DNP-primed spleen cell populations were capable of developing secondary anti-DNP responses to the immunizing antigen, DNP-Ascaris extract (ASC), in parallel transfers utilizing spleen cells not treated with anti-Θ

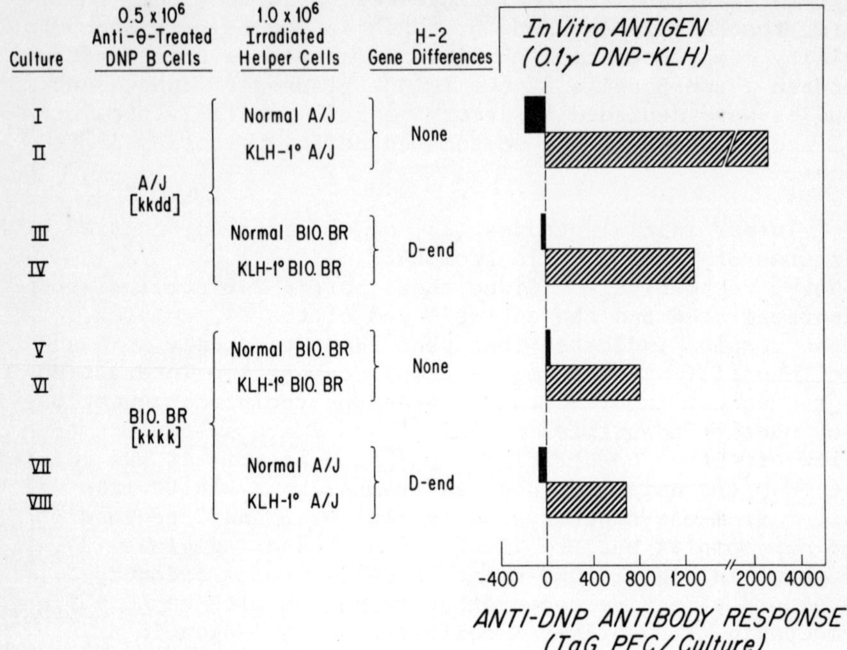

Figure 2. DNP-ASC-primed spleen cells from A/J and B10.BR donors were depleted of T cells by *in vitro* treatment with anti-Θ serum plus complement and then cultured with either irradiated normal or KLH-primed spleen cells in the combinations indicated. Primed donors were immunized with either DNP-ASC in alum or KLH in CFA six months earlier and then boosted with 25 μg of the respective antigen in saline one month prior to culture. Cells were cultured with either no antigen (not shown) or DNP-KLH. The background responses of non-stimulated cultures have been subtracted from the numbers of DNP-specific PFC developed in cultures containing DNP-KLH -- hence, the negative values depicted here. IgG (indirect) DNP-specific PFC responses are shown. Responses in the IgM class (not shown) were parallel (Ref. 9).

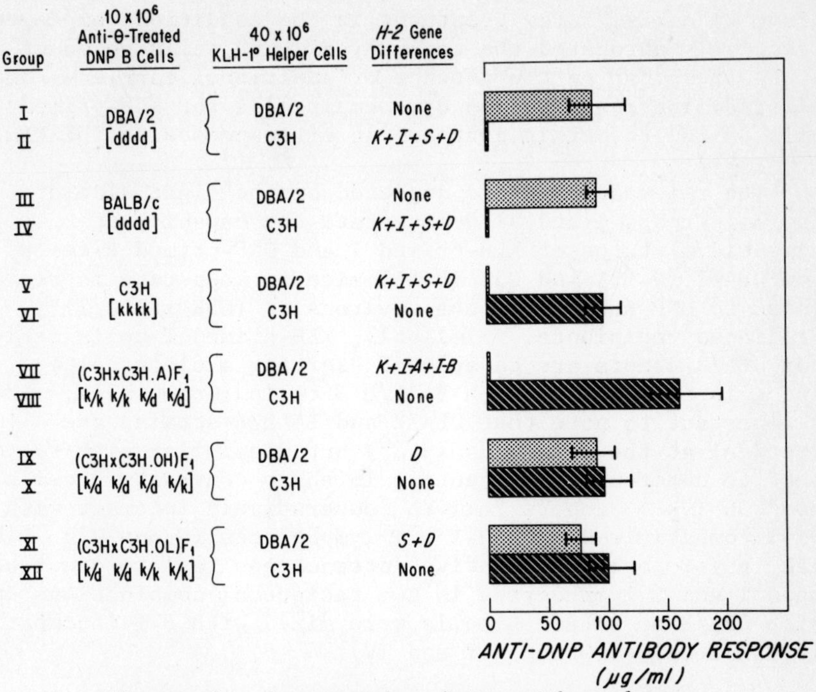

Group	10×10^6 Anti-θ-Treated DNP B Cells	40×10^6 KLH-1° Helper Cells	*H-2* Gene Differences
I	DBA/2 [dddd]	DBA/2	None
II		C3H	*K+I+S+D*
III	BALB/c [dddd]	DBA/2	None
IV		C3H	*K+I+S+D*
V	C3H [kkkk]	DBA/2	*K+I+S+D*
VI		C3H	None
VII	$(C3H \times C3H.A)F_1$ [k/k k/k k/d k/d]	DBA/2	*K+I-A+I-B*
VIII		C3H	None
IX	$(C3H \times C3H.OH)F_1$ [k/d k/d k/d k/k]	DBA/2	*D*
X		C3H	None
XI	$(C3H \times C3H.OL)F_1$ [k/d k/d k/k k/k]	DBA/2	*S+D*
XII		C3H	None

0 50 100 150 200

ANTI-DNP ANTIBODY RESPONSE (μg/ml)

Figure 3. Cooperative interactions between T and B lymphocytes sharing *K* end genes of the *H-2* complex. Recipients for all cell combinations were $(C3H \times DBA/2)F_1$ hybrids. Combinations and strain origins of T and B cells and the relevant genetic differences are indicated. The *H-2* regions of *K*, *I*, *S* and *D* of the strains used are indicated in brackets. Mean serum levels of anti-DNP antibody of groups of four mice on day 7 after secondary challenge with 20 μg DNP-KLH are illustrated. Horizontal bars represent ranges of standard errors. Statistical comparisons between the various groups gave the following results: Groups I and II, Groups III and IV, Groups V and VI, Groups VII and VIII had P values less than 0.001 in all cases; Groups IX and X, Groups XI and XII had P values greater than 0.1 in all cases. (Ref. 11).

serum; 2) Anti-Θ serum treatment in the conditions employed effectively abrogated the capacity of such cells to mount an *in vivo* response in the absence of additional carrier-primed cells; 3) The substitution of normal cells for KLH-primed cells failed to permit development of responses to DNP-KLH.

The relevant data are depicted on the right side of Fig. 3. Groups I and VI demonstrate the capacity of syngeneic mixtures of KLH-primed T and DNP-primed B cells from DBA/2 (H-2^d) and C3H (H-2^k) mice to cooperate in response to DNP-KLH within the environs of (C3H x DBA/2)F_1 irradiated recipients. Similarly, KLH-primed T cells derived from DBA/2 donors are capable of exerting a clear helper effect in cooperating with BALB/c B cells (Group III). It is important to note that DBA/2 and BALB/c strains are identical at the *H-2* locus (H-2^d) but dissimilar with respect to numerous other genes. In sharp contrast, B cells from C3H (H-2^k) donors fail to cooperatively interact with *H-2*-incompatible DBA/2 (H-2^d) T lymphocytes (Group V). Likewise, physiologic cooperative interactions fail to occur between T and B lymphocytes in two reciprocal combinations in which DBA/2 or BALB/c B cells were mixed with *H-2*-incompatible C3H T cells (Groups II and IV).

Groups VII through XII test the ability of DBA/2 (H-2^d) or C3H (H-2^k) helper cells to cooperate with B cells from a series of F_1 hybrids made between C3H and selected C3H congenic mice. The C3H congenic strains carry recombinant *H-2* haplotypes derived from crossovers between the H-2^d and H-2^k parental haplotypes. Very good cooperative responses occurred between C3H carrier primed T cells and hapten-primed B cells derived from all of the C3H F_1 hybrids, in spite of the presence of foreign histocompatibility determinants on these F_1 hybrid cells (Groups VIII, X and XII).

As noted above, DBA/2 KLH-primed T cells failed to effectively cooperate with *H-2*-incompatible DNP-primed C3H B cells (Group V). Similarly, DBA/2 (H-2^d) T cells failed to effectively interact with (C3H x C3H.A)F_1 B cells, although these B cells carry the *I-C*, *S* and *D* regions derived from the H-2^d haplotype (Group VII). In contrast, the same pool of helper T cells from DBA/2 donors were perfectly good helpers in development of secondary anti-DNP responses with hapten-primed B cells from (C3H x C3H.OH)F_1 and (C3H x C3H.OL)F_1 hybrids (Groups IX and XI).

In this complementation experiment, we have demonstrated that one or more *CI* genes that control T-B cell interactions are localized in the *K* end of the *H-2* gene complex. Thus, DBA/2 KLH-primed T cells cooperated with (C3H x C3H.OH)F_1 and (C3H x C3H.OL)F_1 DNP-primed B cells to make a secondary response to DNP-KLH, but not with C3H or (C3H x C3H.A)F_1 DNP-primed cells. It must be emphasized that the carrier-primed DBA/2 T cells are histoincompatible with each of these B cell populations for both non-H-2 and H-2 determinants. The presence of foreign histocompatibility determinants provided by the C3H parent does not therefore prevent successful physiological T-B cell cooperation in F_1 hybrids which have at least one complement of K^d and I^d genes derived from the C3H.OH or C3H.OL parents. However, complementation with D^d, S^d and $I\text{-}C^d$ genes derived from the C3H.A parent fail to complement for successful cell interactions.

The two preceding experiments permit us to draw the conclusion that the histocompatibility genes involved in controlling optimal T-B cell interactions are located to the left of the *S* region of *H-2* -- i.e. somewhere in the *K* and/or *I* region(s). The existence of appropriate inbred and recombinant strains of mice differing at known loci of the *H-2* complex makes it possible to define more precisely which region(s) and/or subregion(s) of the complex contains the relevant gene or genes. The following experiment was designed to answer this question using mixtures of T and B cells from congenic mice A.TL ($H\text{-}2^{t1}$), A.TH ($H\text{-}2^{t2}$), A.AL ($H\text{-}2^{a1}$) A.SW ($H\text{-}2^{s}$), inbred A/J ($H\text{-}2^{a}$) and (A x A.TH)F_1 ($H\text{-}2^{a/t2}$)in *in vitro* cooperative secondary anti-DNP antibody responses (10).

The left side of Fig. 4 depicts the protocol and various combinations of cell mixtures analyzed for cooperative responses to DNP-KLH. The gene regions of the *H-2* complexes are symbolized and the gene region differences among the various combinations are summarized for convenience. The relevant data is depicted on the right side of Fig. 4. Cultures I-IV demonstrate the capacity of syngeneic mixtures of T and B cells from A.TL and A mice to cooperate *in vitro*, and reciprocal mixtures of such cells to interact together despite the existence of gene differences in both the *K* and *S* regions of *H-2* in this combination. Likewise, when gene differences are restricted to only one of these respective regions (*K* or *S*), the capacity for effective T-B cell cooperation remains intact as evidenced by the ability of T

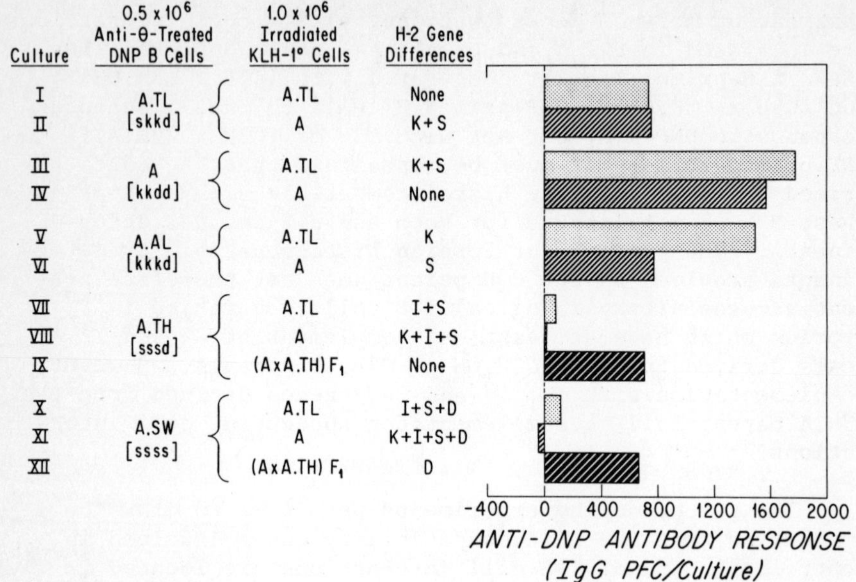

Figure 4. DNP-ASC-primed spleen cells from A.TL, A, A.AL, A.TH and A.SW mice were depleted of T cells by *in vitro* treatment with anti-Θ serum plus complement and then cultured with irradiated KLH-primed spleen cells from A.TL, A or (A x A.TH)F_1 donors in the combinations indicated. Cells were cultured with either no antigen (not shown) or DNP-KLH. The background responses of non-stimulated cultures have been subtracted from the numbers of DNP-specific PFC developed in cultures containing DNP-KLH (hence, the negative value depicted in culture XI). IgG (indirect) DNP-specific PFC responses are shown. Responses in the IgM class (not shown) were parallel (Ref. 10).

---

cells from both A.TL and A donors to interact with B cells from A.AL donors (cultures V and VI). In marked contrast, however, is the inability of either of these primed and functionally intact T cell populations from A.TL or A donors to cooperate with B cells from either A.TH or A.SW mice (cultures VII, VIII, X and XI); in the latter combinations gene differences exist in the *I* region as indicated. The failure of either A.TH or A.SW DNP-primed B cells to respond in these cultures is not a reflection of an incapacity of these B cells to function since irradiated KLH-primed cells from (A x A.TH)F_1 donors were able to provide helper function for A.TH parental cells (culture IX) and for A.SW cells which differ only at genes in the *D* region (culture XII). Moreover, the capacity of A.TH primed cells to develop effective syngeneic cooperative interactions was not inhibited or diminished by the addition of irradiated KLH-primed spleen cells from A.TL donors thereby ruling out a possible suppression mechanism, due to e.g. an allogeneic effect, as an explanation for these findings. Thus, in a syngeneic cooperative control culture response, A.TH cells developed 1253 IgG anti-DNP PFC in the absence of A.TL cells and 1486 anti-DNP PFC in the presence of 1.0×10^6 irradiated KLH-primed A.TL cells (10).

The results of this experiment provide compelling evidence for the existence of the *CI* gene or genes controlling optimal T-B cell cooperative interactions in the designated *I* region of the *H-2* gene complex. This point is particularly emphasized by the inability of A.TL to provide helper T cell function for A.TH or A.SW B cells in which combinations there are gene identities in the *K* region but differences in *I* region genes.

The precise genetic mapping of these genes will require experiments using mixtures of T and B cells from strain combinations with differences and identities at one or more subregions, *Ir-1A*, *Ir-1B* and *I-C*, on the basis of documented cross-overs between definable *Ir* genes and also Ia serological specificities (12). The data presented here indicate that the genes responsible for control of T-B cell interactions in this system are located in the *Ir-1A* and/or *Ir-1B* subregions. This follows from the fact that the A↔B10.BR, A↔A.TL and A↔A.AL combinations, all of which are identical for all genes in *Ir-1A* and *Ir-1B*, were capable of effectively interacting despite the existence of gene differences in the *I-C* subregion. However, despite the fact that the *I-C* subregions of these strains are derived from different paternal haplotypes, they may nevertheless conceivably share genes coded for in the *I-C* subregion which permit effective T-B cell cooperation. Further definition of these possibilities should be forthcoming in the near future.

BIOLOGICAL, BIOCHEMICAL AND IMMUNOLOGICAL PROPERTIES OF A T CELL PRODUCT ACTIVE IN TRIGGERING B LYMPHOCYTES

A major effort in studies on the mechanism of T-B cell interactions has been focused on the identification of various biologically active substances capable of influencing lymphocyte function in antibody responses to different antigens elicited in *in vitro* systems. The demonstration by Dutton et al (13) that supernatants obtained from short-term cultures of histoincompatible mouse spleen cells contained a non-antigen-specific biologically active mediator capable of markedly affecting *in vitro* antibody responses to thymus-dependent antigens provided evidence for the existence of such a possible mediator. In this section we will briefly review our published observations (14) and then present our most recent data on the biological, biochemical and immunological properties of an active moiety produced in supernatants of short-term (24 hours) *in vitro* reactions between T cells specifically activated to foreign alloantigens and the corresponding target cell population. We have termed the factor that we have been studying "allogeneic effect factor" (AEF) since its biological action on *in vitro* antibody responses appear to be identical to the *in vivo* phenomenon known as the allogeneic effect (15).

A. Biological Properties of AEF

The AEF preparations that are the focus of this discussion have been prepared by culturing DBA/2 ($H\text{-}2^d$) T cells (which had been activated for 6 days against (C3H x DBA/2)F_1 ($H\text{-}2^{k/d}$) target lymphocytes in irradiated DBA/2 hosts) for 24 hours with irradiated (C3H x DBA/2)F_1 target spleen cells (14). The culture supernatants from such allogeneic cell mixtures are biologically active in enhancing *in vitro* immune responses when such supernatants are obtained as early as 12 hours after culture initiation of allogeneic cell cultures, display peak activity at 24 hours and thereafter become progressively more suppressive. We have prepared numerous AEF from various genetic mixtures of effector and target cell populations and all appear to behave in analogous fashion biologically. The AEF are active as unfractionated (crude) supernatants or, as will be discussed below, as highly purified fractions obtained by gel and/or ion exchange chromatography.

The principal biological activity of AEF that has been studied in depth is the capacity of this material to functionally replace the requirement for helper T cells in *in vitro* antibody responses. The earlier work of Dutton et al (13) and Schimpl and Wecker (16,17) made it clear that such factors were active in this regard insofar as *in vitro* responses to particulate erythrocyte antigens or haptenated erythrocytes were concerned. Our own studies extended these observations to soluble DNP-protein conjugates in which case AEF can reconstitute helper cell function in responses of T cell-depleted primed spleen cells (14). The strongest evidence that our active AEF acts directly on B cells stems from the capacity of AEF to stimulate B cells exposed to DNP conjugated to the D-glutamic acid, D-lysine (D-GL) copolymer (14). This compound has been demonstrated to be highly tolerogenic for DNP-specific B cells both *in vivo* and *in vitro* under normal circumstances (reviewed in 18,19). However, when administered to appropriately-primed animals during a critical time period after induction of an *in vivo* allogeneic effect, DNP-D-GL can provide a definite inductive stimulus for primary or secondary anti-DNP antibody responses (15,20,21). Since no demonstrable T cell function specific for the D-GL carrier has been demonstrated, these observations provided the strongest indirect proof that the *in vivo* allogeneic effect is mediated by a direct interaction on the responding B cells. The capacity of AEF to permit *in vitro* responses to DNP-D-GL constitutes conclusive evidence, therefore, that the active moiety involved is acting directly on B lymphocytes (14).

B. Biochemical Properties of AEF

The experiments performed thus far on the physicochemical features of AEF indicate that the active component(s) consists of protein and/or glycoprotein which is heat-labile ($56^{o}C$, 1 hour), thereby indicating the importance of tertiary structure to activity and is in the molecular weight range of 30,000 - 45,000 (14,22). Moreover, the active moiety appears to consist of two components associated non-covalently (22).

Initially, crude allogeneic supernatants were fractionated first on Sephadex G-200 yielding multiple peaks of which only one contained active enhancing AEF (14). As shown in Fig. 5, this peak from G-200 was then subjected to chromatography on Sephadex G-100 yielding two fractions of which only one eluting in the range of an insulin marker (m.w. 36,000) was biologically active in triggering B

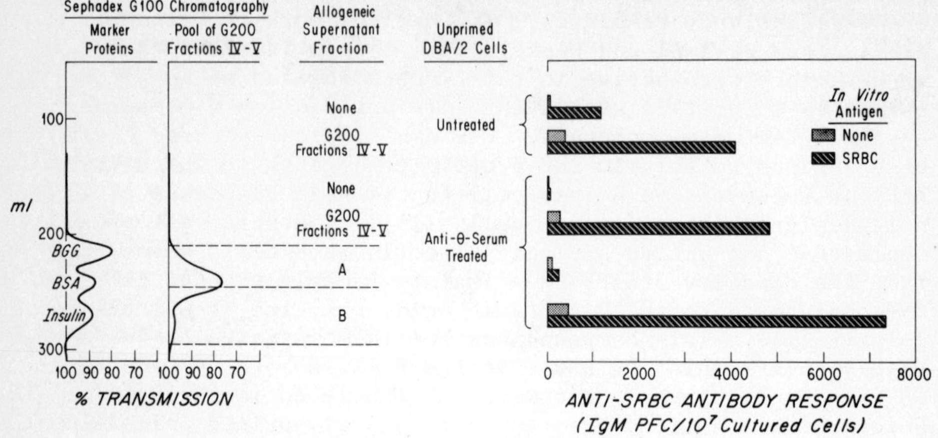

Figure 5. Comparison of activities of unseparated and Sephadex G-100-fractionated AEF on primary anti-SRBC responses of untreated and anti-θ serum-treated DBA/2 spleen cells. Fractions IV and V from G-200 were pooled and subjected to further chromatography on G-100. The elution patterns of this supernatant and the corresponding markers BGG (m.w. 150,000), BSA (m.w. 65,000) and insulin (m.w. 36,000 in hexameric form) are shown on the far left. The primary IgM anti-SRBC responses of untreated and anti-θ serum-treated DBA/2 cells in the presence of the various fractions indicated (50% concentration in reference to the original unseparated supernatant) are shown (Ref. 14).

lymphocyte responses to SRBC (14). On this basis we have estimated the m.w. of AEF to be in the range of 30,000 - 45,000.

The active fraction B (Fig. 5) from Sephadex G-100 was further chromatographed on DEAE cellulose using an exponential gradient from 0.01 - 0.15 M sodium phosphate buffer, pH 8.1. Under these conditions, all of the biologically active material eluted at low salt concentration in a second peak from the column indicating that AEF is homogeneous with regard to charge and that it could be either positive or nearly neutral (22). The active fraction of AEF obtained by DEAE-cellulose chromatography was radio-labelled with ^{125}I by the chloramine-T method and then subjected to electrophoresis on 10% SDS-polyacrylamide gel. The electrophoretic patterns of both unreduced AEF and AEF following reduction with 2-mercaptoethanol are shown in Fig. 6 (22). The patterns were identical and consisted of a large molecular peak which coincided with molecular weight of 47,000 and a smaller peak in the molecular weight range of 11,500 (extrapolated). The molecular weight determinations were made by comparison with parallel gels containing marker proteins with known molecular weights. It should be pointed out, however, that this by no means accurately establishes the molecular weights since the presence of carbohydrate in varying quantities will affect the migration of such a substance in SDS gel. Indeed, the large molecular weight band stains positively with periodic acid Schiff's reagent indicating that it is probably a glycoprotein (22).

The electrophoretic pattern illustrated in Fig.6 is remarkably similar to that observed when solubilized *H-2* antigens are subjected to SDS-acrylamide electrophoresis (23). We were interested, therefore, in determining the biological activity of the two definable molecular species observed. Since the likelihood of recovering biologically active material by elution from SDS-acrylamide gel is extremely low, we attempted to obtain comparable dissociation of AEF into subfractions by chromatography on Sepharose-6B in 6M guanidine HCl. The elution pattern obtained by such chromatography is depicted on the far left panel of Fig. 7 (22). The corresponding biological activities of the tested fractions (after removal of guanidine HCl by dialysis) are shown on the middle and right panels of Fig. 7. Six peaks (II-VII) of UV-absorbing material were demarcated as indicated by the dotted lines. Two heavier molecular weight fractions eluting after the void volume (fractions II and V) and two lighter molecular weight fractions (VI and VII) were tested for activity on *in vitro* primary anti-SRBC antibody responses of untreated (middle panel) and anti-θ serum-treated (far right panel) spleen cells from DBA/2 mice.

As shown in Fig. 7, the addition of unfractionated AEF enhanced the response of untreated spleen cells and fully reconstituted the response of spleen cells depleted of T cells by anti-θ serum treatment. Fraction II from the column substantially enhanced the response of untreated spleen

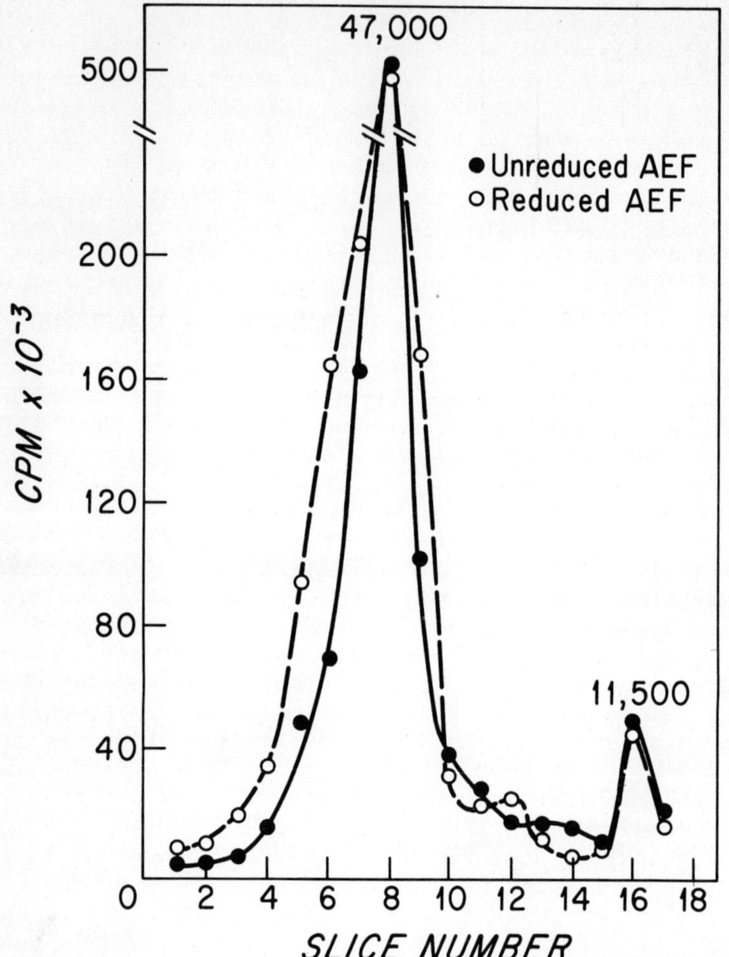

Figure 6. Electrophoretic pattern of AEF on SDS-polyacrylamide gel. The biologically active fraction of AEF purified on Sephadex G-100 followed by chromatography on DEAE-cellulose was radio-labelled with ^{125}I by the chloramine-T method and then subjected to electrophoresis on 10% SDS-polyacrylamide gel either unreduced or following reduction by 2-mercaptoethanol. Gels were cut into 3 mm thick slices and counted in a gamma counter. Molecular weights of the major peaks are indicated (Ref. 22).

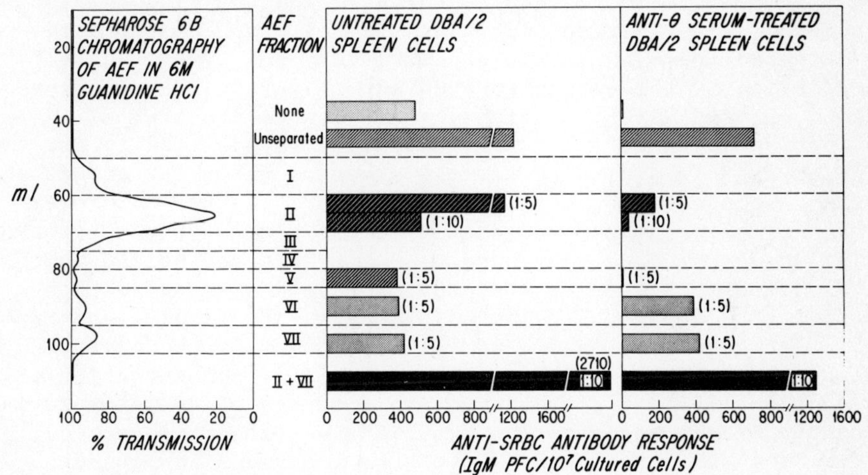

Figure 7. Activities of AEF fractions obtained by chromatography on Sepharose 6B in guanidine-HCl. Biologically active AEF purified by gel chromatography on Sephadex G-100 was chromatographed on Sepharose-6B in guanidine HCl. The elution patterns of this supernatant are shown on the far left panel. The corresponding biological activities of unseparated AEF, the tested fractions (after removal of guanidine-HCl by dialysis) and combinations of fractions II and VII on primary IgM anti-SRBC responses of untreated (middle panel) and anti-θ serum-treated DBA/2 spleen cells (right panel) are shown (Ref. 22).

cells at the 1:5 concentration (around 3-fold) but exerted only a partial effect on anti-θ-treated cells. The 1:10 concentration of fraction II and 1:5 of fraction V had no significant effect on responses of either the intact or depleted cell population. The lighter molecular weight materials in fractions VI and VII exerted no detectable effect on the response of untreated spleen cells but did manifest some activity in reconstituting the responses of the anti-θ-treated cells which was approximately 50% of the activity exhibited by the unfractionated AEF. The striking observation, however, is the effect obtained when fraction II and fraction VII were mixed together prior to addition to the cultures. This mixture exerted a marked enhancing effect on the response of untreated spleen cells (around 5-fold over the normal response) and displayed the highest reconstituting activity on the response of anti-θ-treated cells, which was almost 50% greater than that obtained with unfractionated AEF. It should be noted that: 1) the final concentration of the fraction II and VII components of the mixture was 1:10 (cf. the low activity of the 1:10 concentration of fraction II), and 2) the observed activity of the mixture is substantially greater than the additive effects expected from the biological activity of the individual components themselves (22).

This finding strongly indicates, therefore, that the active moiety of AEF may consist of a bicomponent complex--one heavy and one light--which are associated non-covalently. The variable effects of the individual heavy (fraction II) and light (fraction VI and VII) components on the *in vitro* responses in Fig. 7 deserve some comment. The activity of fraction II predominantly on the intact spleen cell population suggests that this heavier molecule may exert enhancing effects on T lymphocyte function either directly or via effects on macrophages. The capacity of the lighter material in fraction VII to partially reconstitute responses of anti-θ-treated spleen cells while exerting little or no effects on intact spleen cell responses suggests that this molecule by itself exerts little or no effect on T lymphocyte function but some limited influence on B cells. The optimal influence on B cells, however, clearly requires the concomitant presence of the heavy and light components. It is not possible to know from these data whether the heavy and light molecules must become associated in order to function in the manner observed. Studies currently are underway to determine this point.

C. Immunological Properties of AEF

Thus far, we have analyzed the immunological properties of AEF by various immunochemical and functional techniques. Immunochemical analysis has shown that AEF purified on Sephadex G-100 does not react or cross-react with any heterologous antisera directed against immunoglobulin determinants (22). In our initial studies on the activity of AEF, we found that although it did not manifest any specificity for antigens against which the *in vitro* antibody responses were directed, AEF did exhibit some strain-specific properties suggesting a relationship to antigens or gene products coded in the major histocompatibility gene complex (14). Thus, purified AEF from supernatants of DBA/2 ($H\text{-}2^d$) activated T cells, although fully reconstituting B cell responses of DBA/2 and BALB/c mice, only slightly reconstituted responses to SRBC of B cells from C57BL/6 ($H\text{-}2^b$) mice. Moreover, preliminary absorption studies with spleen cell populations have demonstrated that spleen cells from normal DBA/2 mice are considerably effective in absorbing the biological enhancing activity from AEF derived from DBA/2 T cells, whereas cells from strains of other *H-2* haplotypes are not very effective (22).

The aforementioned observations prompted us to explore the relationship of AEF to histocompatibility antigens by functional analysis. Thus, experiments were designed to determine whether immunoadsorbents prepared with antisera reactive with *H-2* determinants would specifically remove the biologically active moiety of AEF. In the first experiments we found that antisera directed against either the entire $H\text{-}2^d$ haplotype or the K-end of $H\text{-}2^d$ would indeed remove the activity of AEF derived from DBA/2 T cells; in contrast, antisera directed against specificities coded by genes in the D-end of $H\text{-}2^d$ failed to absorb AEF activity (24). Recently, investigations in several laboratories using anti-lymphoid cell antisera prepared between recombinant mice differing at genes present in the *I* region of the *H-2* complex identified a new antigen system, which has been termed Ia, coded for by genes in the *I* region; the Ia antigens have been found to exist predominantly on B cells and macrophages and to varying extents on T cells (12,25-29). Accordingly, we considered the possibility that gene products in this region may be involved in regulatory cell interactions in immune responses. The experiment presented in Fig. 8 demonstrates that the active enhancing factor(s) in

AEF can be removed by an immunoadsorbent prepared with an anti-Ia antiserum indicating that, indeed, the biologically active moieties responsible for T-B cell interactions are probably products of genes in the *I* region of the *H-2* gene complex (30). The following antisera were used: 1) B10.A anti-B10--this antiserum contains antibodies reactive with antigens coded by genes in the *I* region of $H\text{-}2^d$(Ia.8) but not with antigens coded by genes in either *K* or *D* regions of $H\text{-}2^d$; 2) (B6A)F_1 anti-B10.D2--this antiserum contains predominantly antibodies reactive with specificity H-2.31 present on cells from animals with the $H\text{-}2^d$ allele; recent analyses have demonstrated the presence in this antiserum also of antibodies reactive with a new Ia specificity (Ia.11) present in $H\text{-}2^d$ (31).

In the experiment shown in Fig. 8, three different concentrations of AEF were directly absorbed independently by immunoadsorbents prepared from (B6A)F_1 anti-B10.D2 and B10.A anti-B10 alloantisera and by an adsorbent prepared from normal B10.A serum. These AEF were then compared to unabsorbed AEF for biological activity on the *in vitro* response to SRBC of DBA/2 B lymphocytes. As shown in Fig. 8, cultures of untreated control whole spleen cells developed primary IgG anti-SRBC responses of around 1200 PFC; anti-θ treatment diminished this response to around 150 PFC. The addition of unabsorbed AEF to such anti-θ serum-treated B cells reconstituted and enriched the response markedly and in a dose-related manner at all three concentrations of AEF employed. The AEF subjected to the adsorbent prepared from normal B10.A serum exhibited virtually identical biological activity. The AEF obtained from the immunoadsorbent prepared from (B6A)F_1 anti-B10.D2 serum retained essentially normal biological activity at the highest concentration (1:5), but the lowest concentration subjected to absorption (1:20) was around 45% lower in activity than the normal serum control. The AEF subjected to the B10.A anti-B10 (anti-Ia) immunoadsorbent, on the other hand, exhibited markedly diminished (80% or more) activity at all three concentrations indicating substantial reactivity of this antiserum with the biologically active component(s) of AEF (30).

The identification of a small molecular weight component which is present in AEF and apparently required for full expression of biological activity (Fig. 7), prompted us to determine the relationship of this component to β_2 microglobulin. The discovery of the association of

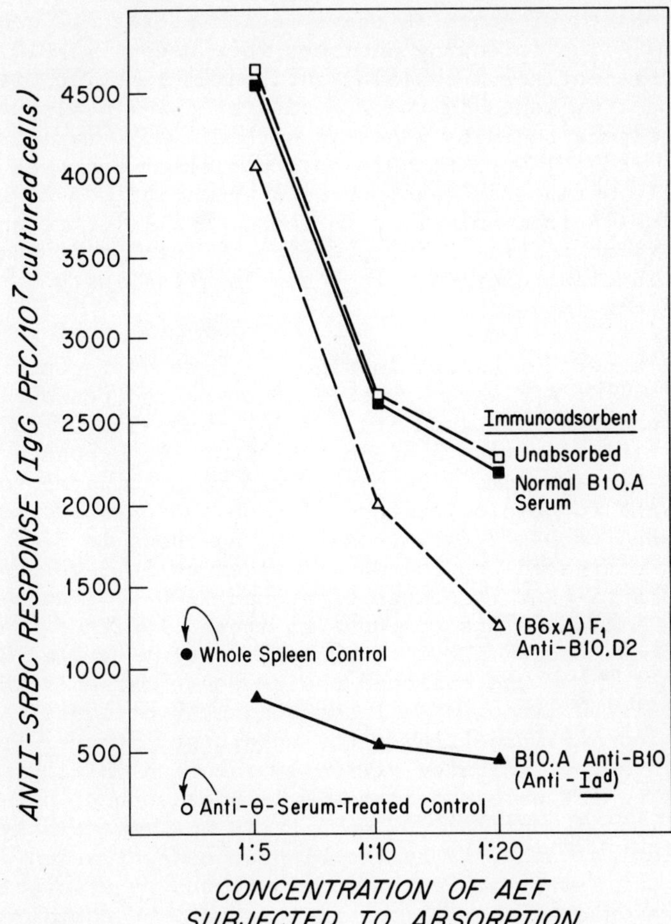

Figure 8. Removal of biological activity of AEF derived from DBA/2 (*H-2*^{d}) T cells by an anti-Ia^d immunoadsorbent. Three different concentrations of AEF were subjected to immunoadsorbents prepared from either normal B10.A serum or from (B6A)F_1 anti-B10.D2 or B10.A anti-B10 (anti-Ia^d) ascites. These AEF were then tested and compared to unabsorbed AEF for activity on the *in vitro* response to SRBC of anti-θ serum-treated DBA/2 spleen cells. Control responses of whole spleen cells and anti-θ-treated cells in the absence of AEF are shown to the left (Ref.30).

β_2-microglobulin with histocompatibility molecules in several species and the demonstration of remarkable homology of its amino acid sequence with the constant homology regions of immunoglobulins have raised intriguing questions concerning the significance and function of this small protein (for review, see 32, 33). In preliminary experiments performed in collaboration with Dr. Howard Grey, we have tested the capacity of antisera directed against a murine β_2-microglobulin-like component to specifically adsorb the biologically active component of AEF. The results of these experiments indicate, indeed, that the activity of AEF can be removed on such immunoadsorbents (34). We are reserving conclusions on these data, however, until evidence is obtained that will establish that the murine cell surface product with which these antisera have been prepared is in fact the homologue of β_2-microglobulin. If such is the case, then our results would indicate that a component in AEF is (or is highly cross-reactive with) β_2-microglobulin. Whether the specificities removed by these latter antisera are present on the heavy or light molecular weight components of AEF (or both) is presently being determined.

We conclude, therefore, that the biologically active enhancing moieties of AEF bear Ia determinants and therefore are most likely composed, at least in part, of gene products of the *I* region of the *H-2* gene complex. The presence of a small protein moiety in the active AEF complex has been demonstrated, and the current data suggest that this may be related to β_2-microglobulin although direct evidence on this point has yet to be obtained. Recent data from other investigators have shown that an antigen-specific T cell product can be adsorbed by immunoadsorbents prepared from antisera directed against the K-end of *H-2* (35). Since such antisera contain antibodies reactive with specificities of both *K* and *I* regions, it is likely that the use of selective anti-Ia sera will yield results consistent with those presented here. Taken collectively, these observations indicate that *I* region gene products may be intimately involved in the mechanism of cell-cell interactions and responsible for the regulation of immune responses.

CONCLUSIONS

The data and observations presented in this paper have shown that the regulatory interactions between T and B lymphocytes in immune responses are governed by products of genes that appear to be located in the *I* region of the *H-2* gene complex. We originally hypothesized, based on data obtained in this system, that there must exist on the surfaces of lymphocytes (and macrophages) certain molecules coded for by genes in the *H-2* complex responsible for permitting effective cell-cell interactions (2,3,6). These molecules, which have recently been termed by us as cell-interaction or *CI* molecules (36), probably are present in varying quantities on T and B lymphocytes and macrophages and are envisaged by us as interacting by homology during the cooperative interactions between such cells. The possible mechanisms by which such molecular interactions may occur have been elaborated upon at length elsewhere (36). The genetic mapping data presented here together with the observations that demonstrate the capacity of anti-Ia antiserum to absorb the biologically active molecule(s) from AEF demonstrate that *CI* molecules are products of genes located in the *I* region of *H-2*.

In closing, it should be noted that the *Ir-1A* and *Ir-1B* subregions where the *CI* genes appear to be mapped by our studies (Fig. 4) are precisely the subregions where all known immune response or *Ir* genes have been mapped (37). However, as discussed at length elsewhere (36), while this suggests an association between Ir and *CI* gene products in lymphocyte function, it does not imply that these are necessarily products of the same gene(s).

ACKNOWLEDGMENTS

We are most appreciative to all of our colleagues who participated with us in the performance of these experiments. We are indebted to Drs. Toshiyuki Hamaoka, David Sachs, and Howard Grey and Miss Mary Graves and Mr. Henry DiMuzio for their invaluable contributions to the accomplishment of these studies. We also thank Ms. Candace Maher for excellent secretarial assistance in the preparation of the manuscript.

The studies reported here were supported by Grants AI-10630 and AI-09920 from the National Institutes of Health. Dr. Armerding is a Research Fellow of the Damon Runyon Memorial Fund for Cancer Research, Inc.

REFERENCES

(1) B. Kindred and D.C. Shreffler. J. Immunol. 109 (1972) 940.

(2) D.H. Katz, T. Hamaoka and B. Benacerraf. J. Exp. Med. 137 (1973) 1405.

(3) D.H. Katz, T. Hamaoka, M.E. Dorf and B. Benacerraf. Proc. Nat. Acad. Sci. 70 (1973) 2624.

(4) A.S. Rosenthal and E.M. Shevach. J. Exp. Med. 138 (1973) 1194.

(5) P. Toivanen, A. Toivanen and O. Vainio. J. Exp. Med. 139 (1974) 1344.

(6) D.H. Katz and B. Benacerraf, in: The Immune System: Genes, Receptors, Signals - Proceedings of the 1974 I.C.N.-U.C.L.A. Symposium on Molecular Biology. eds. E.E. Sercarz, A.R. Williamson and C. Fred Fox. (Academic Press, New York, 1974) p. 569.

(7) D.H. Katz, T. Hamaoka, M.E. Dorf, P.H. Maurer and B. Benacerraf. J. Exp. Med. 138 (1973) 734.

(8) D.H. Katz, T. Hamaoka, M.E. Dorf and B. Benacerraf. J. Immunol. 112 (1974) 855.

(9) D.H. Katz, M.E. Dorf and B. Benacerraf. J. Exp. Med. 140 (1974) 290.

(10) D.H. Katz, M. Graves, M.E. Dorf, H. DiMuzio and B. Benacerraf. J. Exp. Med. 141 (1975) 000.

(11) M.E. Dorf, D.H. Katz, M. Graves, H. DiMuzio and B. Benacerraf. J. Immunol. In Press.

(12) D.C. Shreffler and C.S. David. Adv. Immunol. In Press

(13) R.W. Dutton, R. Falkoff, J.A. Hirst, M. Hoffmann, J.W. Kappler, J.R. Kettman, J.F. Lesley and D. Vann. Prog. Immunol. (1971) 355.

(14) D. Armerding and D.H. Katz. J. Exp. Med. 140 (1974) 19.

(15) D.H. Katz. Transpl. Rev. 12 (1972) 141.

(16) A. Schimpl and E. Wecker. Nature New Biol. 237 (1972) 15.

(17) A. Schimpl and E. Wecker. J. Exp. Med. 137 (1972) 547.

(18) D.H. Katz, in: Immunological Tolerance: Mechanisms and Potential Therapeutic Applications - Proceedings of a conference at Brook Lodge, Michigan, May 1974. eds. D.H. Katz and B. Benacerraf. (Academic Press, New York, 1974) p. 189.

(19) D.H. Katz and B. Benacerraf, in: Immunological Tolerance: Mechanisms and Potential Therapeutic Applications - Proceedings of a conference at Brook Lodge, Michigan, May 1974. eds. D.H. Katz and B. Benacerraf. (Academic Press, New York, 1974) p. 249.

(20) D.H. Katz, J.M. Davie, W.E. Paul and B. Benacerraf. J. Exp. Med. 134 (1971) 201.

(21) D.P. Osborne, Jr. and D.H. Katz. J. Exp. Med. 137 (1973) 991.

(22) D. Armerding and D.H. Katz. Manuscript in Preparation.

(23) J. Silver and L. Hood. Nature. 279 (1974) 765.

(24) D. Armerding, M.E. Dorf and D.H. Katz. Manuscript in Preparation.

(25) C.S. David, D.C. Shreffler and J.A. Frelinger. Proc. Nat. Acad. Sci. 70 (1973) 2509.

(26) V.D. Hauptfield, D. Klein and J. Klein. Science. 181 (1973) 167.

(27) D.H. Sachs and J.L. Cone. J. Exp. Med. 138 (1973) 1289.

(28) G.J. Hämmerling, B.D. Deak, G. Mauve, U. Hämmerling and H.O. McDevitt. Immunogenetics. 1 (1974) 68.

(29) E.R. Unanue, M.E. Dorf, C.S. David and B. Benacerraf. Proc. Nat. Acad. Sci. U.S.A. In Press.

(30) D. Armerding, D.H. Sachs and D.H. Katz. J. Exp. Med.

140 (1975) 000.

(31) D.H. Sachs, C.G. Fathman, J.L. Cone and H.B. Dickler. Transpl. Proc. In Press.

(32) B.A. Cunningham and I. Berggard. Transpl. Rev. 21 (1974) 3.

(33) J.L. Strominger, P. Cresswell, H. Grey, R.H. Humphreys, D. Mann, J. McCune, P. Parham, R. Robb, A.R. Sanderson, T.A. Springer, C. Terhorst and M.J. Turner. Transpl. Rev. 21 (1974) 126.

(34) D. Armerding, H.M. Grey and D.H. Katz. Unpublished Observations.

(35) A.J. Munro, M.J. Taussig, R. Campbell, H. Williams and Y. Lawson. J. Exp. Med. 140 (1974) 1579.

(36) D.H. Katz and B. Benacerraf. Transpl. Rev. 22 (1975) 000.

(37) B. Benacerraf and D.H. Katz. Adv. Cancer Research. 12 (1975) 000.

DISCUSSION

J. QUINTANS: In reference to the A. TH - A. TL experiment how did you exclude an allogeneic effect?

D. H. KATZ: It was not included on that slide; I included the suppression control, but not the controls with normal cells. Normal cells are always used, that is unprimed cells of the various T-cell population donor strains, to control for that possibility in every situation. That is to say that a non-primed T-cell population fails to give a non-specific positive or negative allogeneic effect.

J. QUINTANS: Isn't it surprising, wouldn't you expect an allogeneic effect?

D. H. KATZ: No, because the cells are irradiated and are used in appropriate numbers to circumvent this problem. To obtain an allogeneic effect one would have to use a much larger number of irradiated cells.

M. COHN: I would like to sharpen the differences between Dave Katz and myself on the interpretation of his experiments on the cooperative interactions between histoincompatible T- and B-cells. Now, it is of no use sharpening our differences if we cannot end up with experiments which we both believe will decide which interpretation is correct. Consequently I would like to present a competing interpretation and then suggest two experiments.

The interpretation of the findings, as Dave looks at it, is that they reflect cell-level not population-level events. This is to say that a single T^{c}-cell anti-carrier (BCG or GLT) and a single B^{γ}-cell anti-hapten (DNP) would cooperate in the presence of antigen to give a specific antihapten (DNP) response if they were syngeneic to each other and not if they were allogeneic to each other. He makes the argument that his results cannot be explained by superimposed factors derived from unrelated interactions in the allogeneic situation which create such an insufficiency of cooperating activity that the present B^{γ}-cells cannot be induced. I disagree because this is exactly the explanation I place on the findings.

First I would like to stress that an IgG-anti-DNP response is being measured. An IgG response, as I discussed yesterday, is sharply dependent on the level of cooperating activity. Small differences in the effective level of cooperating activity have large effects on the rate of IgG induction.

Second, the experiments are all performed under conditions where cooperating activity is limiting the B^{γ}-cell response. (See for example Fig. 4 in Hamaoka, Osborne, Katz J.E.M. 137, (1973).

D.H. KATZ: That is not true, as a matter of fact when you go up higher with specific syngeneic cells you get into levels of suppression. In the *in vivo* system if you increase the cells from a carrier primed animal to a much higher number of cells, for example from 50 million to 80 million cells, you do *not* linearly increase the level of cooperative activity.

M. COHN: Yes but that is because when you attempt to increase the cooperating activity by adding more cells you introduce another phenomenon. Now let us consider the experiment in which you analysed an I-difference but did not describe in your presentation. Assume that the irradiated cooperating F1 (A/JXBALB/C) T^{c}_{GLT}-population cannot provide a sufficient level of cooperating activity to permit induction of an IgG anti-DNP response. This for me is particularly profitable because GLT must have a low level of cooperating activity specific for it or an Ir-1 mutational difference would never have been detected. I am implying that a further induction of antigen sensitive t^{c}_{GLT}-cells is required to induce the B^{γ}_{DNP}-cells and this activity cannot be provided by the irradiated Fl (CA) recipient mouse. However, the anti-theta treated splee of a responder has a sufficient number of t^{c}_{GLT}-cells to permit further induction of cooperating anti-GLT activity when present with the Fl T^{c}_{GLT}-population. Consequently the BALB/C responder responds according to the following sequence:

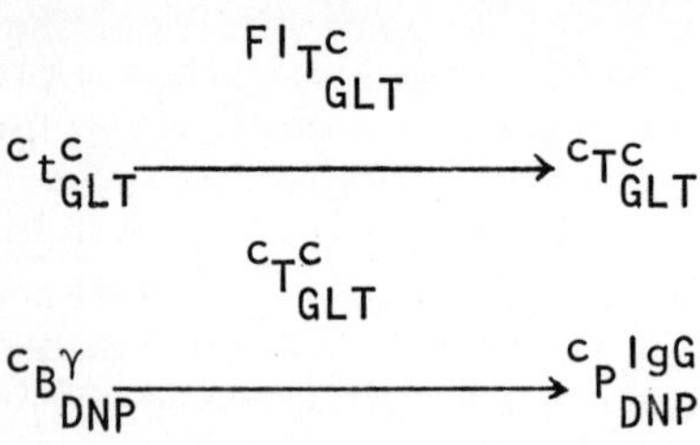

(note: see my contributed paper for meaning of symbols)

However, the non-responder A/J mouse lacking $^{A}t^{c}_{GLT}$ cells, because of the Ir-1 block, does not respond because there is no source of antigen-sensitive t^{c} cells (anti-GLT) to permit further induction of cooperating activity required to induce the $^{A}B^{\gamma}_{DNP}$-cell.

The experiment I propose is to mix the B-cell populations from BACB/C and A/J, $^{C}B^{\gamma}_{DNP}$ + $^{A}B^{\gamma}_{DNP}$, and determine by analyses of allotype whether, when the BALB/C $^{C}B^{\gamma}_{DNP}$-cell responds, the A/J $^{A}B^{\gamma}_{DNP}$-cell also responds. If Dave is correct the A/J B-cell will not respond; if I am correct it will respond. I will bet two bottles of champagne to one, on the outcome of this experiment.

The second part of this study involved the role of I-gene products and is more tricky. Dave insists that suppression cannot be operating to limit the cooperating activity but as you know, a bare assertion is not necessarily the naked truth. His arguments are two fold:

(a) If Fl T^{c}-cells are used in cooperation with parental B-cells, no induced suppression is possible. However, if parental T^{c}-cells are used with Fl B-cells, suppression could be induced but is not found because the latter cooperate normally.

(b) If one mixes the two parental T-cell populations, were suppression to operate they should mutually turn each other off so that no cooperation with either parental B-cell would be possible.

These arguments are insufficient for the following reasons:
1) No quantitative titrations of T vs B have been published and I personally insist on their critical importance throughout these studies. I would like to see quantitatively superimposed induction of FI T-cells vs parental B-cells and parental T-cells vs FI B-cells.
2) Even if these superimposed titrations were not distinguishable because of the obvious large error expressed in those transfer systems, I showed yesterday (see Fig. 7, my paper) that the parental T-cell inhibition of an FI semi-allogeneic response was 5-10 times less than that of an allogeneic response. The reason is obvious. The FI B-cell has less target antigen on its surface than the parental B-cell. Consequently this is not a sufficient contest for the allogeneic situation.
3) I showed (see Fig. 8, my paper) that cooperating activity provides inhibitory activity. Consequently mixing two parental cooperating populations would mask the inhibitory activity, <u>unless quantitative titrations</u> of one against the other were carried out.

The only way to eliminate my arguments is to study cooperative interactions on populations of T- and B-cells which are mutually tolerant (paralyzed-recessive unresponsive) of each other.

Here too I am willing to bet two bottles of champagne to one that mutually tolerant T- and B-cells will cooperate normally across histoincompatibility boundaries.

With the bottles of champagne you will owe me Dave, we can celebrate that immunology has once again become rational.

D. H. KATZ: How many experiments were there?

M. COHN: Two and whats more, you already owe me one bottle from Brighton.

D. H. KATZ: Oh no, you owe me one on that. As a matter of fact, I was going to ask you if that bottle was counted into the bet. Very briefly let me restate the problem as Mel sees it. What he is saying is that if you have mixtures of T- and B-cells (it doesn't matter what the strains are) and you effectively wipe out most, but as he claims not all, of the T-cells by anti-theta serum and complement, you may be left with a few T-cells or precursor T-cells in this population which, in a reaction with an histoincompatible or allogeneic cell population may be stimulated to become effective helper cells. Therefore the response that one sees may reflect the generation of helper cells isogeneic with the B-cell population: He is throwing my own observation back on me because Osborne and I have shown that an allogeneic effect will indeed markedly increase the kinetics and expand the development of helper cells. However, what he is ignoring is that the cell population at issue is an F1 hybrid, and the B-cell population being assayed is the parent. He would have to demand that by some genetic trick this F1 hybrid cell population is going to react against the parental strain haplotype in order to make them develop into effective helper cells. This follows from the fact that we know *in vivo* from our own experiments, and repeated by many others, that while you can make the allogeneic effect work in that direction *in vitro*, you can never make it work *in vivo* where the responding population must be reacted upon in order for the allogeneic effect to be seen. I think that possibility is very unlikely for the following reasons: first, when you effectively treat a cell population with anti-theta serum, you don't even need to lyse them with complement to have virtually all of them removed *in vivo* by the reticulo-endothelial system of the host into which they are transferred. These studies have been done by labelling cells with chromium. Secondly, with an antigen such as the one that Mel has been talking about, which happens to be a DNP derivative of the terpolymer of glutamic acid-lysine tyrosine (GLT), we have never been able to induce in a responder animal, even with an allogeneic effect, helper T-cells for GLT in an adoptive primary response within 7 days, which is the time course of these experiments. In fact, it is exceedingly difficult to get adoptive primary responses to this type of relatively weak antigen unless you use sufficient numbers of spleen cells that have *not* been depleted of T-cells in the adoptive recipient. I think this argues very strongly against the possibility Mel has raised. The mixed B-cell experiment is now to take a mixture of the parent which is a respondent and a B-cell population from a non-responder which is histoincompatible with it (and which would differ by immunoglobulin allotypes) and measure which allotype antibody is being produced. I agree, that would be a very nice control to do and we haven't done it. I would be willing therefore, to take you up on a bet of the champagne on that one. So we have one bottle of champagne on this experiment and you owe me one already from Brighton, so you'll owe me two at the next meeting.

B. A. CUNNINGHAM: In most cases in which a molecule is associated with β_2-microglobulin, the peak for β_2-microglobulin tends to be much higher than the one you showed. Do you believe that the relatively small amount that you see is a technical problem?

D. H. KATZ: I think so, yes.

B. A. CUNNINGHAM: If this is an Ia or Ir gene product should not it also be expressed in B-cells? Have you cultured B-cells to look for the same factor?

D.H. KATZ: Yes, as a matter of fact we're doing experiments of that type right now to find out whether there is homology between the molecules we are talking about; but we first want to determine if we can get biologically active ones from the B-cell surface- that is not known at present. It is known that Ia is present in very large quantities on the B-cell surface. But I should point out also that the Ia on the B-cell surface that has been extracted by detergent procedures does not conform to the molecular characteristics of the heavy component of AEF that I described. It may be that AEF is a form of Ia from T-cells that is molecularly different or is in association with some factor, perhaps a receptor, and that Ia extracted from B-cells with detergent may no longer be associated with the factor. I do not have the answer.

B. A. CUNNINGHAM: You seem to be getting activity from guanidine extracted materials which is generally difficult to do. The procedure could make a difference in comparing other systems. Also, it might be interesting to try a totally different type of cell, even nonlymphoid cells, to see if the same cell surface components are expressed on these cells.

D. H. KATZ: You mean activating them by non-clonal mitogens or simply incubating them to see if you can extract off the factors from such cells because many of these antigens are expressed on other cells. That is a good point. In fact, we recently obtained a tumor from Bruce Chesebro from Montana that is producing large quantities of this particular Ia specificity, (Ia.8) and we are in the process of trying to extract these molecules to find whether they have any biological activity.

H. WHITTEN: Dr. Katz, what is your opinion of Noel Warner's suggestion that the Ir product may be comprised, in part, of some type of Fc receptor and do you know if Fc receptors co-cap with anti H-Z antisera?

D.H. KATZ: That point is controversial. There may be some relationship between the Ia antigens, which may or may not reflect gene products of the immune response type, and Fc receptors. The current knowledge about this is that an anti-Ia reaction with B-cells inhibits the capacity of the Fc receptor to bind aggregated gamma globulin (the Dickler and Sachs experiment). That experiment is open to several interpretations. An interesting suggestion is that perhaps the Fc receptor could be the site on the B-cell which, if in fact these products do have a β_2-microglobulin-like component associated with them for B-cell differentiation, may be the receptor for the β_2-component of this type of product. This suggestion is intriguing and should be experimentally testable.

H. WHITTEN: It is conceivable that the immunoglobulin binding product released from activated T-cells is some type of Fc receptor which comprises part of your AEF and that your receptor B-cell acceptor site is β_2-microglobulin.

D.H. KATZ: Perhaps.

THE ROLE OF THYMOSIN AND THE ENDOCRINE THYMUS ON THE ONTOGENESIS AND FUNCTION OF T-CELLS*

A. L. GOLDSTEIN, G. B. THURMAN, G. H. COHEN, and J. A. HOOPER
Division of Biochemistry
University of Texas Medical Branch, Galveston, Texas

INTRODUCTION

Recent studies in immunobiology point to an important regulatory role for the endocrine thymus in the ontogenesis and function of the mammalian lymphoid system (1). The thymus influences host immunity through its secreted hormone thymosin (and perhaps other hormones) which may act _in situ_ and/or peripherally to induce the maturation and differentiation of thymic-dependent (T) lymphocytes (2). The subnormal levels of thymosin detected in the blood of humans with certain diseases and with aging (3) may lead to immunological deficiencies similar to those observed after experimental thymectomy in animals. Studies in progress suggest that thymosin insufficiencies may indeed contribute towards the development of various primary and secondary immunodeficiency diseases in man. Using a newly developed _in vitro_ E-rosette assay (4, 5) a number of disease states have already been identified that are characterized in part by thymosin insufficiencies. These studies implicate a role for thymosin in the etiology of cell-mediated immunodeficiencies. Thymosin abnormalities have been noted in patients with various cancers, with certain autoimmune diseases, with disease states commonly associated with aging, with severe viral infections, and with severe burns (4-7).

In this paper we review some of the most recent developments in the biology of thymosin as they relate to the ontogenesis, function and senescence of T-cells in a number of animal models _in vitro_ and _in vivo_. In addition, we discuss the effects of thymosin

*These studies were supported, in part, by grants from The John A. Hartford Foundation, Inc., and the National Cancer Institute (CA 14108 and CA 15419).

in vitro on lymphocytes purified from the blood of patients with a variety of primary and secondary immunodeficiency diseases as well as describe our initial clinical experiences with thymosin administered *in vivo*.

CHEMICAL PROPERTIES OF THYMOSIN USED IN PHYSIOLOGICAL STUDIES

The method of Goldstein *et al.* (8, 9) as modified recently by Hooper *et al.* (10) was used to prepare the partially purified calf thymosin fraction 5 and the more purified thymosin fraction 8 employed in the studies to be described. Thymosin fraction 5, the hormone preparation used for most of the biological studies to date, contains at least 11 heat-stable acidic peptides and proteins with molecular weights that range from 1, 200 to 14, 000. It is not yet known whether all of the biological activity ascribed to thymosin resides within a single molecular species or whether there exists a family of thymus-specific molecules which act in concert to endow the host with its normal complement of immunity (10, 11).

The first thymosin molecule to be purified to homogeneity was thymosin fraction 7 (10). Recently we have improved the isolation procedure to increase the yields and quality of the purified protein which is now termed thymosin fraction 8 (11). Fraction 8 is a heat-stable acidic polypeptide. Amino acid analysis indicates the presence of approximately 108 amino acid residues per molecule. Thymosin contains one residue of histidine, one cysteine and no tryptophan. Carbohydrate, lipid and nucleotide are absent.

The suggestion that several biologically active factors are present in fraction 5 comes from recent observations that not all preparations of thymosin fraction 8 are as active as less pure fractions when tested in some of the *in vitro* systems presently under investigation (10). This decreased specific activity may reflect chemical modification of the molecule, the existance of several biologically active thymic factors or the removal of an active component or cofactor during the purification procedure.

ROLE OF THYMOSIN IN THE ONTOGENESIS AND FUNCTION OF T-CELLS

A. Developmental Studies

Studies primarily in mice have demonstrated that a functional thymus gland is required at birth to induce the maturation of immunologically competent lymphocytes (T-cells) (c. f. 12). As diagrammed in Figure 1, removal of the thymus within the first 24 hours of birth prevents the development of cell-mediated immunity

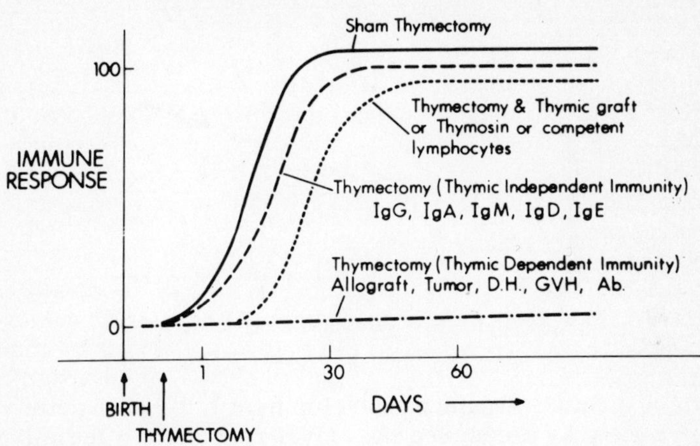

Fig. 1. Effect of thymosin, thymic grafts and competent lymphocytes on immunity in neonatally thymectomized mice.

in mice. Following neonatal thymectomy, mice as well as several other mammalian species usually succumb to overwhelming infection and a wasting disease (c. f. 12). Studies with partially purified bovine thymosin reveal that this hormone can act in lieu of the thymus gland and reduce the incidence of wasting disease and death due to neonatal thymectomy (9, 13) and can partially reconstitute cell-mediated immune responses (9, 14). Illustrated in Fig. 1 is the finding that deficient cell-mediated immunity may also be reconstituted by transplantation of a thymic graft or competent lymphocytes.

In other developmental studies, thymosin administration was shown to accelerate the normal ontogenesis of T-cells in the spleen with regard to their ability to elicit a graft-versus-host (GVH) reaction. Three day old CBA/Wh mice were injected intraperitoneally with thymosin (fraction 3) or with calf spleen fraction 3 and 24 hours later the spleens were removed and cell suspensions were prepared. These cells were then injected intravenously into lethally irradiated (800R) B6AF1/J mice and the capacities of the spleen seeking cells to elicit a GVH were compared to control cells from mice treated with calf spleen fraction 3 using a previously described assay (15). Fig. 2 shows that thymosin treatment

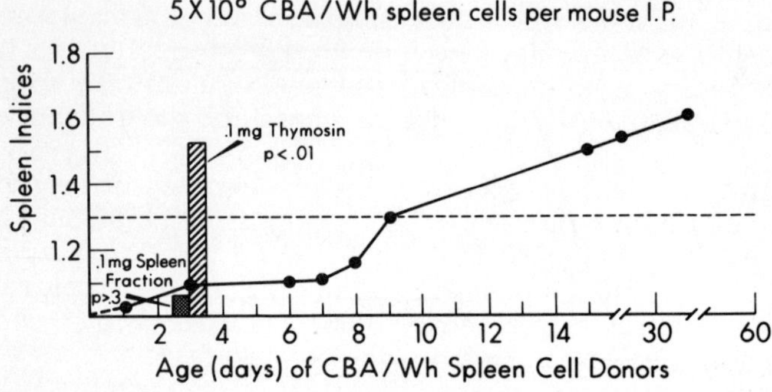

Fig. 2. Thymosin enhanced development in vivo of cell-mediated immunity as measured by a GVH response in lethally irradiated (800R) B6AF1/J mice.

significantly increased the capacity of spleen cells to elicit a GVH. As indicated by the solid line, mouse spleen cells normally do not develop the capacity to elicit a good GVH reaction (spleen index >1.3) until the second week post birth.

Similarly, as seen in Fig. 3, thymosin fraction 3 could be

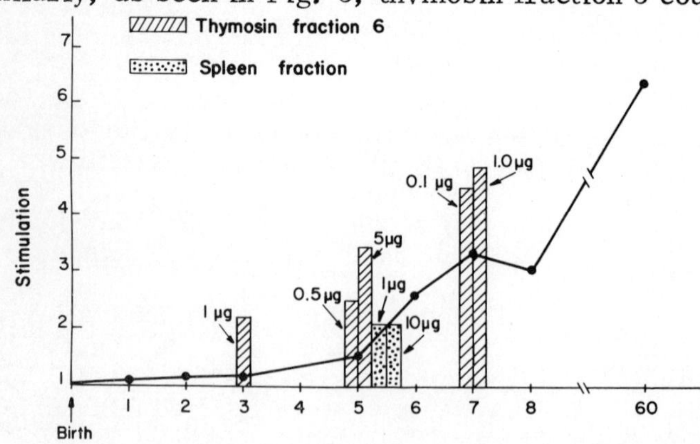

Fig. 3. Effect of thymosin on ontogenesis of PHA responsivity in CBA/Wh spleen cells.

shown in newborn mice to accelerate the development of responsiveness of spleen cells to PHA (a T-cell mitogen) when tested in vitro. Twenty-four hours after thymosin administration, spleen cell suspensions were prepared and incubated with PHA for 48 hours. The spleen cells were pulsed with tritiated thymidine during the last 24 hours of incubation and the amount of radioactive thymidine incorporated into cells was used as a measure of PHA-induced blastogenesis. As indicated by the solid line in Fig. 3, the capacity of spleen cells from newborn animals to respond well to PHA normally does not develop until the second week of life.

Thymosin treatment accelerates the development of resistance to virus-induced tumors in mice. The administration of thymosin fraction 3 to neonatal CBA/Wh mice innoculated with Moloney sarcoma virus (MSV) prolongs host survival (Fig. 4) and accelerates the regression of the resulting virus-induced rhabdomyosarcoma (16). Newborn mice, in contrast to adult mice, do not have the capacity to reject a tumor induced by MSV injection. In CBA/Wh mice the resistance to progressive MSV induced tumor growth develops between the 2nd and 3rd week of life. An amount of MSV that would kill 80-90% of the mice if introduced at day 14 will kill only 40-50% of the animals if introduced at day 21 post-parturition. The administration of thymosin from birth significantly reduces the incidence of MSV induced tumor death in CBA/Wh mice (Fig. 4). In contrast, similarly prepared calf liver and spleen afford no protection.

B. T-Cell Function in Normal and Immunodeficient Mice

For many years it was thought that the thymus gland, whatever its role, added nothing significant to the quality of health in the adult (c. f. 17). This erroneous conclusion was based on two observations: first, that adult thymectomy had no immediately obvious effect on the physiology of the thymus-deprived animal and second, that at puberty, the thymus gland atrophies, leaving only a trace of its former existance as a stromal epithelial structure.

The first observation made by early workers in this field was incorrect. As illustrated in Fig. 5, very dramatic cellular changes and responses do occur after adult thymectomy in the mouse, as well as in other species. We now know that the failure to detect physiological changes soon after thymectomy of the adult was due to the presence of long-lived thymus-derived (T) cells in the circulation that, despite the absence of the thymus, could continue to carry the "immunological burden" until they wore out at a much later time. The life spans of these T-cells have been estimated to be over 100 days in rodents (17) and perhaps several years in humans (18). This time frame did not meet with the

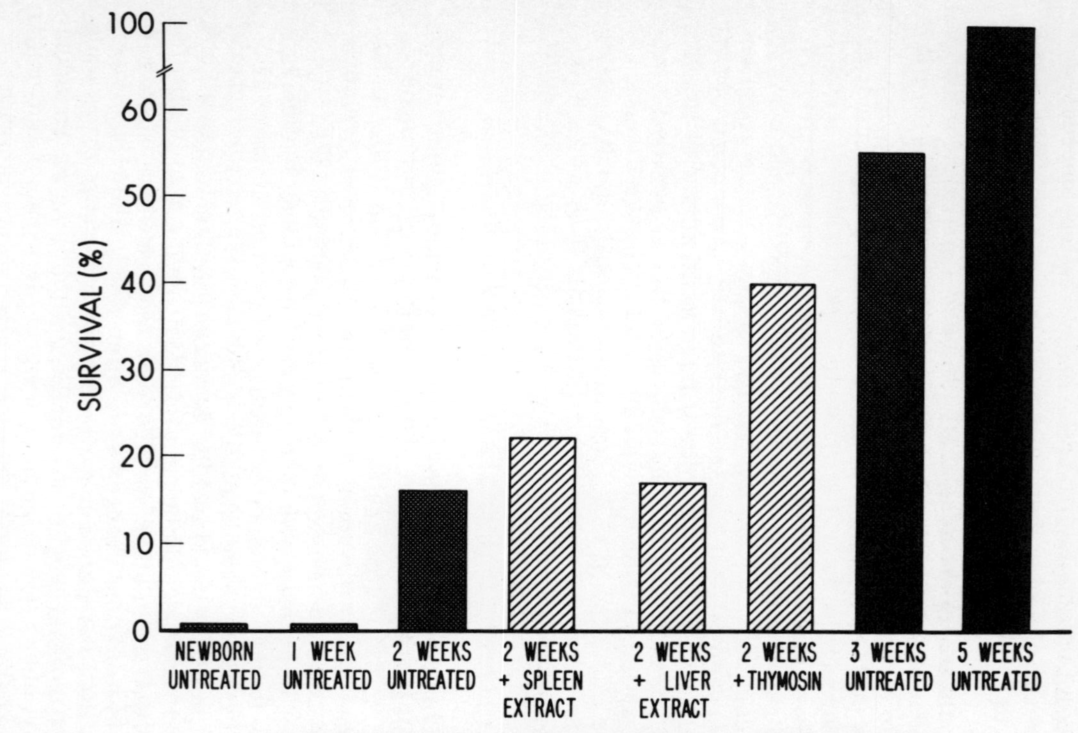

Fig. 4. Development of resistance to progressive tumor growth in CBA/Wh mice innoculated with MSV and treated with thymosin. [From Zisblatt et al. (16).]

patience of the early thymologists and hence the gradual depletion of T-cells and slow progressive loss of immune function went unnoticed. This delayed loss of in vivo responsivity of cell-mediated and humoral immunity following adult thymectomy is depicted in Fig. 5. Using more sensitive in vitro assays developed in recent years, however, it has been possible to demonstrate dramatic changes in immunological competence of lymphoid cell populations following adult thymectomy. These changes include decreased

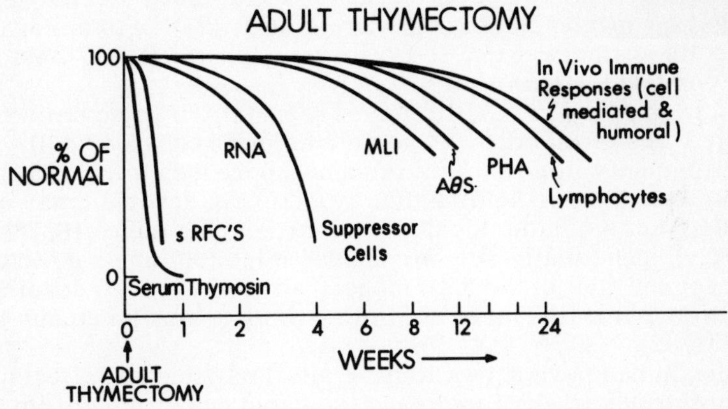

Fig. 5. Decay of T-cell and metabolic functions after adult thymectomy in the mouse.

capacity of lymphoid populations from adult thymectomized mice to respond in vitro to PHA (19), decreased capacity of lymphocytes to undergo a mixed lymphocyte reaction (MLR) (20), and significantly decreased numbers of peripheral lymphocytes containing T-cell marker antigens such as the Thy-1 (θ) (21).

Within 2 to 4 weeks post-adult thymectomy there is also a decrease in the number of suppressor-like T-cells (22) that is preceeded by a decreased capacity of thoracic (23) and peripheral lymph node cells (24) to incorporate radioactive uridine into RNA. Within 1 week after thymectomy, Bach et al. were able to observe a decrease in the number of spontaneous rosette-forming cells in the spleen (25). This decrease in spontaneous rosette-forming cells is the earliest known cellular change that occurs after adult thymectomy in the mouse. Still earlier, within hours after adult thymectomy, there is a detectable decrease in serum thymosin-like activity (26). We have found that short-term incubation with thymosin in vitro or treatment in vivo can reconstitute the populations of spontaneous rosette-forming cells and serum thymosin-like activity lost after adult thymectomy (9).

It is apparent from recent studies in cellular immunology that T-cells are heterogenous and belong to any one (or more) of several distinct classes presumably reflecting various stages of maturation. Recent findings suggest that thymosin may act on at least three distinct classes of lymphoid cells as illustrated in Fig. 6: pre-thymic cells, post-thymic cells, and more mature thymosin-sensitive cells (cortisone-sensitive thymocytes). One of the most interesting new findings is the observation that thymosin causes thymocytes to be converted in vitro into more mature T-cells with the capacity to elicit in vitro a MLR (27) or to act as "killer" cells against P-815Y($H-2^d$) mastocytoma cells (S. Waksal, personal communication).

In addition to the reconstitution of neonatally thymectomized mice, it has been found that thymosin treatment enhances cell-mediated immunity in normal or immunosuppressed mice. Thymosin administration promotes tumor rejection in several types of immunodeficient animals, including tumor bearing mice (16, 28) and rats (29), genetically athymic "nude" mice (30) and corrects T-cell abnormalities in the NZB mouse, an animal which develops an autoimmune-like disease similar to lupus erythmatosus in humans (31, 32).

Thymosin has been shown to have similarly marked effects on T-cell populations in vitro including the rapid conversion of immature mouse lymphoid cells into more mature T-cells which acquire distinctive T-cell marker antigens at their surface (6, 7, 33, 34) and specialized functions. In vitro studies with the genetically thymusless "nude" mice have shown that incubation with thymosin restores the capacity of spleen cells to produce a graft-versus-host response (36), and to elicit a mixed-lymphocyte reaction in vitro (S. Waksal, personal communication).

THYMUS DEPENDENT SENESCENCE OF IMMUNITY IN MAN

It is generally recognized that the two most critical periods of life, with regard to health, occur shortly after birth and after the sixth decade of life. Our cell-mediated immune function does not achieve maximum competence until about the time of puberty and then it undergoes a sharp decline with age. There is increasing support for the concept that the waning of thymic dependent cell-mediated immunity is importantly related to the etiology of diseases such as cancer, autoimmune disorders and infectious diseases, the incidences of which increase with age as illustrated in Fig. 7. Recent studies by Bach et al. (38) using a rosette bioassay and by Schulof (39) and Goldstein et al. (3) using a rosette and crude radioimmunoassay have shown that thymosin or thymosin-like activity in the blood of humans decreases precipitously with

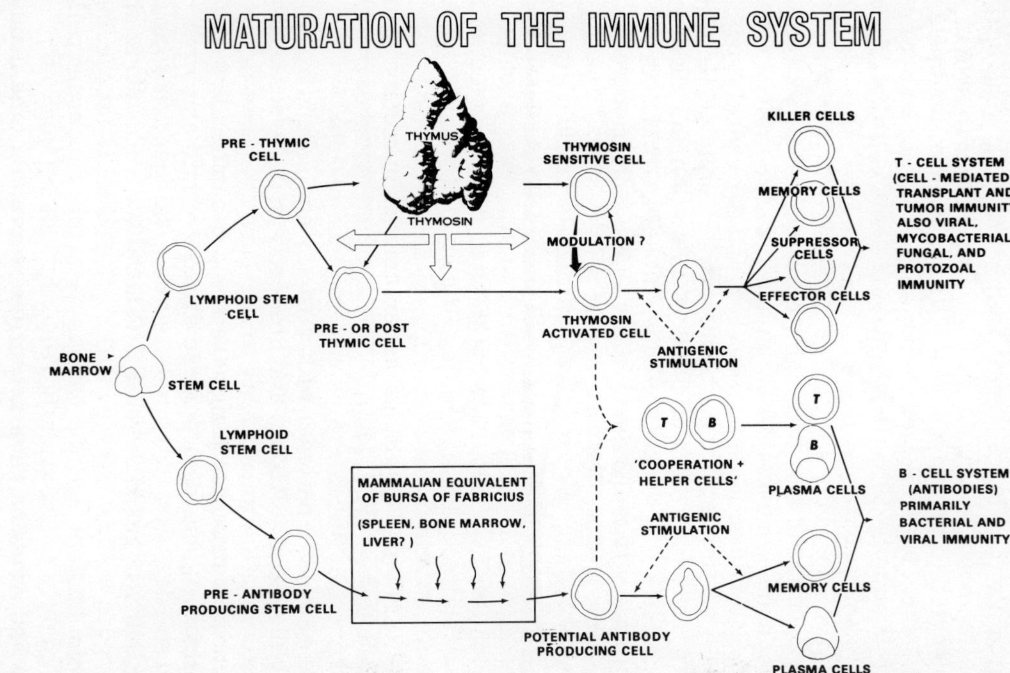

Fig. 6. Maturation of the immune system.
[From Goldstein et al. (3).]

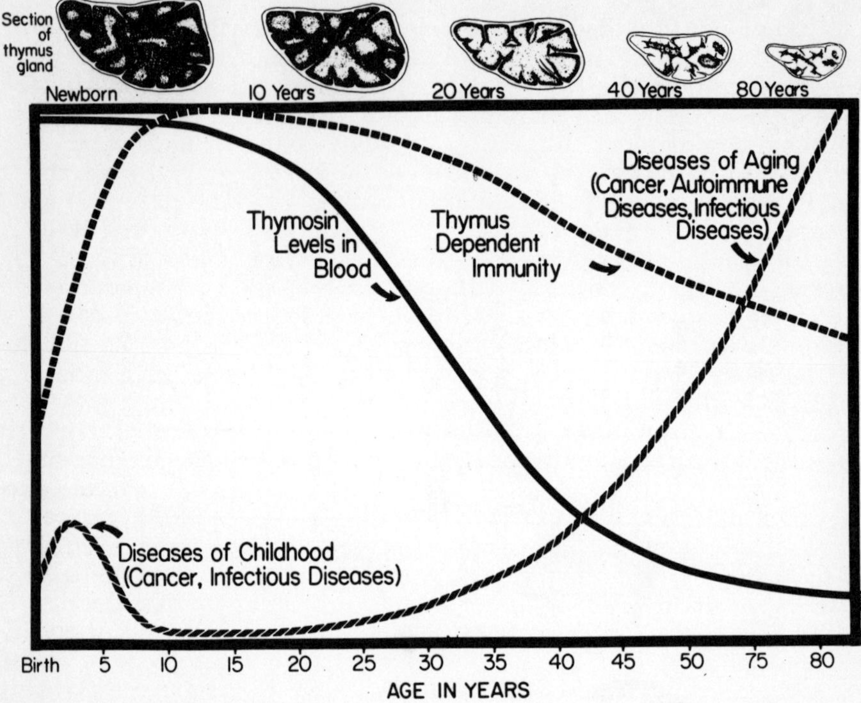

Fig. 7. Thymus dependent senescence of immunity in man. [From Goldstein et al. (11).]

age and is altered in patients with primary and secondary immunodeficiency diseases. Studies are presently in progress to develop a quantitative radioimmunoassay to measure thymosin in the blood and to detect the precise changes that occur during the aging process and thymic-dependent disease states.

FIRST CLINICAL TRIALS WITH THYMOSIN

A. In vitro Studies

Wara and Ammann have recently observed that the number of total E-rosettes formed by peripheral blood lymphocytes obtained from patients with immunodeficiency diseases but not from normal individuals can be increased in vitro after incubation with thymosin (4). This observation has led to the development of a new in vitro test for identification of patients with possible thymosin-dependent immunodeficiency diseases. The method for this assay is outlined in Fig. 8.

Other similar studies have shown that incubation of peripheral blood lymphocytes with thymosin increases the number of E-rosette forming cells (T-cells) from patients with a variety of serious clinical disorders including thymic hypoplasia (4, 5, R. Hong, personal communication), ataxia telangiectasia (4, 5), Wiscott-Aldrich (4, 5), lupus erythmatosus (4, 5), cancer (6, 7, E. Hersh and P. Chretien, personal communication), virus infection (5) and severe burns (6). Some of the relevant data are shown in Table 1.

Thymosin does not appear to influence the number of E-rosette forming cells from patients with combined-immunodeficiency disease, where the defect is apparently at the level of a stem cell deficiency. Thymosin has a marked effect on the lymphocytes from certain cancer patients as well as those from most patients with thymic hypoplasias.

The Wara-Ammann E-rosette assay has been particularly useful in identifying immunodeficient patients who may be candidates for thymosin therapy *in vivo*. Patients whose E-rosettes are elevated by incubation with thymosin *in vitro* appear to have greater than normal numbers of "thymosin-sensitive" precursor T-cells in the blood. The failure to increase the number of E-rosettes with thymosin *in vitro* in other patients may indicate that the patients have adequate endogenous levels of thymosin or that they have a thymosin-independent disorder (e. g., stem-cell deficiency). As can be seen in Table 1, not all cancer patients have lymphocytes that respond to thymosin *in vitro*. In other studies not reported here (6) we have observed that in severely burned children, T-cell function is aberrent and that thymosin added *in vitro* to peripheral blood lymphocytes can significantly increase the number of total E-rosettes. Most recently Harris *et al.* (personal communication) have found that lymphocytes from the majority of patients with chronic uremia studied respond to thymosin treatment *in vitro*, which suggests the possibility of a defect at the endocrine level of the thymus.

In summary, the effect of thymosin on E-rosettes suggests that a defect in thymosin secretion and/or release may exist in individuals having a wide variety of disorders and that populations of thymosin responsive lymphoid cells circulate in the blood. Although the origin of these thymosin-sensitive cells in humans is not known, studies by Touraine and coworkers indicate that they may originate in the bone-marrow compartment (37). Previous studies in our laboratory have identified a population of thymosin-responsive bone marrow cells in mice that can be induced to differentiate into more mature T-cells (15, 33).

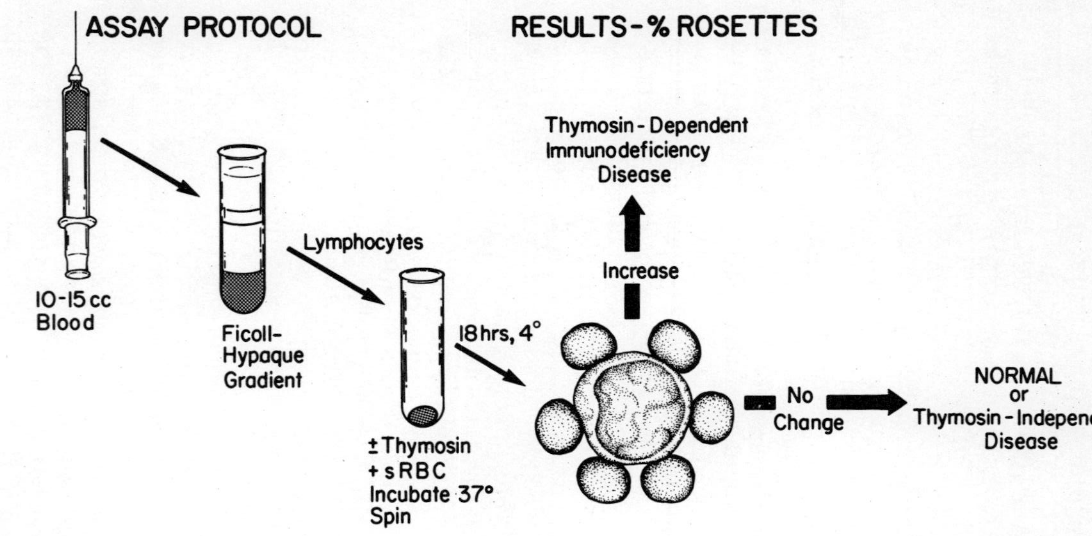

Fig. 8. Wara-Ammann E-rosette bioassay. [From Goldstein *et al.* (11)].

TABLE 1

Effect of Thymosin (Fraction 5) on Human T-Cell Rosettes of Immunodeficient Patients

Investigators, Disease and Number of Patients	Base-line	Thymosin Treatment	Significant Increase
D. Wara (4, 5) and A. Ammann*			
Normals (20)	50-65%	45-65%	-
Thymic hypoplasia	20%	45%	+
DiGeorge syndrome	25%	49%	+
Thymic hypoplasia and successful thymus transplant	32%	38%	-
Ataxia telangiectasia	27%	43%	+
Wiskott-Aldrich syndrome	28%	45%	+
Combined immunodeficiency	17%	20%	-
R. Hong*			
Normals (4)	43-76%	46-60%	-
DiGeorge syndrome	30%	54%	+
Lupus erythmatosus	59%	75%	+
Cartilage hair	10%	20%	+
E. Hersh and L. Schafer*			
Normals	50-70%	N. T.	
Lung carcinoma (3)	21-35%	45-51%	+
P. Chretien and T. Fehniger*			
Normals (20)	55-80%	50-80%	-
Lung carcinoma (29)	25-70%	40-90%	+
Pelvic cancer (7)	35-65%	50-75%	+
H. Sakai et al. (7)			
Normals (8)	34-71%	43-72%	-
Lung carcinoma (undifferentiated adenocarcinoma)	24%	42%	+
Hodgkin's disease, IV-B	34%	47%	+

TABLE 1 (continued)

Investigators, Disease and Number of Patients	Base-line	Thymosin Treatment	Significant Increase
Acute lymphocytic leukemia	35%	52%	+
Acute myelomonocytic leukemia	23%	54%	+
Disseminated melanoma	23%	37%	+
Stem cell leukemia (complete remission)	71%	74%	-
Endometrial carcinoma (no metastasis found)	61.5%	70%	-
Acute myelogenous leukemia	2%	17%	+
M. Scheinberg et al. (40)			
Normals (8)	58-67%	58-69%	-
Active systemic lupus erythmatosis (6)	23-47%	35-72%	+
Inactive systemic lupus erythmatosis (5)	52-70%	59-71%	-
Rheumatoid arthritis (5)	60-69%	58-67%	-
J. Montgomery*			
Normal	66%	68%	-
Combined immunodeficiency	10%	8%	-

*personal communications

B. *In vivo* Studies in Humans

On the basis of the well-documented physiological effects of thymosin in a variety of animal models and the completion of extensive toxicity studies with thymosin fraction 5 in mice and dogs, clinical trials have been initiated at a number of medical centers in the United States. The first clinical trial of thymosin was initiated by Drs. Arthur Ammann and Diane Wara at the University of California Medical Center in April 1974 (5). The patient was a 5 year old female with thymic hypoplasia and hyper-immunoglobulinemia A. Following therapy with 1 mg of thymosin per kg body weight per day, T-cell rosettes rose significantly and delayed-type skin responsivity to a number of antigens became positive. There was also marked clinical improvement which included increased appetite, decreased stools and weight gain. On cessation of thymosin administration, T-cell rosettes fell to pre-treatment levels. Maintenance of near normal numbers of T-cell rosettes in the blood and partial reconstitution of immunological competence was achieved with the administration of 1 mg per kg body weight of thymosin on a weekly basis. The incidence of infection was significantly reduced. A small number of other patients with primary immunodeficiency diseases being treated with thymosin are presently under study.

Phase I trials in terminal cancer patients have been recently initiated. The major objectives of the Phase I study is to determine (1) the maximum tolerable dose of thymosin, (2) the quantitative and qualitative toxicity of thymosin, (3) if thymosin effects the reconstitution of immunodeficiency diseases associated with malignancy, and to determine if thymosin produces a response rate in disseminated malignancy. Fifteen patients have now received thymosin in doses ranging from 1 mg per m^2 to 350 mg per m^2 for 7 days. To date the patients have tolerated thymosin administration well and there is no indication of toxicity. In addition the majority of patients have responded to thymosin therapy with a significant increase in the number of T-cells (E-rosettes in the blood) and have demonstrated a general tendency for conversion of skin tests from negative to positive.

C. Proposed Sites of Action of Thymosin

Our working hypothesis concerning the basic sites of thymosin action is diagrammed in Fig. 9. Our studies indicate that thymosin can act on bone marrow-derived or -dwelling primitive stem cell populations (Pre-T) as well as on more mature T-cells (T_1) which may transiently reside within the thymus gland. The short time period required for thymosin to convert a primitive lymphoid cell into a more mature T-cell suggests that thymosin probably

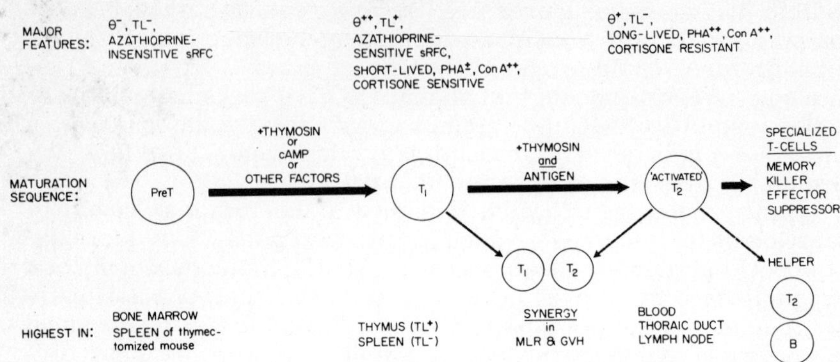

Fig. 9. Hypothetical sites of thymosin action in murine thymic (T) cell maturation [From Cohen et al. (27)]

derepresses or activates a cell that is already genetically programmed for T-cell differentiation. As depicted in Fig. 9, precursor T-cells can be induced by thymosin, cyclic AMP, or other factors both specific and non-specific to express T-cell surface (6, 7, 33, 34) and functional characteristics (15, 27, 33, 35).

Most recently we have shown that thymosin can act in vitro in the presence of antigen to facilitate the differentiation of immature thymocytes toward full immunological function as mature T_2 cells in the MLR. These studies by Cohen and her associates (27) suggest that thymosin can drive a T_1 cell to a T_2 state in vitro.

Recent in vivo studies by Dauphinee and coworkers (31) on NZB mice have demonstrated that a subpopulation of thymosin-activated cells, the so-called "suppressor" or "regulator" cells, is dependent upon the endocrine thymus for their maturation. We have suggested that the thymosin-dependent suppressor cells exert fine control over other subpopulations of T- and B-cells and may be directly implicated in the etiology of the autoimmune disease in NZB mice and by analogy, perhaps in humans.

Interestingly, we have observed that addition of thymosin to more mature populations of T-cells (lymph node cells and spleen cells) under the appropriate conditions actually suppresses the MLR response (27). This observation has led us to hypothesize that enhancement or suppression of an immunological response may depend upon the ratio of less mature T_1 cells to more mature T_2 cells that are in intimate contact at the time of antigenic challenge (11). Thus, the so-called suppressor cells may be qualitatively similar to other specialized T-cells, and may represent the end result of excessive generation of T-cells (T_2?) whose development and life span are dependent upon thymosin. It is possible that immunosuppression due to stress or pathogen invasion may result in thymosin-stimulated overproduction of T-cells, which, in turn, could proceed to suppress other T- and B-cell functions. Waldmann and his associates have reported evidence for the possibility that in common variable hypogammaglobulinemia there is excessive production of suppressor T-cells which presumably prevents maturation of B-cells (41).

During the aging process, hypothymic function may result in secretion of less thymosin which in turn could lead to a decrease in the optimal number of suppressor T-cells and consequent loss of regulatory control over other vital T- and B-cell populations. This loss of control perhaps is a causal factor in the appearance of "maverick" auto-aggressive lymphoid cells with the onset of autoimmune disease. Studies by Dauphinee et al. (31) and Bach et al. (42) on NZB mice indeed demonstrate that the disappearance of thymosin is correlated with the appearance of the autoimmune disease syndrome in mice. Loss of suppressor T-cell function might also permit increased proliferation of other T- and B-cells and may thus be a factor in the production of blocking antibodies and development of certain lymphoid cell malignancies.

Although the exact mechanism by which thymosin activates lymphoid T-cells has not been defined, ongoing studies suggest that an adenyl cyclase mediated mechanism may be involved (P. Naylor, C. Camp and A. L. Goldstein, in preparation; P. Chretien, personal communication). Our increased understanding of the molecular biology of these basic control mechanisms of the T-cell system should contribute significantly to the development of new approaches for enhancing the immunological function of patients having disorders associated with aberrant thymic-dependent function.

REFERENCES

(1) N. Trainin, Physiol. Rev., 54 (1974) 272.

(2) A. L. Goldstein and A. White, in: Contemporary Topics in Immunobiology, eds. A. J. S. Davies and R. L. Carter (Plenum Publishing Co., New York, 1973) p. 339.

(3) A. L. Goldstein, J. A. Hooper, R. S. Schulof, G. H. Cohen, G. B. Thurman, M. C. McDaniel, A. White and M. Dardenne, Fed. Proc., 33 (1974) 2053.

(4) D. W. Wara and A. J. Ammann, Ann. N. Y. Acad. Sci. (In press).

(5) D. W. Wara, A. L. Goldstein, W. Doyle and A. J. Ammann, New England J. of Med., 292 (1975) 70.

(6) A. L. Goldstein, D. W. Wara, A. J. Ammann, H. Sakai, N. S. Harris, G. B. Thurman, J. A. Hooper, G. H. Cohen, A. S. Goldman, J. J. Costanzi and M. C. McDaniel, Trans. Proc. (In press).

(7) H. Sakai, J. J. Costanzi, D. F. Loukas, R. G. Gagliano, S. E. Ritzmann and A. L. Goldstein, Cancer (In press).

(8) A. L. Goldstein, F. D. Slater and A. White, Proc. Natl. Acad. Sci., 56 (1966) 1010.

(9) A. L. Goldstein, Z. Guha, M. M. Zatz, M. A. Hardy and A. White, Proc. Natl. Acad. Sci., 69 (1972) 1800.

(10) J. A. Hooper, M. C. McDaniel, G. B. Thurman, G. H. Cohen, R. S. Schulof and A. L. Goldstein, N. Y. Acad. Sci. (In press).

(11) A. L. Goldstein, G. B. Thurman, G. H. Cohen and J. A. Hooper, in: Biological Activity of Thymic Hormones, ed. D. W. van Bekkum (Kooyker Scientific Publications, 1975) (In press).

(12) R. A. Good and A. E. Gabrielson, eds., The Thymus in Immunobiology Structure, Function and Role in Disease (Hoeber-Harper, New York, 1964).

(13) Y. Asanuma, A. L. Goldstein and A. White, Endocrinology, 86 (1970) 600.

(14) A. L. Goldstein, Y. Asanuma, J. R. Battisto, J. Quint, M. A. Hardy and A. White, J. Immunol., 104 (1970) 359.

(15) A. L. Goldstein, A. Guha, M. L. Howe and A. White, J. Immunol., 106 (1971) 773.

(16) M. Zisblatt, A. L. Goldstein, F. Lilly and A. White, Proc. Natl. Acad. Sci., 66 (1970) 1170.

(17) J. R. Little, G. Brecker, T. R. Bradley and S. Rose, Blood, 19 (1962) 236.

(18) R. E. Buckton and M. C. Pike, Nature, 202 (1964) 714.

(19) J. M. Johnston and D. B. Wilson, Cell. Immunol., 1 (1970) 430.

(20) L. C. Robson and M. R. Schwarz, Transplantation, 11 (1971) 465.

(21) M. Schlesinger and I. Yron, Israel J. Med. Sci., 5 (1969) 445.

(22) M. M. Zatz and A. L. Goldstein, J. Immunol., 110 (1973) 1312.

(23) W. O. Reike, Science, 152 (1966) 535.

(24) Y. Asanuma and A. White, Endocrinology, 89 (1971) 413.

(25) J. F. Bach, M. Dardenne and A. J. S. Davies, Nature, New Biology, 231 (1971) 110.

(26) J. F. Bach, M. Dardenne and M. A. Bach, Transplant. Proc., 5 (1973) 99.

(27) G. H. Cohen, J. A. Hooper and A. L. Goldstein, Ann. N. Y. Acad. Sci. (In press).

(28) M. A. Hardy, M. Zisblatt, N. Levine, A. L. Goldstein, F. Lilly and A. White, Transplant. Proc., III (1971) 926.

(29) B. A. Khaw and A. H. Rule, Br. J. Medicine, 28 (1973) 288.

(30) G. B. Thurman, A. Ahmed, D. M. Strong, M. O. Gershwin, A. D. Scheinberg and A. L. Goldstein, Trans. Proc. (In press).

(31) M. J. Dauphinee, N. Talal, A. L. Goldstein and A. White, Proc. Natl. Acad. Sci., 71 (1974) 2637.

(32) M. E. Gershwin, A. Ahmed, A. D. Steinberg, G. B. Thurman and A. L. Goldstein, J. of Immunol., 113 (1974) 1068.

(33) J. F. Bach, M. Dardenne, A. L. Goldstein, A. Guha and A. White, Proc. Natl. Acad. Sci., 68 (1971) 2734.

(34) M. P. Scheid, M. K. Hoffman, K. Komuro, U. Hammerling, J. Abbott, E. A. Boyse, G. H. Cohen, J. A. Hooper, R. S. Schulof and A. L. Goldstein, J. Exp. Med., 138 (1973) 1027.

(35) B. Wolf, Ann. N.Y. Acad. Sci. (In press).

(36) B. Lowenberg, H. T. M. Nieuwerkerk and D. W. van Bekkum, in: Annual Report 1972, The Radiobiological Institute, Rijswijk, The Netherlands (1972) p. 105.

(37) J. L. Touraine, E. Touraine, G. S. Incefy and R. A. Good, Ann. N.Y. Acad. Sci. (In press).

(38) J. F. Bach, M. Dardenne, M. Papiernik, A. Barois, P. Levasseur and H. LeBregand, Lancet, 2 (1972) 1056.

(39) R. S. Schulof, Tex. Rep. Biol. Med., 30 (1972) 195.

(40) M. A. Scheinberg, E. S. Cathcart and A. L. Goldstein, (Submitted)

(41) T. Waldmann, S. Broder, M. Durm, M. Blackman, R. M. Blaese and W. Strober, Lancet, II (1974) 609.

(42) J. F. Bach, M. Dardenne and J. C. Salomon, J. Clin. Exper. Immunol., 14 (1973) 247.

DISCUSSION

I. SCHEINKEIM: Not being a cellular immunologist, I am surprised at the bewildering array of activities this group of molecules has. Do you obtain an increase in specific activity for all or only some of these functions when you purify? Do they copurify, or do you lose some?

A. L. GOLDSTEIN; As I indicated in my opening remarks we have found an increase in specific activity as we purify. However in some of the bioassays we have found that fraction 8 is not as active as fraction 5. From studies in progress it looks as if the biological activity ascribed to thymosin may reside in several chemically distinct peptides which may act in concert to endow the host with its normal complement of immunity.

S. TAYLOR: I was very interested in your observations about the patient with Hodgkins disease being treated with thymosin. Can you give us any information about his in vivo or in vitro responses following this treatment?

A.L. GOLDSTEIN: We have treated approximately 15 cancer patients so far with thymosin daily for 7 days, including some Hodgkins patients. In the majority of these patients there has been an increase in E-rosettes as well as a tendency of skin tests that were previously negative to a battery of skin sensitizing antigens to become positive. PHA and MLR responses have remained low. We do not know if longer thymosin treatment will increase these responses. I might add that Heather, the first patient to receive thymosin, has been treated for ten months and her PHA and MLC responses still remain low in spite of the increase in her E-rosettes and her positive skin responsivity.

L. HERTZENBERG: Would you clarify the relationship between thymosin in the various assays that you and others have used and the thymic humoral factor that Dr. Trainin has been studying with respect to the developmental sequence of T-cells? Also, how does the amount of thymosin fraction 5 injected in the nude mouse experiments compare with the amount of thymosin which you would expect to be produced in mice with intact thymuses during the same time period?

A.L. GOLDSTEIN: With regard to the first question, Trainin's THF is a relatively heat stable acidic peptide with a lower molecular weight (about 3,000) than thymosin, fraction 8. The biological activities seen with thymosin and THF are similar in some systems and different in others. For example, in a system equivalent to our MLR, I believe that THF must be removed from the cell cultures in order to see the conversion of thymocytes into cells that will respond in the MLR. In contrast, thymosin can remain in the culture medium throughout the course of the 5 day incubation. With regard to the amount of thymosin --the answer to this must await the development of a good radioimmune assay so that we can determine the levels in blood.

L. HERZENBERG:: My understanding of Trainin's factor is that it may very well work on the pre T-cell going to a thymocyte, whereas yours works on a thymocyte going to a more mature cell.

A.L. GOLDSTEIN: Thymosin fraction 5 appears to work on a pre T-cell as well as a more mature T-cell. Critical analysis of the cell populations must wait until the day that the cellular immunologists get together and purify and characterize the heterogenous T-cell populations.

N. GRANT:: I am curious about the mixture that you are using for the clinical studies. In fraction 5, you say you have at least 11 acidic proteins. Why haven't you fractionated them and given a single species or are they all required to obtain the clinical effect?

A.L. GOLDSTEIN: We hope to characterize each of these molecules. The partially purified thymosin fraction 5 was the first fraction that we felt (on the basis of our animal studies) contained all of the biological potency of the intact thymus gland. So it was the first one to be tested clinically. I think it is only a matter of time before we have enough of the purified thymosin to complete toxicity studies and initiate clinical trials with the purified hormone or hormones.

E.A. KABAT: Can you get thymosin out of any tissues other than thymus?

A. L. GOLDSTEIN: Yes, we have seen some activity in other tissues, like spleen and liver. The important point is that, pound for pound, there is more in the thymus than in any other tissue we have studied.

C. H. CHANG: : I have two questions. The first follows from Dr. Kabat's question. Can antibody against thymosin stand up to extensive adsorption by extracts of normal tissues other than thymus? Also, have you attempted to administrate anti-thymosin antibody to developing animals at various early stages to see if it causes any defect in the development of the immune response system?

A. L. GOLDSTEIN: The answer to your second question is no. With regard to your first question, we have recently raised an antibody to thymosin fraction 6 that is thymus specific and does not cross-react with other tissue extracts that we have studied.

B.B. LEVINE: In view of the amino acid composition have you tried the effect of polyglutamic acid or any other synthetic peptide in this system? Does it have a thymosin-like effect?

A. L. GOLDSTEIN: Perhaps Dr. Cohen can answer that question.

G. COHEN: We did try polyglutamate and polyaspartate in the MLR with negative results.

IMMUNOREGULATION BY T CELLS

RICHARD K. GERSHON

YALE UNIVERSITY, SCHOOL OF MEDICINE, DEPARTMENT OF PATHOLOGY

INTRODUCTION

As do most stories, the T cell story has two sides to it; these cells act to turn on immune responses and they also act to turn them off (1). This observation has led to the formulation of what has been called (only somewhat facetiously) "the second law of thymodynamics" which states that "for every helper T cell effect, there is an equal and opposite suppressor effect" (2). The law was formulated with "helper" preceding "suppressor" because, in most cases the discovery of helper effects preceded the discovery of suppression. Recently, some reports have appeared of T dependent suppression of immunological functions which were not previously thought to depend on T helper cells (3,4). The reciprocal of the "second law of thymodynamics" would predict that such helper functions exist. I would like to discuss the available evidence in support of this notion. In addition, I would like to discuss a corollary of the "second law" stated above: that those immune responses which do not require or utilize helper T cells do not require or utilize suppressor T cells for their regulation.

To begin, it would seem to be useful to briefly summarize those immunological situations in which suppressor T cells have been shown to play a regulatory role.

I. IMMUNOLOGICAL TOLERANCE

a. DIRECT: SUPPRESSION BY T CELLS

Certain states of acquired immunologic tolerance have been shown to be "infectious" in that cells from putatively tolerant animals can cause normal cells to become specifically unresponsive (6-17). This specific suppressor phenomenon is totally thymic dependent in both its inductive and effector phases. (Specific suppressor T cell effects have been demonstrated with cells from non-tolerant animals as well (18-27)). They are operative in high and low zone tolerance, affect antibody and cell-mediated responses, can be activated by soluble or particulate antigens, and can exhibit hapten or carrier specificities. Some investigators have been unable to show "infectious" suppression by mixing tolerant and normal cells which may suggest that suppressor T cells are not active in all types of tolerance (28,29). However, in one case where cells from tolerant animals failed to produce "infectious suppression" in mixture type experiments, it was also impossible to break tolerance by adoptive transfer of normal cells into the tolerant animals (28). Although the reasons for this failure were not determined, it is possible that suppressor cells were involved. For reasons not entirely clear it is always much easier to demonstrate suppression by transferring cells into a suppressive environment than by transferring the suppressor cells into a new or neutral environment (1,30,31).

b. INDIRECT: T CELL DEPENDENCE OF SPECIFIC B CELL UNRESPONSIVENESS

Presentation of antigen to B cells which are incapable of responding by antibody production, due to the removal of T cells, fails to induce a state of tolerance (27,32-36). In several instances the same antigen presentation produced a state of specific B cell unresponsiveness if T cells were present during the induction period (27,32,35,36). Although these results are compatible with the notion that B cell tolerance depends on suppressor T cell activity, there are a number of discordant results and complicating factors which may make such an interpretation hazardous. I will discuss this point in greater detail below (see 1-Thymus dependence of B cell differentiation).

II. ANTIGENIC COMPETITION

Antigenic competition, the phenomenon by which inoculation of one antigen non-specifically interferes with the subsequently induced immune response to a second antigen, has been shown to be thymus dependent (37-38). Thus, a modest reduction of an animal's T cell complement, which does not greatly affect its antibody response, can abrogate antigenic competition. This phenomenon, like immunological tolerance, was shown to be an active immunosuppressive event. Normal cells added to an animal in which antigenic competition is occurring become inactivated, and subjected to the milieu effect (31,37-39). Antibody production is not required for this effect, since passively administered antibody to the first (competing) antigen may inhibit antibody production against this antigen, while allowing the competitive event to occur undampened (40). It is important to emphasize that this non-specific thymus-dependent form of suppression has not been shown to be directly mediated by a T cell produced factor; the indirect participation of thymus dependent macrophages has been implicated in some cases (41). Further, it has not been conclusively demonstrated that the T cell (or the T dependent macrophage) makes a factor which is directly suppressive. Feldmann has suggested the possibility of an indirect suppression produced by the occupancy (saturation) of essential cooperating sites on macrophages by T cell helper factors, induced by and specific for the first antigen (42).

More recently, several new types of non-specific T cell dependent suppression have been described which are probably related to antigenic competition and which suggest that activated T cells do release factors which directly suppress other immunologically competent cells.

1. MITOGEN ACTIVATED T CELLS

Subpopulations of Con A activated T cells release a highly immunosuppressive factor (43-46). Studies of its mode of action make it seem highly unlikely that it works by blocking macrophages; there is a considerable latent period after it is added to culture before its suppressive effect is seen (46). Similar latencies have been noted in other studies on suppressor T cells (6,47-48). This delay in action of suppressor T cell factors could explain why transient immune responses are often seen during tolerance induction.

2. CULTURED T CELLS

Educated thymic T cells cultured for a 6-8 hour period with the specific antigen used for education acquire the ability to suppress the specific response of normal cells, as well as non-specific responses, if specific antigen is present (49). The "specific" effect of a non-specific suppressor cannot be explained by a macrophage saturation mechanism. Interestingly, during the 6-8 hour cultivation period the educated T cells release a specific cooperating factor into the supernatant. The relationship of the loss of this factor from the cultured cells to the appearance of the suppressors is unclear but appears to be a fruitful area for investigation. It has previously been suggested that suppressor activity can be masked by "contrasuppressor" activity (50). This may be a case where suppressor activity is unmasked by loss of contrasuppression.

3. SPLEEN SEEKING T CELLS

Splenic and thymic T cells which localize in the spleen can exert a pronounced suppressive effect on ongoing immune responses in the lymph nodes (2,47,51). T cells harvested from lymph nodes do not appear to have similar suppressive effects when they localize in the spleen, suggesting that this effect may be mediated by a distinct T cell subpopulation rather than being a microenvironmentally induced phenomenon (2,51). Another argument against microenvironmental induction is the ability of antigen activated splenic T cells to suppress <u>in vitro</u> responses, while lymph node T cells from the same animal help the response (52-54). This <u>in vitro</u> effect of splenic T cells appears to have the same specificity and induction requirements as the educated cultured T cells described above.

The observation that spleen seeking T cells exert immunosuppressive effects may be particularly revelent to <u>tumor immunology</u>. The immunosuppressive role of the spleen in the response to tumors has been well established, although the mechanism by which it exerts its immunosuppressive influence is unknown (reviewed in 55). Suppressor T cells have been shown to modulate the immune response to tumors (56-59). That they may be the important regulatory cells in the spleens of tumor bearing mice is suggested by the bidirectional nature of the splenic regulation; that is the effect of splenectomy on the immune response to a tumor graft depends to some extent on the size of the graft (60). (See section VII below on feedback regulation). Thus, the spleen has been shown to suppress the response to large tumor grafts and increase the response to smaller grafts.

III AUTOIMMUNITY

4. Monier and Allison have reviewed evidence suggesting that T cells may have a prophylactic role in prevention of autoimmune disease (61-63). In particular, T cell depletion may hasten and increase the appearance of autoantibodies and autoimmune diseases in some strains of mice, rats and chickens. Inoculations of normal T cells may delay or prevent their occurrence. In addition, spleen cells from

young but not older NZB mice may exert a suppressive effect on GVH responses (64). Older NZB mice are highly prone to develop autoimmune disease. Their thymic T cells have also been noted to be deficient in immuno regulatory functions (65). Lastly, it has recently been recognized that thymusless nude mice are particularly prone to develop autoantibodies (66-68).

IV CLASS SPECIFIC T CELL SUPPRESSION

Tada and his associates have reported that the homocytotrophic dinitrophenyl (DNP) antibody response of rats immunized with DNP-Ascaris could be increased by a number of maneuvers which deplete T cells (69-72). This enhanced response could be rapidly abrogated by the inoculation of thymocytes from syngeneic rats hyperimmunized to either Ascaris or DNP-Ascaris, whereas cells from rats hyperimmunized to DNP-bovine serum albumin (BSA) were without effect. These experiments virtually rule out antibody as a causative agent as the carrier (ascaris) immune cells were suppressive while anticarrier antibody was not. In addition, the same carrier specificity for T cell suppression was shown as had previously been shown for T cell help. Kishimoto and Ishizaka have shown similar class specific antibody suppression *in vitro* (73).

V AUGMENTATION OF THYMUS INDEPENDENT IMMUNE RESPONSES

There are some antigens which fail to activate any demonstrable helper T cell activity in normal animals (1,74). The immune response to these antigens can be augmented by a variety of means which reduce the T cell complement (75-76). The augmented response may be diminshed by restoration of thymocytes (76). These observations appear to be at odds with the "second law" I have discussed above, in that it would seem at first glance that there is a suppressor effect without a helper effect. I will discuss why I think this is not the case below. (See 4-Thymus dependence of immunoaugmentation produced by thymus deprivation).

VI CONTROL OF GENETICALLY DETERMINED IMMUNOLOGICAL UNRESPONSIVENESS

A gene or genes closely linked to those which determine histocompatibility has (have) been shown in a number of species to determine the capacity to make an immune response to certain well-defined antigens (77). In at least one such case, the basis for this form of specific immunological unresponsiveness has been shown to be that the T cells of non-responder animals have an inordinate propensity to become tolerant to the antigen in question (78). This form of tolerance in addition to the others detailed above has been shown to be governed by suppressor T cells (79).

VII FEEDBACK REGULATION

a) From T cells

T cells respond to antigen with a circumscribed period of DNA synthesis (80,81). The amount of DNA synthesized, as well as the duration of the period of DNA synthesis, is determined in part by regulatory interactions between the responding cells (47,81-84). Non-antigen responsive T cells may also regulate the response in a fashion which suggests that they recognize signals from the responding cells; that is the same population of non-antigen responsive regulatory cells can act to augment low responses and suppress higher responses (2,47,82-84).

b) From B cells

B cell products, in particular antibody, can both inhibit or augment immune responses (85). At least some of these regulatory functions are mediated indirectly by T cells (86), which seem to be able to sense the level of B cell activity and regulate the subsequent antibody response in a fashion quite similar to the way they regulate the response of other T cells (87).

VIII REGULATION OF NON-ANTIGEN INDUCED EVENTS

1. ALLOTYPE SUPPRESSION

Allotype suppression, in which exposure of the neonate to antibody against allotypic determinants on its own immunoglobulins suppresses production of those immunoglobulins, has been found to exhibit T cell dependence in some circumstances (3).

2. IMMUNOGLOBULIN PRODUCTION

Peripheral blood B cells from humans with common variable hypogammaglobulinemia fail to make significant amounts of any immunoglobulin when cultured with pokeweed mitogen, while cells from normal controls do (4). Mixtures of cells from different normal controls respond to pokeweed quite normally, while mixtures of normal and hypogammaglobulinemic cells fail to respond. The suppressing cell in the peripheral blood of the hypogammaglobulinemic patients was shown to have T cell characteristics.

It has also been shown that bone marrow cells from chickens rendered agammaglobulinemic by bursectomy and irradiation contain similar suppressor cells although their T cell origin is less well established in this case (88). It is of note however, that the richest source of allotype suppressor T cells is the mouse bone marrow (89). This may be related to the fact that the bone marrow is where the action is or, more interestingly, it may that there is a subpopulation of bone marrow seeking T cells with a special function of regulating B cell differentiation.

DISCUSSION

In the brief review I have presented above I raised 3 main points I would like to discuss in greater detail.

1. The apparent T cell dependence of B cell tolerance
2. Augmentation of the response to seemingly thymus independent antigens by T cell deprivation.
3. T cell regulation of non-antigen induced events

To relate these observations to the "second law of thymodynamics" and its corollary (see introduction) I offer the following set of hypotheses: (1) that non-antigen induced B cell differentiation is in part under T cell control; (2) that those B cells whose differentiation is not influenced by the thymus are less thymus dependent in both responsiveness and tolerance induction; (3) that there is no such thing as a thymus independent antigen and (4) that augmentation of responses to those antigens classically classed as thymus independent, by thymus deprivation, is thymus dependent.

1. THYMUS DEPENDENCE OF B CELL DIFFERENTIATION

There is as far as I know only one direct piece of published evidence in support of this contention. Cells and extracts from the thymus have been shown to significantly enhance non-specific immunoglobulin production of in vitro cultured bone marrow cells (90).

Indirect evidence comes from comparisons of bone marrow functions of nude thymusless mice with those of normal mice. When newborn mice are given large doses of anti-gamma M antibody they remain agammaglobulinemic as long as they continue to receive treatment (91). Almost immediately after the cessation of treatment normal mice start making immunoglobulin. It takes a considerably longer time for immunoglobulin to be produced after cessation of such treatment of nude mice (92).

Another indirect bit of evidence comes from studies attempting to induce tolerance in T deprived B cell populations. As I mentioned above (section I-b) several workers have failed to be able to do this. On the other hand it seems to be an easily accomplished phenomenon with standard antigens in nude mice. (It should be noted that some special antigens, like DNP conjugated to a polymer of dextrorotary amino acids (DNP‿DGL) (93) or conjugated to mouse immunoglobulin (94) or red blood cells (95) and injected into mice, seem to be able to induce direct B cell tolerance quite easily; these antigens are extremely weak immunogens). There are several possible explanations for this discrepancy. One which has been championed by Mitchell is that thymus-deprived mice contain some residual T cells (which they surely do) which act to prevent tolerance induction (96). This explanation is unlikely for the following reason. We gave thymus deprived mice up to 13 injections of 2×10^9 sheep red cells (SRBC) before reconstituting them with T cells without producing B cell tolerance (32,50). Mitchell produced B cell tolerance with one injection in nudes. Surely the first 12 injections of SRBC would have made the residual T cells of our thymus deprived mice tolerant and thus the basis for the difference in results would appear to reside in the B cell population.

2. THYMUS INDEPENDENT B CELLS

The argument that the difference in susceptibility to tolerance induction between nude and conventional thymus deprived mice is due to a B cell difference secondary to a thymic influence on bone marrow differentiation, implies the existence of sub-populations of B cells. There is evidence for the existence of a B cell line in conventional mice which both makes antibody, and becomes tolerant without T cell help (32,50). Tolerance induction in this B cell line does not diminish the thymus dependent response to the antigen in question, suggesting a functional difference in the two (thymus dependent and independent) B cell lines. Other evidence that these two B cell lines are different has been deduced by Playfair in limiting dilution type experiments (97). More recently Jennings and Rittenberg (personal communication) have shown that the antibody response to DNP of cultured mouse cells peaks at a certain antigen dose. When the optimal amount of DNP on a thymus dependent carrier is present, the addition of DNP on another thymus dependent carrier does not augment the response. However, when the DNP is added on a thymus independent carrier the anti-DNP response increases. In fact the thymus dependent and independent responses often are additive.

Thus, there is ample evidence to alert us to the possibility that there are sub-populations of B cells with different requirements for T cell help in both triggering and tolerance induction. The thymus independent B cell has been called B_1 and the dependent one B_2 (97). Other differences between B_1 and B_2 and evidence that B_1 precedes B_2 both phylo- and ontogenetically has been recently summarized (1). The new suggestion I am putting forth here is that the B_1 to B_2 maturation path is in part thymus dependent, both in normal differentiation and also when driven by exogenous antigen.

3. THYMUS INDEPENDENT ANTIGENS

The concept of a thymus independent B cell makes the term "thymus independent antigen" ambiguous. To some people the term implies that the immune response of normal animals to that antigen is devoid of a thymus dependent component. As has already been pointed out, some so-called thymus independent antigens (such as polymerized flagellin (POL)) are excellent stimulators of T cells and elicit a significant B_2 type response in normal but not in thymus-deprived animals. Thus this type of antigen is a good activator of both B_1 cells and T cells. Another type of "thymus independent antigen" such as the purified polysaccharide antigen of type III pneumococcus (SIII) elicits only a B_1 type of response in both normal and thymus deprived recipients. The majority of antigens lie in between these extremes, being less good stimulators of B_1 cells than POL and less poor stimulators of T cells (and/or B_2 cells) than SIII. Thus, thymus dependency applies directly to the type of B cells activated and only indirectly to the stimulating antigen.

There is an excellent reason why antigens like SIII should activate suppressor T cells and be good stimulators of B_1 cells (98). Polysaccharide antigens are heterophilic in nature and thus many strange cross reactions are seen with antibodies raised against them. Red blood cells are rich in these antigens and thus often react with so-called natural antibodies. Thus, if B_2 cells participated in the response to antigens like SIII mothers would tend to have IgG antibodies, which cross the placenta and react with the fetal red cells. One can easily see the survival value to the species in selecting a mechanism which prevents this from occurring. It apparently was easier to select for suppression of the B_2 response than against the presence of polysaccharide antigens on red cells. However, apparently there also is survival value to having antibodies directed against these antigens, which are also commonly found on pathogenic bacteria. This is probably one of the important reasons why the primitive B_1 response has remained with us; to help make 19 S antibodies which will not cross the placenta.

4. THYMUS DEPENDENCE OF IMMUNO-AUGMENTATION PRODUCED BY THYMUS DEPRIVATION

The reason that ALS treatment augments the response to SIII is almost certainly because reduction of the T cell complement decreases the action of suppressor T cells, allowing helper T cells whose activity is suppressed in normal animals, to boost the response (48). Thus, total thymus deprivation should prevent augmentation. It appears that this is what occurs since homozygous nude mice (Nu/Nu) and their heterozygous littermates which have a thymus (Nu/+) make the same magnitude response to SIII (99). After ALS treatment, which eliminates recirculating T cells (T_2)(100), the SIII response of the Nu/+ mice is markedly enhanced while the response of the Nu/Nu mice is unchanged (99). Should anyone care to interpret this observation as indicating that T_2 cells act as suppressors of a more sessile (T_1) helper, I remind them that reconstitution of ALS treated mice with lymph node cells (which is a source rich in T_2 cells) furthur augments the response while reconstitution with thymus (T_1) cells is suppressive (76). It is most likely that a complex series of interactions between several T cell subpopulations determines whether the net outcome will be suppression or help (see section VII above). More direct evidence for the existence of SIII specific helper cells has recently been presented (101). In any case this appears to be an instance where the discovery of a suppressor effect preceded the discovery of a helper effect and not a contradiction of the "second law of thymodynamics".

Relation to genetic control

A situation which seems to be similar to the response to SIII in all mice occurs in mice with the $H-2^k$ haplotype in their response to a synthetic amino acid polymer, (T,G)-A--L. These mice have no thymus-dependent component in their response to this antigen (102). In addition, an ongoing graft versus host response (GVHR) greatly augments the primary response (103). This GVHR augmentation of a primary response, "allogeneic effect" (104), also works on the SIII response (105) but not on the primary response to antigens which activate helper T cells (106). The lack of a thymic dependent response in another system (GAT as antigen in mice with the $H-2^q$ haplotype) regulated by so-called Ir genes has been shown to be due to suppressor T cell activity, as mentioned above, although it has not yet shown for the (T,G)-A--L system. Also, very recent evidence indicates that GAT specific helper cells can be raised in non-responder mice, by the same techniques which raise SIII helper cells (107,108). If the (T,G)-A--L and GAT systems prove to be analogous the response to SIII in any mouse and the response to (T,G)-A--L in mice with the $H-2^k$ haplotype will also be analogous. Thus, the genetic requirements for stimulation of B_1 and B_2 cells will probably turn out to be another distinguishing difference between these types of B cells.

Since the B_1 response to SIII of mice with a normal complement of T cells is no different than that of their thymusless counterparts, it seems probable that suppressor T cells do not play a major role in B_1 regulation. There is evidence for thymus independent regulation of the thymus independent response to (T,G)-A--L (109). Thus if C3H mice are immunized with (T,G)-A--L on day 0, and lethally irradiated and reconstituted with normal spleen cells on day 7, the newly inoculated spleen cells cannot respond to furthur immunization with (T,G)-A--L. The same spleen cells respond quite well if the (T,G)-A--L immunization is omitted on day 0. Thymus deprivation of the hosts does not in anyway diminish the specific radiation resistant suppressive environment induced by the (T,G)-A--L immunization, nor does removal of the T cells from the added spleen cells reduce their ability to be suppressed. We are at present testing whether this thymus independent regulation alters the response of the thymus dependent response to (T,G)-A--L conjugated to methylated BSA.

In summary, I am suggesting that those immunological functions which are initiated or helped by T cells are not abandoned by the T cell once they get going. They remain under T cell control and their shutoff is as thymus dependent as is the other aspects of their response. In addition there are components of the immune response which turn on and shut off without T cell help.

I hope the evidence I have marshalled in defense of the "second law of thymodynamics--that for every helper T cell effect there is an opposing suppressor effect" will serve as a useful framework from which a better understanding of T cell regulation may be forthcoming. I certainly hope that I have not generated sufficient heat to drive the story of T cell regulation to one of maximum chaos and thus lay the foundations for a "third law of thymodynamics".

REFERENCES

(1) R.K. Gershon, in: Contemporary Topics in Immunobiology vol. 3, eds, M.D. Cooper and N. Warner (Plenum Press, New York, 1974) p. 1.

(2) R.K. Gershon, in: The Immune System: Genes, Receptors, Signals, eds. E. Sercarz, A. Williamson and C.F. Fox (Academic Press, New York 1974) p. 471.

(3) L.A. Herzenberg, and L.A. Herzenberg, in: Contemporary Topics in Immunobiology, vol. 3, eds. M.D. Cooper and N. Warner (Plenum Press, New York 1974) p. 41.

(4) T.A. Waldmann, M. Durm, S. Broder, M. Blackman,

R.M. Blaese, and W. Strober, Lancet, II (1974) 609.
(5) R.K. Gershon, and K. Kondo, Immunology 21 (1971) 903.
(6) P.J. McCullagh, J. Exp. Med. 132 (1970) 916.
(7) M. Zembala, and G.L. Asherson, Nature 244 (1973) 227.
(8) G. Weber, and E. Kolsch, Eur. J. Immunol. 3 (1973) 767.
(9) G.L. Ada, and M.G. Cooper, in: Immunological Tolerance: Mechanisms and Potential Therapeutic Applications, eds. D.H. Katz and B. Benacerraf (Academic Press, New York 1974) p. 87.
(10) P. Baker, P.W. Stashak, D.F. Amsbaugh, and B. Prescott, J. Immunol. 112 (1974) 2020.
(11) A. Basten, J.F.A.P. Miller, J. Sprent, and C. Cheers, J. Exp. Med. 140 (1974) 199.
(12) H.N. Claman, T. Phanuphak, and J.W. Moorhead, in: Immunological Tolerance: Mechanisms and Potential Therapeutic Applications, eds. D.H. Katz and B. Benacerraf (Academic Press, New York 1974) p. 123.
(13) R. Huchet and M. Feldmann, Eur. J. Immunol. 4 (1974) 768.
(14) B.H. Waksman, in: Immunological Tolerance: Mechanisms and Potential Therapeutic Applications, eds. D.H. Katz and B. Benacerraf (Academic Press, New York 1974) p. 431.
(15) B.T. Rouse and N.L. Warner, J. Immunol. 113 (1974) 904.
(16) I. Zan-Bar, D. Nachtigal, and M. Feldmann, Cell Immunol. 10 (1974) 19 (and personal communication).
(17) R. Zinkernagel and P. Doherty in: Immunological Tolerance: Mechanisms and Potential Therapeutic Applications, eds. D.H. Katz and B. Benacerraf (Academic Press, New York 1974) p. 403.
(18) W. Droege, Current Titles in Immunology, Transplantation and Allergy 1, (1973) 95 and 131.
(19) W. Droege, in: The Immune System: Genes, Receptors, Signals, eds. E. Sercarz, A. Williamson and C.F. Fox (Academic Press, New York 1974) p. 431.
(20) M. Feldmann, Nature New Biol. 242 (1973) 84.
(21) M. Feldmann, Eur. J. Immunol. 4 (1974) 660.
(22) M. Feldmann, Eur. J. Immunol. 4 (1974) 667.
(23) T.Y. Ha, and B.H. Waksman, J. Immunol. 110 (1973) 1290.
(24) K. Okumura, and T. Tada, Nature New Biol. 245 (1973) 180.
(25) T. Tada, in Immunological Tolerance: Mechanisms and Potential Therapeutic Applications, eds. D.H. Katz and B. Benacerraf (Academic Press, New York 1974) p. 471.
(26) C.J. Elson and R.B. Taylor, Eur. J. Immunol. 4 (1974) 682.
(27) H. Waldmann, and A.J. Munro, Eur. J. Immunol. 4 (1974) 410.

(28) J.M. Chiller and W.O. Weigle, J. Immunol. 110 (1973) 1051.
(29) D.W. Scott, in: Immunological Tolerance: Mechanisms Potential Therapeutic Applications, eds. D.H. Katz and B. Benacerraf (Academic Press, New York 1974) p.503.
(30) J.M. Dwyer, and F.S. Kantor, J. Exp. Med. 137 (1973) 32.
(31) R.H. Waterston, Science 170 (1970) 1108.
(32) R.K. Gershon, and K. Kondo, Immunology 18 (1970) 723.
(33) G.E. Roelants and B.A. Askonas, Nature New Biol. 239 (1973) 63.
(34) J.M. Davie and W.E. Paul, J. Immunol. 113 (1974) 1439.
(35) J.M. Phillips-Quagliata, D.O. Bensinger, and F. Quagliata, J. Immunol. 111 (1973) 1712.
(36) R.B. Taylor and C.J. Elson, in: Immunological Tolerance: Mechanisms and Potential Therapeutic Applications, eds. D.H. Katz and B. Benacerraf (Academic Press, New York 1974) p. 203.
(37) R.K. Gershon, and K. Kondo, J. Immunol. 106 (1971) 1524.
(38) J-C Monier, Controle par le Thymus et les Cellules T., des Phenomenes D'Auto-Immunisation et de Competition Antigenique (Ediprim, Lyon 1972).
(39) J.S. Menkes, R.S. Hencin, and R.K. Gershon, J. Immunol. 109 (1972) 1052.
(40) R.K. Gershon, and K. Kondo, J. Immunol. 106 (1971) 1532.
(41) O. Sjoberg, Clin. Exp. Immunol. 12 (1972) 365.
(42) M. Feldmann, J. Exp. Med. 136 (1972) 737.
(43) R.W. Dutton, J. Exp. Med. 136 (1972) 1445.
(44) R.R. Rich, and C.W. Pierce, J. Exp. Med. 137 (1973) 649.
(45) R.W. Dutton, J. Exp. Med. 138 (1973) 1496.
(46) R.R. Rich and C.W. Pierce, J. Immunol. 112 (1974) 1360.
(47) R.K. Gershon, E.M. Lance, and K. Kondo, J. Immunol. 112 (1974) 546.
(48) P.J. Baker, B. Prescott, P.W. Stashak, D.F. Amsbaugh in: The Immune System: Genes, Receptors, Signals, eds. E. Sercarz, A. Williamson and C.F. Fox (Academic Press, New York 1974) p. 415.
(49) M.J. Taussig, Nature 248 (1974) 236.
(50) R.K. Gershon, in: Immunological Tolerance: Mechanisms and Potential Therapeutic Applications, eds. D.H. Katz and B. Benacerraf (Academic Press, New York 1974)p.441.
(51) C-Y. Wu, and E.M. Lance, Cell. Immunol. 13 (1974) 1.
(52) H. Folch and B.H. Waksman, J. Immunol. (1974) 127.
(53) H. Folch and B.H. Waksman, J. Immunol. (1974) 140.
(54) S.S. Rich and R.R. Rich, J. Exp. Med. 140 (1974) 1588.
(55) R.K. Gershon, Isr. J. Med. Sci. 10 (1974) 1012.

(56) J.M. Kirkwood and R.K. Gershon, Prog. Exp. Tumor Res. 19 (1974) 757.
(57) A.J. Treves, C. Carnaud, N. Trainin, M. Feldmann and I.R. Cohen, Eur. J. Immunol. 4 (1974) 722.
(58) T. Umiel and N. Trainin, Transplantation 18 (1974) 244.
(59) A. Schwartz and R.K. Gershon (in preparation).
(60) J.J. Nordlund and R.K. Gershon, J. Immunol. In Press.
(61) J-C. Monier, Controle par le Thymus et les Cellules T., des Phenomenes d'Auto-Immunisation et de Competition Antigenique (Ediprim, Lyon 1972).
(62) A.C. Allison, in: Contemporary Topics in Immunobiology vol. 3, eds. M.D. Cooper and N. Warner (Plenum Press, New York 1974) p. 227.
(63) A.C. Allison, in: Immunological Tolerance: Mechanisms and Potential Therapeutic Applications, eds. D.H. Katz and B. Benacerraf (Academic Press, New York 1974)p. 25.
(64) J.A. Hardin, T.M. Chused, and A.D. Steinberg, J. Immunol. 111 (1973) 650.
(65) M.J. Dauphinee, and N. Talal, Proc. Nat. Acad. Sci. 70 (1973) 3769.
(66) E.M. Pantelouris, Proc. 1st Int. Workshop on Nude Mice eds. J. Pygaard and C.O. Poolsen. (Fisher Verlag, Stuttgart 1974) p. 235.
(67) J-C. Monier, M. Sepetjian, J.C. Czyba, J.P. Ortonne, and J. Thivolet, Proc. 1st Int. Workshop on Nude Mice eds. J. Pygaard and C.O. Poolsen. (Fisher Verlag, Stuttgart 1974) p. 243.
(68) L. Morel-Maroger and J-C. Salomon, Proc. 1st Int. Workshop on Nude Mice eds. J. Pygaard and C.O. Poolsen. (Fisher Verlag, Stuttgart 1974) p. 251.
(69) T. Tada, M. Taniguchi, and K. Okumura, J. Immunol. 106 (1971) 1012.
(70) T. Taniguchi, and T. Tada, J. Immunol. 107 (1971) 579.
(71) L. Okumura, and T. Tada, J. Immunol. 106 (1971) 1019.
(72) L. Okumura, and T. Tada, J. Immunol. 107 (1971) 1682.
(73) T. Kishimoto and K. Ishizaka, J. Immunol. 112 (1974) 1685.
(74) J. Kruger, and R.K. Gershon, J. Immunol. 108 (1972) 581.
(75) R.S. Kerbel, and D. Eidinger, Eur. J. Immunol. 2 (1972) 114.
(76) P.J. Baker, P.W. Stashak, D.F. Amsbaugh, B. Prescott, and R.J. Barth, Immunology 105 (1970) 1581.
(77) B. Benacerraf, and H.O. McDevitt, Science 175 (1972) 273.
(78) R.K. Gershon, P.H. Maurer, and C.F. Merryman, Proc. Nat. Acad. Sci. 70 (1973) 250.
(79) B. Benacerraf, J.A. Kapp, and C.W. Pierce, in:

Immunological Tolerance: Mechanisms and Potential Therapeutic Applications, eds. D.H. Katz and B. Benacerraf (Academic Press, New York 1974) p. 507.
(80) A.J.S. Davies, Transpl. Rev. 1 (1969) 43.
(81) R.K. Gershon and S.A. Liebhaber, J. Exp. Med. 136 (1972) 112.
(82) R.K. Gershon, P. Cohen, R. Hencin, and S.A. Liebhaber, J. Immunol. 108 (1972) 586.
(83) R.K. Gershon, S.A. Liebhaber, and S. Ryu, Immunology 26 (1974) 909.
(84) R.K. Gershon, in: Immunological Tolerance: Mechanisms and Potential Therapeutic Applications, eds. D.H. Katz and B. Benacerraf (Academic Press, New York 1974)p.413.
(85) J.W. Uhr and G. Moller, Adv. Immunol. 8 (1968) 81.
(86) R.K. Gershon, M.S. Mitchell, and M.B. Mokyr, Nature 250 (1974) 594.
(87) R.K. Gershon, S. Orbach-Arbouys and C. Calkins, Proc. 2nd Int. Cong. Immunology. In Press.
(88) R.M. Blaese, P.L. Weiden, I. Koski and N. Dooley, J. Exp. Med. 140 (1974) 1097.
(89) L.A. Herzenberg and C.M. Metzler, in: Immunological Tolerance: Mechanisms and Potential Therapeutic Applications, eds. D.H. Katz and B. Benacerraf (Academic Press, New York 1974) p. 519.
(90) K. Okumura, S. Nobukata and M. Kern, J. Immunol. 113 (1974) 2027.
(91) A.R. Lawton and M.D. Cooper, in: Contemporary Topics in Immunobiology, vol. 3 eds. M.D. Cooper and N. Warner (Plenum Press, New York 1974) p. 193.
(92) D.D. Manning and J.W. Jutila, Cell Immunol. 14 (1974) 453.
(93) D.H. Katz, in: Immunological Tolerance: Mechanisms and Potential Therapeutic Applications, eds. D.H. Katz and B. Benacerraf (Academic Press, New York 1974)p. 189.
(94) Y. Borel and M. Aldo-Benson, in: Immunological Tolerance: Mechanisms and Potential Therapeutic Applications, eds. D.H. Katz and B. Benacerraf (Academic Press, New York 1974) p. 333.
(95) J.A. Hamilton, J.F.A.P. Miller and J. Kettman, Eur. J. Immunol. 4 (1974) 268.
(96) G.F. Mitchell, in: Immunological Tolerance: Mechanisms and Potential Therapeutic Applications, eds. D.H. Katz and B. Benacerraf (Academic Press, New York 1974) p. 283.
(97) J.H.L. Playfair, Nature New Biol. 231 (1971) 149.
(98) P.E. Byfield (personal communication).
(99) P.J. Baker, W.H. Burns, B. Prescott, P.W. Stashak and

D.F. Amsbaugh, in: Immunological Tolerance: Mechanisms and Potential Therapeutic Applications, eds. D.H. Katz and B. Benacerraf (Academic Press, New York 1974)p. 493.
(100)M.C. Raff, and H. Cantor, in: Progress in Immunology ed. B. Amos (Academic Press, New York 1971) p. 83.
(101)H. Braley-Mullen, J. Immunol. 113 (1974) 1909.
(102)G.F. Mitchell, F.C. Grumet and H.O. McDevitt, J. Exp. Med. 135 (1972) 126.
(103)J. Ordal and F.C. Grumet, J. Exp. Med. 136 (1972) 1195.
(104)D.H. Katz, W.E. Paul, E.A. Goidl, and B. Benacerraf, J. Exp. Med. 133 (1971) 169.
(105)P.E. Byfield, G.H. Christie and J.G. Howard, J. Immunol. 111 (1973) 72.
(106)D.H. Katz, Transpl. Rev. 12 (1972) 141.
(107)J.A. Kapp, C.W. Pierce and B. Benacerraf, Proc. 9th Leukocyte Culture Conf. (Academic Press, New York) In Press.
(108)R.K. Gershon, P.H. Maurer and C. Merryman (in preparation).
(109)J. Ordal, S. Smith, F.C. Grumet and R.K. Gershon (in preparation).

ACKNOWLEDGEMENTS

My research has been funded by USPHS grants CA-08593 from the NCI and AI 10497 from the NIAID. I am also pleased to acknowledge the contributions of my many colleagues who helped in the work reported, who are annotated in the references.

DISCUSSION

A.L. GOLDSTEIN: I have two questions with regard to the model in which you looked at the effects of spleenectomy on survival of mice given a tumor challenge with large and small tumor loads. If you get rid of your short-lived T-cells by adult thymectomy what do you see? Secondly, have you given back to your spleenectomized animals spleen cells, spleen grafts or irradiated spleen,or spleen stroma? In other words is the regulation you see due to a humoral factor being elicited by the spleen or is it due to a cellular event?

R. K. GERSHON: Adult thymectomy has produced some interesting effects. We don't have enough data to tell you precisely what it does but I can tell you that it does not act as spleenectomy does. Second, putting back cells taken from the spleen is a difficult type of experiment to do. If you fractionate the cells by putting them into an irradiated animal and retrieve the cells that migrate to the spleen, the spleen seeking T-cells go to the liver and gut rather than to another immunological organ when put into a spleenectomized animal. I think a good idea, as you suggest, is putting in spleen grafts. Bob Taub has done some very interesting work with spleen grafts but he has not reported the bi-directional effects we find; he finds that spleen grafting is a very immunosuppressive event.

R. W. LONGTON: The evidence you have presented suggests that there may be two regulating sites on the membrane, one which activates and the other which suppresses T-cell activity.

R. K. GERSHON: Yes, that is a possibility and I have thought about it. However, I know of no definitive evidence for or against it. It is rather difficult evidence to get until one has the appropriate molecules in hand. An alternative possibility is that a single receptor may have a different allosteric response to simple amino acid changes in the molecule that is coming to the cell. One could have an Fc fragment, let us say of IgT, in which a simple amino acid change results in a change of signal from go to stop.

C. BELL: I was interested in your speculation that there might be cell help in T-independent antigens, for instance in the SIII polysaccharide response. I believe that an immunoregulation must exist and operate to control the level of response to the T-independent antigens but that the regulatory event, and perhaps the immunoregulators, are different from these involved in the response of T-dependent antigens. What activators besides T-cell help, which is apparently not required in B-cell activation by strict T-independent antigens, will be required to give an IgG response. My second question pertains to suppression effects noted in responses of B-cell to T-independent antigen or high concentration of mitogen. Since you can not have T-cell dependent suppressor effects, what is the mechanism operative in this kind of suppression?

R. K. GERSHON: I'll answer your second question first. I made the point that T-independent responses are T-independently regulated. We havn't worked on the response to S III but we have worked on the thymus independent response to TGAL and shown non-T suppressor cells which shut off the response to TGAL very nicely. No one has shown that the presence of T-cells diminishes in any way the T-independent response. Since the thymus seems to be a late comer in the immune response and those systems that evolved prior to the thymus were already very well regulated, it may be only those systems which developed in the post-thymic period that require the thymus to be initiated and are T-cell regulated. The answer to the first question is that if you immunize appropriately so that you get helper cells to S III, then you will get a very nice IgG response. I also should mention that the elegant experiments of Kapp, Pierce and Benacerraf, and also some experiments that we did with Merryman and Maurer, show that if non-responder mice (to the antigen GAT) are immunized with the GAT on methylated bovine serum albumin a sufficient number of times then GAT specific helper cells appear in these non-responder animals.

M.M. SIGEL: I was under the impression that ALS in Phil Baker's work did in fact increase the response to S III. Didn't you just say that there was no T-cell regulation with this antigen?

R. K. GERSHON: Well Baker's interpretation and mine, and this is another point I was trying to make, is that ALS augments the response because it allows the helper T-cell to work. If you give too much ALS you don't augment the response. If you give ALS to a T-deprived animal you don't augment the response. A totally T-deprived animal and a normal animal make the same response, it is only a partially T-deprived animal that makes an increased response. There has been a tremendous controversy for at least three years between Baker and James Howard in England. Howard doesn't get any increase in the S III response by thymus deprivation. That's probably because he takes away all the T-cells. If he would just partially thymus deprive his animal he might get the augmented response.

E. W. LAMON: You indicated briefly that T-cells could become suppressor cells in the presence of antigen-antibody complexes in antibody excess. I wonder if there is a situation where you can rigorously rule out the participation of antibody binding by an FC receptor to the T-cell. For example, if you took a T-suppressor population and depleted it of B-cells and then protease treated the cells, do they maintain their suppressor functions?

R. K. GERSHON: I haven't tried that. In our studies all the mixtures were done together. If antibody is added to a population of memory T-cells, the memory makes the T-cells refractory to antibody mediated- as well as T-cell mediated-suppression. That is, memory T-cells will respond to antigen at a level of antibody that normal T-cells will not. If now normal T-cells are added they wipe out the response of the memory T-cells. If you take away the antibody and then add normal T-cells, they help the response. Do you follow?

E. W. LAMON: Yes, but I don't think you answered the question.

M.M. SIGEL: To answer your point, experiments in our laboratory indicate that complexes of IgM antibody, but not IgG, and antigen will turn off T-lymphyocytes in cell mediated reactions as determined by stimulation with PHA.

E. W. LAMON: They will turn off the lymphocytes?

M.M. SIGEL: Yes, inhibit lymphocyte responses.

E. W. LAMON: That's interesting because we have evidence in our lab that IgM coated tumor cells will induce thymus cells to be cytotoxic.

R. K. GERSHON: I tried to show this bi-directional regulation and to point out that if you want to skew the system to help or to suppress you have to do the particular maneuver which will help one or the other. One of the important things is to determine what the maneuvers are and this is why I suggest that there really isn't a suppressor T-cell; there is a cell which responds to a number of things including the molecular nature of the antigen; when all these things come together the T-cell decides whether to suppress or help.

A. GHAFFAR: Am I right in thinking that there was a contradiction in your two answers to the suppression of polysaccharide response. On the one hand you said that thymus independent antigens are not regulated by T-cells ---

R. K. GERSHON: There is a B-1 type of cell which will respond to any antigen without T-cell help and this cell is regulated without T-cell participation. There is another type of B-cell (B-2) which makes high affinity antibody of the gamma G type; this cell will not respond to any antigen without T-cell help and it is the response that is T-cell regulated. Ordinarily S III stimulates only B-1 cells because it also stimulates suppressor T-cells which suppress helper T-cells. When you eliminate a few T-cells then you get T-cell help, and you get a B-2 response to S III.

A. GHAFFAR: As far as I remember, Baker demonstrated an enhancement of IgM response rather than enhancement of any other class. James Howard has tried his best to get an IgA or IgG subclass response to pneumococcal polysaccharide, but he has not succeeded in demonstrating any response other than IgM. We have tried to repeat Baker's work but we have not been able to show any enhancement with anti-lymphocytic globulin. However, one does get some enhancement with the whole anti-serum, which is rather peculiar.

R. K. GERSHON: Your reporting of Baker's work is not precisely correct. He does get IgG responses. Secondly he has found that if you take away too many T-cells you do not get any augmentation. In your work in James' lab, in which you use ALS to get rid of T-cells, you probably have too few T-cells. If you were to use less ALS, and use it the way Phil Baker does, you would probably get augmentation. People have now obtained augmentation of the S III response by means that produced partial T-cell depletion other than by using ALS. Furthermore, Baker has shown that when he takes animals that have been partially T-cell deprived and adds back to them more T-cells of a certain type he increases the response. The effect depends on which T-cell he adds.

A. GHAFFAR: This is what is surprising. Thymus is the main organ from which Baker gets his suppressor T-cells and yet the removal of the thymus does not cause an increase in the immune response to polysaccharide. With regard to your comment about getting rid of all the T-cells - we have tried several ALG preparations down to a dilution of 1:100 but were unable to increase the immune response to the polysaccharide using the globulin preparation. When we do obtain an enhancement with ALS it can not be suppressed by the administration of thymocytes.

R. K. GERSHON: I have one comment. You are not unique in being amongst those people who have looked for suppressor effects and have been unable to find them. I think only time will tell whether or not they are really there or whether you just can't find them.

CONTROL OF GROWTH OF MAMMALIAN CELLS

ROBERT W. HOLLEY and IAN S. TROWBRIDGE
The Salk Institute
Post Office Box 1809
San Diego, California 92112

Abstract: Factors that control the initiation of DNA synthesis in mouse embryo 3T3 cells and in small lymphocytes are reviewed. It is concluded that a wide variety of different substances can be active. Many of these substances presumably act on the cell membrane. The possible roles of cyclic nucleotides and membrane properties are discussed.

Mouse Embryo 3T3 Cells

The growth of 3T3 cells in culture is dependent on serum (1). The cell density attained is proportional to the serum concentration in the culture medium, even up to concentrations in excess of 30% serum (1). The high serum requirement of these cells is responsible for their low saturation density, and it is this property that has drawn attention to 3T3 cells as having a controlled, "normal" growth behavior. A high serum requirement is probably representative of only certain aspects of normal growth, but it does provide an opportunity to study serum factors that can control growth.

Studies of the growth regulatory functions of serum with 3T3 cells have indicated that the functions are complex (2, 3). Serum factors are required for "survival", for initiation of DNA synthesis and for continued growth.

The serum factors that are required for the initiation of DNA synthesis are of particular interest because of the key role that initiation of DNA synthesis plays in growth. The serum requirement of the cells is highest during that part of the cell cycle prior to the initiation of DNA synthesis. Lowering the serum concentration in the medium, to 0.2% for example, arrests the growth of even sparse 3T3 cells in the G_1 (or G_o) phase of the cell cycle. Raising the serum concentration reinitiates DNA synthesis and growth.

Fractionation of serum has shown that a combination of at least four different serum factors is required to replace serum in stimulating the initiation of DNA synthesis in quiescent 3T3 cells (3). Three of the four serum fractions can be replaced by pure materials (3). The pure factors are: (a) the fibroblast growth factor (FGF) of Gospodarowicz, a new hormone isolated from pituitary glands and brain (4, 5), (b) insulin, and (c) a glucocorticoid such as hydrocortisone or dexamethasone. Interactions between the pure factors are shown in Fig. 1. The presence of a low concentration of one factor, for example FGF, greatly increases the activity of a second factor, insulin, and vice versa.

The same combination of four factors promotes the initiation of DNA synthesis both in sparse quiescent 3T3 cells and in confluent quiescent cells, the former in fresh low serum medium and the latter in high serum that has been depleted by growth of the cells (3). This indicates that quiescent 3T3 cells are subject to the same growth controls whether the cells are sparse or confluent.

Requirements for the different factors appear to vary with the cell culture conditions and with the particular 3T3 cell clone. In our experience, a variety of 3T3 cell clones respond to the four factors. By varying the culture conditions and the cell clone, one can observe initiation of DNA synthesis by one or a combination of these factors. The quantitative differences observed between the different 3T3 cell clones may be due to differences in the expression or

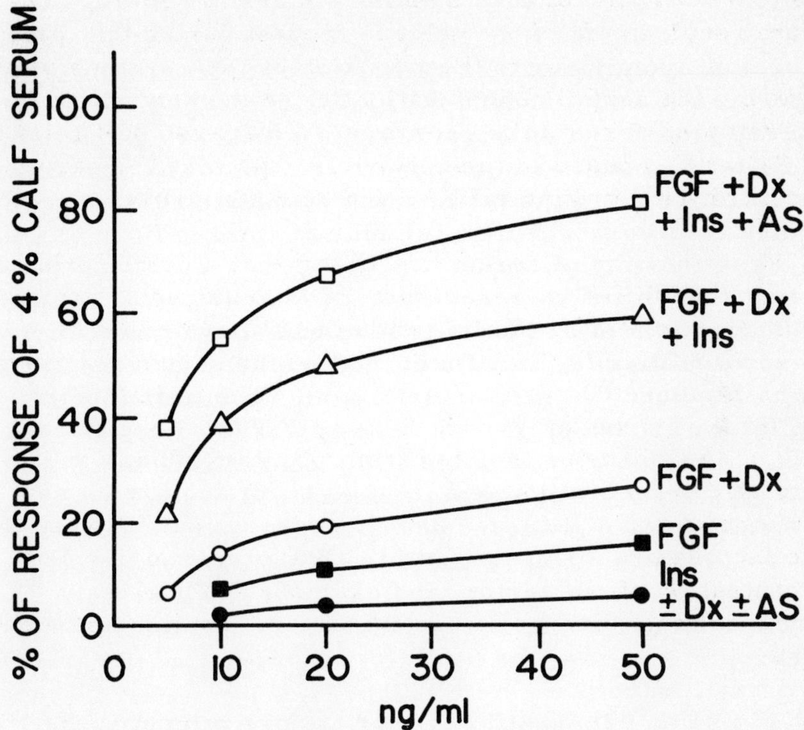

Fig. 1. Initiation of DNA synthesis by known factors. The figure gives the percentage replacement of 4% calf serum achieved by: (solid circles) insulin, either alone or with added dexamethasone and/or heated ammonium sulfate fraction of mouse serum; (solid squares) varying concentrations of FGF alone; (open circles) varying concentrations of FGF plus 0.4 μg/ml dexamethasone; (open triangles) FGF plus 50 ng/ml insulin plus 0.4 μg/ml dexamethasone; (squares) FGF plus 50 ng/ml insulin plus 0.4 μg/ml dexamethasone plus 0.2 mg/ml protein from the heated (10 min at 100°) 50-70% ammonium sulfate fraction of mouse serum. (From ref. 3.)

affinities of hormone binding sites, to differences in the retention or destruction of hormones, or to still other causes.

The stimulation of 3T3 cells by a combination of factors (FGF, insulin and a glucocorticoid) is similar to the stimulation of growth and differentiation of mammary gland cells by prolactin, insulin and glucocorticoid (6, 7, 8). There are also similarities to the factors that stimulate DNA synthesis in chick embryo fibroblasts (9) and rat embryo fibroblasts (10), as well as other cells.

The growth of 3T3 cells is also subject to control by the concentrations of certain of the common nutrients in the culture medium. In medium with a high concentration of serum, the growth of the cells can be arrested in the G_1 (or G_0) phase of the cell cycle if the concentrations of amino acids or glucose or phosphate are reduced to low levels in the medium (11). A subsequent increase in the concentration of the nutrient that is limiting leads to the re-initiation of DNA synthesis and growth. Results in the literature (cf. 12, 13) suggest that many different low molecular weight nutrients have the potential of controlling the growth of mammalian cells.

Preliminary information is available on the actions of the various factors that control the growth of 3T3 cells. Both FGF and insulin stimulate movement of 3T3 cells on the surface to which the cells are attached (Holley and Klinger, unpublished). Combination of FGF and insulin, especially with the further addition of the other two factors required for maximum DNA synthesis, gives the greatest stimulation of movement.

FGF and insulin also stimulate the uptake of low molecular weight nutrients by the cells (11). Again a combination of factors is most active (Hilborn, unpublished).

FGF has been found to increase the activity of guanylate cyclase in isolated vesicles prepared from 3T3 cell plasma membranes and insulin lowers the activity of adenylate cyclase (14). These effects are consistent with the observed rise in the intracellular concentration of cyclic GMP and fall in cyclic AMP in quiescent 3T3 cells immediately after the intact cells are stimulated by serum (15).

It is also of interest that immediately after G_1-arrested cells are stimulated to grow by the addition of a nutrient the intracellular concentration of cyclic GMP rises and that of cyclic AMP fall in these cells. This has been observed with quiescent 3T3 cells that have been arrested in G_1 (or G_0) by limitation of phosphate or amino acids in the medium (16). Apparently growth control by limitation of low molecular weight nutrients also involves changes in intracellular cyclic nucleotide levels.

Lymphocytes

The small lymphocytes of the peripheral lymphoid tissues are non-dividing cells arrested in the G_1 (or G_0) phase of the cell cycle. The molecular details of the initiation of growth of these cells can be studied in vitro since primary lymphocyte cultures can be induced to synthesize DNA, divide and differentiate by exposure to a variety of nonspecific mitogens (17). This provides a simple system for study, since the mitogens act in the absence of serum (18). Calcium ions appear to be essential for mitogenesis (19).

The biochemical events that occur when lymphocytes respond to mitogen stimulation are strikingly similar to those that take place following the initiation of growth in 3T3 cells. Within an hour after stimulation, increases in the transport of glucose (20, 21), amino acids (21-23), phosphate (24), calcium (19, 21, 25), and potassium ions (26, 27) can be detected.

One of the earliest metabolic changes after lymphocytes are stimulated by mitogens is a rapid, transient increase in the intracellular concentration of cyclic GMP (28). Within twenty minutes after exposure to mitogen the intracellular level of cyclic GMP increases to a value at least ten-fold higher than that found in resting cells. Within another thirty minutes the intracellular cyclic GMP level in stimulated lymphocytes falls to less than three-fold higher than in unstimulated cells but does not decline further during the next twenty-four hours (29). Most recent studies show that, in contrast to cyclic GMP, the intracellular level of cyclic AMP remains relatively unchanged after mitogen stimulation.

The prolonged modest increase in intracellular cyclic GMP levels, observed after stimulation of lymphocytes as well as mouse embryo 3T3 cells, may resolve the paradox that although the maximum increase in cyclic GMP levels is transient, removal of mitogen four hours after initial stimulation results in a complete inhibition of mitogenesis and even after ten to eighteen hours partial inhibition of the mitogenic response (30-34). It may be that continued exposure to mitogen is required to maintain the small long-term increase in intracellular cyclic GMP concentration, and that this may be essential for the mitogenic response.

Although presently no evidence is available, it is tempting to speculate, by analogy with the effects of serum and FGF on fibroblasts, that mitogens increase intracellular cyclic GMP levels in stimulated lymphocytes by activation of a guanylate cyclase located in the lymphocyte plasma membrane.

From a comparison of the metabolic changes that occur in lymphocytes and fibroblasts after stimulation, it seems that all cells may share a common pathway leading to the initiation of DNA synthesis and that the differences between differentiated cells in their response to various growth stimuli lies in the way in which they recognize and respond to external signals received at their cell membranes. Because lymphocytes respond to purified plant lectins with well-characterized molecular structures and known sugar-binding specificities, lectin-induced lymphocyte mitogenesis is a particularly favorable system in which to study the translation of an external stimulus into the intracellular metabolic changes that culminate in the initiation of growth. Even with these inherent advantages it is clear from the present rate of progress that more information is needed about the structure and properties of the lymphocyte plasma membrane. Some pertinent observations have been made, however, which will contribute to the final solution to the problem. For example, since lectins that have been insolubilized on agarose beads (35) or plastic dishes (36) are mitogenic, and their activity can be inhibited by the appropriate sugar inhibitor, it is probable that the interaction of a mitogenic lectin with glycoproteins on the lymphocyte cell surface is sufficient to trigger growth. Plant lectins with defined sugar specificities that are presently known to stimulate peripheral thymus dependent (T) lymphocytes bind either α-D-glucosyl and α-D-mannosyl residues or carbohydrate residues related to N-acetyl-D-galactosamine (see refs. 37 and 38). One possible interpretation of this is that these lectins bind to a specific glycoprotein on the T lymphocyte surface with a carbohydrate moiety to which both classes of lectins can bind. The mitogenic activity of lectins at a concentration at which only a small proportion of the maximum number of lectin molecules are bound is consistent with this hypothesis if the lectin-glycoprotein interaction that triggers mitogenesis is of a higher affinity than the interaction of the lectins with the majority of the cell-surface glycoproteins. The failure of soluble T cell mitogens to stimulate peripheral thymus independent (B) lymphocytes that possess the necessary intracellular machinery for growth as evidenced by their response to lipopolysaccharide, and that bind the mitogenic plant lectins to the same extent as T cells, can be explained if the specific glycoprotein is either modified or found at a much lower concentration on B cells. This explanation is not necessarily inconsistent with the observation that insolubilized concanavalin A stimulates B cells (36). In this light a search for a glycoprotein, which interacts with both groups of plant lectins, and which is found on peripheral T cells and possibly on thymocytes but not on peripheral B cells may prove fruitful. The technology for such a search is now available (39-41), and recent results have led to the identification of two T cell-specific glycoproteins which bind concanavalin A and which may be of interest in relationship to mitogenesis (41; Bevan, Weissman & Trowbridge, unpublished results).

DISCUSSION

It is clear from even this brief summary that the growth of mammalian cells can be controlled by many different substances. Mouse embryo 3T3 cells and a number of other cultured cells grow in response to polypeptide hormones, as well as in response to the addition of low molecular weight materials under certain conditions. Small lymphocytes which *in vivo* proliferate in response to antigens, can also be stimulated *in vitro* by various plant lectins and by calcium ions, as well as by other materials. The variety is striking.

One possible explanation is that quiescent cells can be in various metastable states from which they can be displaced in multiple ways. The actions of the different mitogens could then be totally unrelated to each other. If so, a search for a common mechanism of mitogenesis will go unrewarded.

Alternatively, the variety of mitogens may correspond to multiple facets of a complicated but uniform mechanism. All of the high molecular weight mitogens may act on the cell membrane, perhaps activating the internal mechanism that is activated by hormones in those cells that have hormone receptor sites.

From this viewpoint, it is of interest that the intracellular cyclic nucleotide levels correlate with the growth rate of the cell (15, 28, 29) and cyclic nucleotides are known to be intimately involved in hormone action (42). Also intriguing are changes in the transport and permeability properties of the membrane that are associated both with mitogenesis (12) and hormone action (43).

Whether the changes in membrane properties and intracellular cyclic nucleotide levels are direct or indirect effects of mitogenic stimulation is not clear. It may be impossible to distinguish between these alternatives in work with intact cells. However, it is now possible to study the actions of mitogens on the isolated plasma membranes of the target cells. Investigations with these simplified systems may help to elucidate the sequence of early events that follow stimulation by mitogens.

In addition to the many mitogens that act at the cell surface, a wide variety of low molecular weight materials can also initiate DNA synthesis and growth under certain laboratory conditions. Amino acids are a common example. Although the tendency among biologists is to discount the importance of this type of observation, it is worth noting that serum concentrations of many of these substances as well as of the hormones can be close to the concentrations that are observed to control growth in the laboratory. The fact that uptake of low molecular weight materials is influenced by mitogens suggests that natural growth control of mammalian cells may involve low molecular weight materials also. Thus, it is possible that the complicated interaction of many different growth-controlling factors, observed in the laboratory, may actually represent the natural state (44).

REFERENCES

(1) R. W. Holley and J. A. Kiernan, Proc. Nat. Acad. Sci. US 60 (1968) 300.

(2) D. Paul, A. Lipton and I. Klinger, Proc. Nat. Acad. Sci. US 68 (1971) 645.

(3) R. W. Holley and J. A. Kiernan, Proc. Nat. Acad. Sci. US 71 (1974) 2908.

(4) D. Gospodarowicz, Nature 249 (1974) 123.

(5) D. Gospodarowicz, J. Biol. Chem. (1974), in press.

(6) W. G. Juergens, F. E. Stockdale, Y. J. Topper and J. J. Elias, Proc. Nat. Acad. Sci. US 54 (1965) 629.

(7) A. S. Mukherjee, L. L. Washburn and M. R. Banerjee, Nature 246 (1973) 159.

(8) E. M. Rivera, Endocrinol. 74 (1964) 853.

(9) H. M. Temin, R. W. Pierson, Jr. and N. C. Dulak, in: Growth, Nutrition, and Metabolism of Cells in Culture, ed. V. I. Cristafalo and G. Rothblat (Academic Press, New York, 1972) p. 50.

(10) R. Hoffmann, H.-J. Ristow, J. Veser and W. Frank, Exptl. Cell Res. 85 (1973) 275.

(11) R. W. Holley and J. A. Kiernan, Proc. Nat. Acad. Sci. US 71 (1974) 2942.

(12) R. W. Holley, Proc. Nat. Acad. Sci. US 69 (1972) 2840.

(13) R. W. Holley, J. H. Baldwin and J. A. Kiernan, Proc. Nat. Acad. Sci. US 71 (1974) 3976.

(14) P. S. Rudland, M. Hamilton, R. Hamilton, D. Gospodarowicz and W. Seifert, (1975), submitted for publication.

(15) W. Seifert and P. S. Rudland, Nature 248 (1974) 138.

(16) W. Seifert and P. S. Rudland, Proc. Nat. Acad. Sci. US (1974), in press.

(17) Transplantation Reviews, Vol. 11, Lymphocyte Activation by Mitogens, ed. G. Möller (Munksgaard, Copenhagen, 1972).

(18) A. Coutinho, G. Möller, J. Andersson and W. W. Bullock, Eur. J. Immunol. 3 (1973) 299.

(19) V. C. Maino, N. M. Green and M. J. Crumpton, Nature 251 (1974) 324.

(20) J. H. Peters and P. Hausen, Eur. J. Biochem. 19 (1971) 509.

(21) R. Averdunk, Hoppe-Seyler's Z. Physiol. Chem. 353 (1972) 79.

(22) J. Mendelsohn, A. Skinner and S. Kornfeld, J. Clin. Invest. 50 (1971) 818.

(23) K. J. van den Berg and I. Betel, Exptl. Cell Res. 66 (1971) 257.

(24) M. E. Cross and M. G. Ord, Biochem. J. 124 (1971) 241.

(25) R. B. Whitney and R. M. Sutherland, Cell. Immunol. 5 (1972) 137.

(26) M. R. Quastel and J. G. Kaplan, Exptl. Cell Res. 63 (1970) 230.

(27) J. E. Kay, Exptl. Cell Res. 71 (1972) 245.

(28) J. W. Hadden, E. M. Hadden, M. K. Haddox and N. D. Goldberg, Proc. Nat. Acad. Sci. US 69 (1972) 3024.

(29) J. Watson, J. Exptl. Med. (1974), in press.

(30) A. E. Powell and M. A. Leon, Exptl. Cell Res. 62 (1970) 315.

(31) A. Novogrodsky and E. Katchalski, Biochim. Biophys. Acta 228 (1971) 579.

(32) K. Lindahl-Kiessling, Exptl. Cell Res. 70 (1972) 17.

(33) M. D. Stein, H. J. Sage and M. A. Leon, Exptl. Cell Res. 75 (1972) 475.

(34) R. M. Pauli and B. S. Strauss, Exptl. Cell Res. 82 (1973) 357.

(35) M. F. Greaves and S. Bauminger, Nature New Biol. 235 (1972) 67.

(36) J. Andersson, G. M. Edelman, G. Möller and O. Sjöberg, Eur. J. Immunol. 2 (1972) 233.

(37) I. S. Trowbridge, J. Biol. Chem. 249 (1974) 6004.

(38) G. L. Nicolson, Int. Rev. Cytol. 39 (1974) 89.

(39) D. Allan, J. Auger and M. J. Crumpton, Nature New Biol. 236 (1972) 23.

(40) M. J. Hayman and M. J. Crumpton, Biochem. Biophys. Res. Commun. 47 (1972) 923.

(41) I. S. Trowbridge, P. Ralph and M. J. Bevan, Proc. Nat. Acad. Sci. US (1975), in press.

(42) G. A. Robison, R. W. Butcher and E. W. Sutherland, Cyclic AMP (Academic Press, New York, 1971).

(43) O. H. Petersen, Experientia 30 (1974) 1105.

(44) J. Short, R. F. Brown, A. Husakova, J. R. Gilbertson, R. Zemel and I. Lieberman, J. Biol. Chem. 247 (1972) 1757.

ACKNOWLEDGMENT

This research was supported in part by the American Cancer Society (#BC30A), The National Cancer Institute (CA11176) (NO1-CP-33405), and the National Science Foundation (GB 32391X). R. W. H. is an American Cancer Society Professor of Molecular Biology.

DISCUSSION

A. WHITE: Have you had the opportunity to examine the possible activity of any of the somatomedins in your system? Secondly, are the requirements that you have demonstrated for growth of 3T3 cells required for growth of other cell lines? Finally, I don't think you mentioned whether the acrylamide gels you showed were for the total solubilized proteins of the cells or just the plasma membrane proteins?

R.W. HOLLEY: The gels were for the total solubilized proteins from the cells. The somatomedins which were tested possibly correspond to the insulin part of our requirement. They are more active by themselves than insulin is, but the FGF effect is clearly synergistic with them. Gospodarowicz has been studying the FGF on many cell lines and finds it active on a great variety of things.

H. HEINIGER: What happens to your 3T3 cells if you add serum from which the lipid fraction has been removed?

R.W. HOLLEY: If one extracts the serum with chloroform-methanol one finds the activity either in the particulate fraction or the aqueous layer. The lipid fraction is actually toxic so that one really cannot say whether there are important lipids there or not. There are suggestions that 3T3 cells can respond to lipids. Some cells certainly do respond to lipids. We have a curious cell which arrests in G_1 or Go when it runs out of essential fatty acids and all you have to do in order to initiate DNA synthesis and growth is to add linoleic acid.

M.M. SIGEL: Your 3T3 cells, of course, respond to nutritional factors and they are possibly also regulated by some factor which may bear on the β2-microglobulin. In contrast, lymphocytes usually are considered to be mainly responsive to antigens and mitogens and people ignore the nutritional millieu of the lymphocyte. When different laboratories compare their data they do not address themselves to the important point of the differences in sera used as supplements which can inhibit or amplify lymphocyte proliferation and thereby alter quantitatively the degree or net amount of response to mitogenic stimulation. For example, rabbit serum has a different effect from human serum or fetal calf serum.

RESTRICTED CLONAL RESPONSES: A TOOL IN UNDERSTANDING ANTIBODY SPECIFICITY

E. HABER, M.N. MARGOLIES, L.E. CANNON, AND M.S. ROSEMBLATT
Departments of Medicine and Surgery
Massachusetts General Hospital and Harvard Medical School

INTRODUCTION

There remains little reason now to doubt the hypothesis that myeloma proteins are representative of the population of elicited antibodies. Not only are antigens bound at a clearly defined site in the Fab portion of the molecule as lucidly and convincingly demonstrated in x-ray crystallographic studies of myeloma protein-hapten complexes (1,2), but there is accumulating evidence of structural identity between certain antigen-binding myeloma proteins and antibodies elicited by conventional immunization (3,4). The most convincing studies bearing on the latter point include the demonstration of cross-reactivity of idiotypic antibodies between phosphorylcholine-binding myeloma proteins and elicited antibodies to phosphorylcholine containing antigens in mice (5). The important question to be answered, however, is whether or not the diversity in variable region sequences seen among myeloma proteins both with respect to sequences participating in the binding of antigen (hypervariable regions) or the distribution of other variable region sequences ("framework residues") is truly representative of what is to be found in elicited antibodies. It has long been apparent that the set of myeloma proteins induced in mice by hydrocarbon carcinogens (6) reflect a very different distribution of isotypes (features common to all members of the species) from those found in the normal mouse serum. While the marked dominance of IgA myelomas has been attributed to the site of installation of the carcinogen, the peritoneum, there is no *a priori* reason for denying that other selective factors may not also operate during the process of neoplastic induction.

Largely on the basis of an examination of myeloma proteins, both with respect to their amino acid sequence and the nature of antigen binding, a hypothesis of limited diversity in variable region primary structure has become current. The amino terminal sequences of both light and heavy chains of human myeloma proteins may be arranged conveniently into "subgroups" or sets on the basis of apparent linked substitutions (7). Such sets are less apparent among mouse kappa chains although the principal of subgroups has become accepted as an important cornerstone on which to build hypotheses of antibody diversity. The number of subgroups have been used to estimate the minimal number of germ line genes responsible for variable regions. An important question that must be asked continually is whether these apparent subgroups are representative of the population of elicited antibodies or in some way are an artefact of the very process that selects myeloma proteins. The ambiguities of amino acid sequence studies of heterogeneous populations of serum antibodies do not permit this question to be addressed rigorously.

Studies of both the amino acid sequence and the binding properties of myeloma proteins lead to an impression of limited diversity. The interesting discoveries of Richards and colleagues (8), which indicate that the capacious antibody combining site may bind several different haptens of differing specificities has led to a revival of Talmage's hypothesis (9) which allows for a very small number of antibodies to account for the recognized wide spectrum of specificity of the immune response. If, indeed, the apparent specificity of the immune response is generated by selection of multifunctional antibodies capable of binding a given antigen from a relatively small population of total antibodies, the number of combining site structures which must be postulated to exist is sharply limited. Contributing in a very major way to the perception of a relatively simple immunological potential (i.e., a relatively small number of possible antibodies), were the observations showing idiotypic cross-reactivity among independently induced or discovered myeloma proteins (5) which demonstrated similar antigen binding specificities. Even more persuasive was the demonstration not only of idiotypic cross-reactivity among a set of mouse myeloma proteins binding phosphorylcholine, but also marked similarity or identity in amino acid sequence of proteins secreted by independently induced tumors which have an identical spectrum of hapten binding as well as identical or similar amino acid sequences (10). The demonstration that the response to phosphorylcholine immunization in the BALB/c mouse may be monoclonal and that the elicited antibody largely cross-reacts with idiotypic antibodies to this set of myeloma proteins serves neatly to cap the concept of a quite simple immune response. Such data have been employed by theorists to estimate the number of germ line variable genes and from such estimates to build hypotheses which support the concept of as few as 100 heavy chain and 100 light chain germ line genes with perhaps a 10-fold increase in each, allowable by somatic mutation (11). Cohn and colleagues admit, however, (11) that the hypothesis will stand or fall on the number of germ line V genes expressed in a way that can be selected upon somatically and that the only likely way to obtain such information is through amino acid sequence analysis.

In this report, amino acid sequence data from elicited antibodies will be examined in order to determine whether or not the impression of the relative simplicity of the immune response gained from study of myeloma proteins with antigen binding characteristics can be supported. Antibodies of course, are also subject to selection, but the nature of selection may well be different from that bearing on myeloma tumors. While the data are as yet sparse, they suggest an order of complexity of the immune response, particularly a diversity in hypervariable regions among antibodies specific for relatively simple antigens that challenges models dependent upon a small number of variable region genes.

The intrinsic heterogeneity of the immune response has impeded detailed structural analysis of elicited antibodies and led to the extensive interest in products of myeloma tumors. More recently, however, it has been shown that immunization with bacterial vaccines may result in a restricted antibody response in which the several species of antibody may be readily separated by conventional means (12,13). Less frequently, the immune response to other antigens or even hapten-protein conjugates (14,15) results in a sufficiently homogeneous antibody so that extensive sequence analysis may be performed. Improved methods for separating more complex mixtures such as isoelectric focussing (16) have also been successfully employed to allow limited structural analysis of a heterogeneous antibody population. Monoclonal and biclonal responses in rabbits immunized with pneumococcal polysaccharides are sufficiently frequent so that sophisticated methods of fractionation appear no longer to be needed.

The kinds of information that may be uniquely addressed with elicited antibodies include:

1) How large is the set of variable region sequences from which a single antigen may select a complementary antibody? The diversity of the set of "framework" residues utilized in response to any given antigen bears importantly on the number of variable region genes, whether inherited or somatically generated.

2) An examination of the evolution of the immune response in a single animal by assessing the structural relationship of antibodies appearing at the same time or sequentially (18,19). One might thereby obtain insight as to whether or not structural changes in hypervariable regions occur by somatic mutation (11).

3) Whether or not there is evidence for inheritance of the sets of hypervariable region sequences which an animal requires to respond to a given antigen (20).

4) A unique opportunity in the rabbit to sort out the problem of inheritance of a limited number of variable region heavy chain allotypes in relation to a large number of hypervariable regions (21).

5) To assess the complexity of the immune response to a set of relatively simple antigens in order to approach the question of how many binding sites can be synthesized to accomodate a simple antigen. One cannot readily obtain a library of myelomas binding a given antigen while this can be predictably accomplished by immunization.

6) To determine the structural basis of cross-reactivity to related antigens, such as pneumococcal type III and VIII polysaccharides which have cellobiuronic acid as a common determinant.

METHODOLOGIC APPROACH

The production of pneumococcal polysaccharide antibodies has been discussed previously (19). Fractionation of antibodies by affinity chromatography or isoelectric focussing was thought necessary (22), but it now appears that in most instances antibodies may be purified from a single antiserum using ion exchange chromatography on DEAE cellulose.

The general approach to amino acid sequence analysis has emphasized the isolation of large peptides, either tryptic peptides obtained from light or heavy chains after blocking lysines with citraconic anhydride (23), or cyanogen bromide peptides from heavy chains. A marked increase in sensitivity of automatic sequenator methodology regularly permits sequence analyses extending between 40 and 58 steps utilizing between 50 and 150 nanomoles of a light chain or large peptide. Both large and small peptides are analyzed using an aqueous 0.1 M Quadrol program (24). The analysis of smaller tryptic peptides is additionally facilitated by modification with Braunitzer's reagent (25). Complete sequences of light chain variable regions including information on ordering of peptides have been obtained through the use of tryptic fragments obtained from blocked and unblocked chains, as well as the products of acid cleavage at the switch region (26), without the necessity of applying other enzymes in many instances.

RESULTS

Amino Terminal Sequences

We have now been able to cull 60 sequences from the amino terminal region of the light chain derived from various rabbit antibodies of different specificities. There are 20 antibodies specific for pneumococcal polysaccharides obtained in our own laboratories and those of others, as well as antibodies specific for streptococcal polysaccharides and hapten-protein conjugates (14,15,17,18, 21,22,27-41).

Fig. 1 shows a variability plot for the first 22 residues. As will be seen later, the chains are of different lengths, but in order to construct this plot, they were aligned by the invariant sequence Thr-Gln-Thr-Pro from positions 5 to 8. As reported previously (22), there is evidence of marked hypervariability at the amino-terminus of these chains in comparison to human and mouse chains. The degree of hypervariability in this region approaches that seen in two other hypervariable regions of the light chain to be discussed subsequently. In addition to the marked hypervariability at the amino terminus, it is remarkable that there is far more uniformity in the amino-terminal segment of the chain than previously observed in human or murine light chains (42).

The degree of uniformity of these sequences is evidenced by the observation that of the N-terminal 23 positions, 10 positions appear absolutely invariant, positions 5-8, 15, 18-21, and Cys 23. Furthermore, those sequences associated with the b_4 allotype demonstrate an invariant glycine at position 16 and ca. 90% of these sequences display invariance at positions 10,11, and 17 (serine, valine, and glycine, respectively). The glycine reported

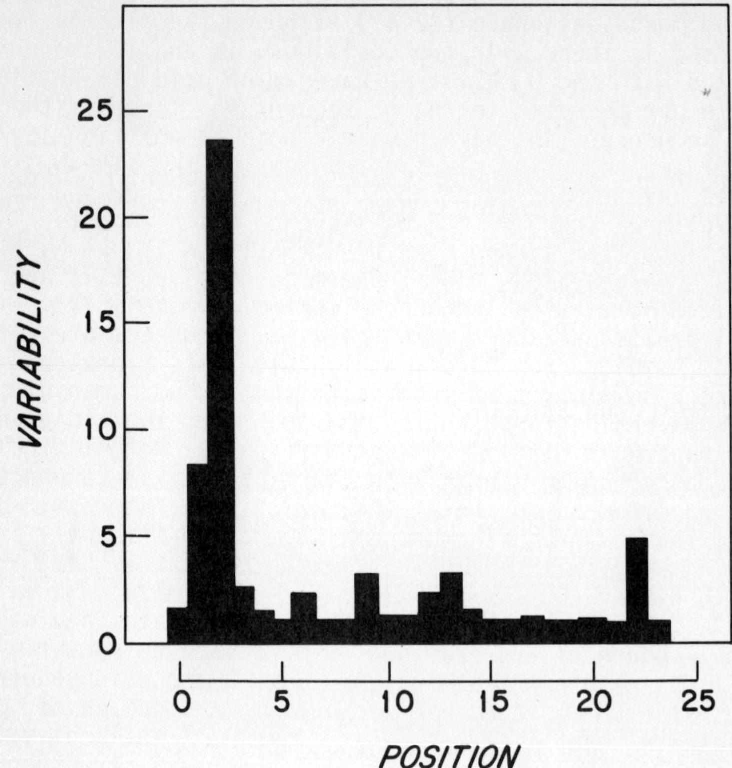

Fig. 1. Hypervariability plot of amino terminal 20 residues of rabbit antibody light chain based on the method of Wu and Kabat (42). Data are taken from 50 sequences (44).

at position 17 in 49 of 53 rabbit sequences is not found in human and mouse sequences (42,43) although the alternative, Asp or Asx, is found. In two positions, 11 and 16, sequences associated with the b_9 allotype have amino acid alternatives which are not detected in the b_4 sequences. Three of the five b_9 sequences (40) have glutamic acid at position 16, the other two reporting glycine and four of the five b_9 sequences have threonine at position 11, the other sequence having valine. There is one b_9 sequence which reports serine at position 11 and glycine at position 16, however.

The homology among rabbit pneumococcal Type VIII and Type III amino terminal sequences is approximately 78%. When all published rabbit amino-terminal sequences are compared, homology is approximately 75%. This represents a far greater homology than seen among the set of human or mouse kappa chains reported to date and makes the assignment of subgroups within this set difficult. Mathematical analysis of grouping within amino-terminal rabbit sequences will be reported subsequently (44). It is of interest, however, that all rabbit sequences have a significantly greater homology with human Ag (VκI, approximately 54%) than with either CUM (VκII 39%) or TI (VκIII 35%) (43).

In Fig. 2, groups of two or more light chains having identical sequences are examined with respect to specificity. It is apparent that the very same amino acid sequence for the first 20 residues may be found in antibodies of very different specificities. For example, 2 antibodies to pneumococcal polysaccharide Type VIII, one to a streptococcal polysaccharide and an antibody to the hapten-protein complex Ap-BGG, share identical sequences.

As noted previously, if the amino terminal segments of the chain are aligned by invariant residues, the length of the polypeptide chains may differ by two residues at their amino-terminal ends. Table 1 analyzes the relationship between chain length and specificity of the antibody. It can be seen that the distribution of chain lengths among light chains derived from specific antibodies and light chains from nonimmune immunoglobulins do not differ significantly except for a bias toward shorter chain lengths among light chains derived from antibodies to streptococcal vaccines. It should be noted that in the latter instance, rabbits were obtained from a relatively highly inbred group (21,35), in contrast to the animals immunized with pneumococcal and other antigens. These observations suggest that the chain length at the amino-terminal end is not correlated with antibody specificity. Fig. 3 lists the sequences of amino-terminal segments of the light chain derived from six

```
Specificities(a)          Position
                          0                   5                   10                  15                  20
             Prototype(b) ALA ASP ILE VAL MET THR GLN THR PRO SER SER VAL SER ALA ALA VAL GLY GLY THR VAL THR ILE LYS

Pneu 3 (1),
Strep C (1)               ------------------------------------ ALA ------------------------------------------------ ASX

Pneu 8 (2),                                           c
Pneu 3 (3)                [ ] --- VAL --------------------- ALA ---------- GLU(c) PRO --------------------------

Strep C (1),                                          c
Strep Av (1)              [ ] ALA LEU --- LEU ------------- ALA ------------------------------------------------

Pneu 8 (2),
Strep A (1),
Ap-BGG (1)                [ ] ALA TYR ASP ------------------------------------------------------------------------

Pneu 8 (1),
Pneu 2 (1)                [ ] [ ] ALA --- LEU ----------------------------------------------------------------

Strep C (1),                                                 d
Strep Av (1),             [ ] [ ] ------------------------------- LYS --- VAL PRO ------ ASX ---------------- ASX
Rp-BGG (1)
```

Fig. 2. Identities among amino terminal sequences from light chains of different antigen specificities, each isolated in a different animal. Numbers in parentheses are the number of chains of a given specificity having the indicated sequence. Sequences are from (17,18,21,29,31,32,33,34,35,40,44). Numbering in this and subsequent figures is based on human $V_{\kappa}I$, Ag.

a) Rp-BGG = p-arsanilate diazotized to bovine gamma globulin.

Ap-BGG = p-aminophenyltrimethylammonium chloride diazotized to bovine gamma globulin.

b) Prototype is derived by taking the most frequently occurring amino acid alternative at each position from 60 sequences examined.

c) Some sequences report GLX.

d) One sequence reports an unidentified residue (27,44).

TABLE 1

N-TERMINAL LIGHT CHAIN
LENGTH VERSUS ANTIBODY SPECIFICITY

SPECIFICITY	CHAIN LENGTH[A] 24	23	22	NO. OF SEQUENCES EXAMINED
NONIMMUNE	0.20	0.70	0.10	—
PNEU 8	0.09	0.82	0.09	11
PNEU 3	0.25	0.63	0.12	8
STREP C	0.21	0.47	0.32	19
STREP AV	0.40	0.40	0.20	5
STREP A	0.00	0.50	0.50	4
HAPTENS	0.00	0.60	0.40	5

A) Chain length is relative to an invariant cysteine at position 23. Data from nonimmune light chains is extrapolated from (38). The numbers given are the proportions of the total number of chains for the indicated specificity which have a given chain length.

```
Antigen  ID          Position
                     0                   5                        10                       15                       20
          Prototype^a ALA ASP ILE VAL MET THR GLN THR PRO SER SER VAL SER ALA ALA VAL GLY GLY THR VAL THR ILE LYS

Pneu 8
         ( -5    [ ] — VAL ———————————————— ALA ——————————————————————————————————
 2388    { -2Aa  [ ] — PRO — LEU ——————————— PRO ————————————————————————————————————————
         ( -C    [ ] ALA TYR ASP ————————————————————————————————————————————————
         ( -B    [ ] ALA TYR ASP —————————————————————————————————————————————————————————
 3322    ( -A    [ ] [ ] ALA — LEU ——————————————————————————————————————————————————— SER
         ( -3    [ ] — VAL ———————————————— ALA ———————— GLU PRO ————————————————————————
 2348    ( -2Aa  [ ] ALA LEU ————————————————

Strep C
         ( -1    [ ] ALA PHE GLX ————————X ———— ALA ———— THR — PRO ————————————————————————
 2461    { -1a   [ ] ALA ALA GLX LEU ————X ———— ALA ———————— GLX PRO ————————————————————————
         ( -1b   [ ] ALA LEU — LEU ——————X ———— ALA ————————————————————————————————————————
         ( -1    [ ] [ ] — LEU ————————————————————— THR (?) ———————— GLU ———————————————— ASN
 2869    ( -2    [ ] ALA VAL — LEU ——————————————————————— (?) ————————————————————————— ASN
         ( -I    [ ] [ ] VAL ——————————————————————————— THR ———————————— GLU ———————————————— ASN
 4153    ( -II   [ ] [ ] VAL ——————————————————————————— THR LYS ———————— GLU ———————————————— ASX
```

Fig. 3. Amino-terminal sequences of 6 sets of light chains, each set isolated from a single rabbit; references for chains are as follows: 2388, 3322 (28), 2348 (29), 2461 (21), 2869, 4153 (40).

a) Prototype is derived as in Fig. 2. A line denotes identity with the prototype, GLX, ASX, and —X denote unidentified acid or amide. (?) denotes unidentified residue and [ ] denotes a deletion.

antisera, each containing two or three homogeneous antibodies elicited by the same antigen. In each instance the antibodies were obtained at the same time during the course of immunization. These data indicate that a single animal may produce as many as three antibodies differing in amino-terminal sequence and chain length in response to immunization with the same antigen and confirm earlier observations from our own laboratory (22,29) as well as those of others (21).

Light Chain Hypervariable Regions

Essentially complete amino acid sequences of variable regions are now available on seven rabbit antibody light chains (15,33,34,36), including three from our laboratory (31), as well as partial sequences on several others (28,31). Fig. 4 shows a hypervariability plot generated from these data. In addition to the hypervariability of the amino-terminal three residues discussed previously, there appear two additional nodes of hypervariability in the region of residues 30 to 32 and 91 to 97. It should be noted that substantial variations in sequence length also occur in these regions. In comparison to the data obtained by Wu and Kabat from an analysis of human κ chains (42), there does not appear to be a hypervariable region between residues 50 and 56 in the rabbit light chain. Indeed, there is considerable uniformity of amino acid sequence in this area.

In Fig. 5 we have tabulated the structures of the first hypervariable region in detail. Five antibodies specific for Type III pneumococcal polysaccharide, three for Type VIII polysaccharide, one for streptococcus C and one for azobenzoate-BGG are compared. Cysteine 23 is used for alignment; glutamine 24 is invariant in all the sequences examined. Position 25 may be either alanine, serine, or threonine. Position 26 is serine except in one chain, the antiazobenzoate antibody. Position 27 is either glutamic acid, glutamine or lysine. Position 28 is serine in all chains but one, 3374, in which asparagine is found. Three alternatives are found at position 29, all functionally homologous side chains: isoleucine, valine or leucine. Significant hypervariability as determined both by the plot (Fig. 4) and by scanning of Fig. 5 begins at position 30, which has five alternatives, position 31 which has four, and position 32 which has seven among 10 sequences. The hypervariable region appears to end before an invariant leucine at position 33, a residue also seen in all human κ

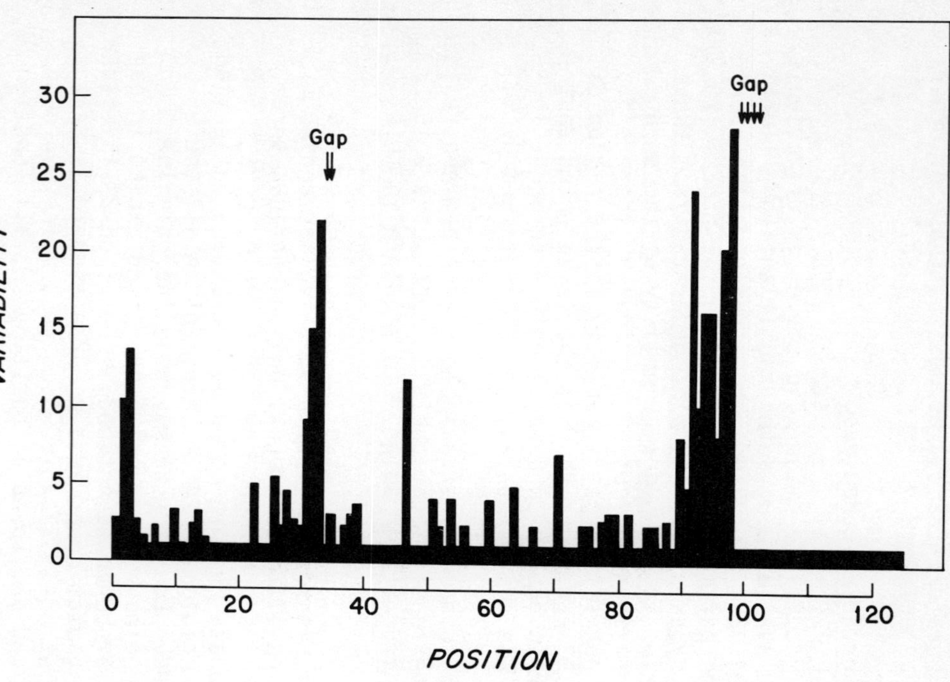

Fig. 4. Hypervariability plot of rabbit antibody κB light chains according to the method of Wu and Kabat (42). Data beyond residue 23 are reported in references (15,31,33, 34, and 36).

	23	24	25	26	27	28	29	30	31	32	32A	32B	33	34	35	36	37	38	39	40
Pneu 3 3374	[Cys]	Gln	Ala	Ser	Gln	Asn	Ile	Asp	Ser	Trp	---	---	Leu	Ala	Trp	Tyr	Gln	Gln	Lys	Pro
Pneu 3 3368	—	—	—	—	Glu	Ser	(—)	Gly	Asn	Glu	---	---	—	—	—	—	—	—	—	—
Pneu 3 3381	—	—	—	—	Glu	Ser	—	Ser	Asn	—	---	---	—	—	—	—	—	—	—	—
Pneu 3 BS-5	—	—	—	—	—	Ser	—	Tyr	Asn	Gly	---	---	—	—	—	—	x	x	—	—
Pneu 3 BS-1	—	—	—	—	—	Ser	—	Tyr	—	Gly	---	---	—	—	—	—	x	x	—	—
Pneu 8 3315	—	—	Ser	—	—	Ser	Val	Tyr	Glu	Asn	Gly	Arg	—	Ser	—	Phe	—	—	—	—
Pneu 8 3322A	—	—	—	—	—	Ser	Val	Tyr	Asn	Asn	(Asn)	( )	—	—	—	—	—			
Pneu 8 3322B	—	—	—	—	—	Ser	Leu	Thr	Asn	Gln	Tyr	---	—	—	—					
Strep C 4135	—	—	Thr	—	—	Ser	—	—	Asp	Tyr	---	---	—	Ser	—	—	—	—	—	—
AZBGG 2717	—	—	Ser	Thr	Lys	Ser	—	Tyr	Asx	Asx	Asx	Tyr	—	—	—	—	—	x	—	—

Fig. 5. Sequence around the first hypervariable region of rabbit antibody light chains. Data are from (15,28,31,33,34,36). A line denotes identity with the uppermost sequence, (—) denotes residues identified by a single criterion, ( ) designates an unidentified residue, --- denotes a deletion. Numbering and other symbols are as in Fig. 2.

chains (43). Seven of the chains examined in this region have a hypervariable region segment length of three residues as defined by the invariant leucine at position 33. However, 3322B has an additional amino acid and 3315, 3322A and 2717 have two additional amino acids prior to the invariant leucine. Thus the hypervariable region length is 3 to 5 residues in the chains examined thus far. Position 34 is either alanine or serine and position 35 is an invariant tryptophan also found in all human κ chains. The sequence subsequent to residue 35 shows very little variability.

It is of interest to note that the hypervariable region sequences in the five Type III specific antibodies are identical with respect to chain length in this region but differ in sequence. The three Type VIII specific antibodies differ in both sequence and length in this hypervariable region. With the data presently available it is difficult to draw a correlation between hypervariable sequence and/or length with antibody specificity in this region.

Fig. 6 depicts the sequence information available for rabbit antibody light chains from positions 47 to 62. This includes the second hypervariable region as defined by Wu and Kabat in human and murine light chains. It is apparent immediately not only from Fig. 4 but from a careful examination of the actual sequence data that there is very little variability in this portion of these sequences. Residue 49 is invariant. Residue 50 has three alternatives but one of these occurs five times. Residue 52 is invariant. Residue 53 has three alternatives but one is dominant. Residue 54 is invariant. Residue 55 is alanine in all but one chain. Residues 56, 57, and 58 are invariant. Residue 59 has two alternatives, and residues 60 through 62 are invariant. Apparently then, rabbit antibody light chains do not display a second hypervariable region.

The third hypervariable region, identified in Fig. 4, is examined in detail in Fig. 7. Cysteine 88 is a constant feature of all rabbit antibody light chains as it is in human and murine light chains. Position 89 has three or four alternatives, 90 three alternatives. Ninety-one is a position of greater hypervariability with six alternatives; 92 has four or five alternatives; 93 six alternatives; 94 six alternatives; 95 four alternatives; 96 begins a region of the sequence of extreme hypervariability and differences in chain length. Phenylalanine 98 begins an invariant sequence for the rest of the light chain. If position 91 is said to begin the hypervariable region and phenylalanine

	47	48	49	50	51	52	53	54	55	56	57	58	59	60	61	62
Pneu 3 3374	Leu	Ile	Tyr	Arg	Thr	Ser	Thr	Leu	Ala	Ser	Gly	Val	Pro	Ser	Arg	Phe
Pneu 3 3368	—	—	—	—	Ala	—	Lys	—	—	—	—	—	Ser	—	—	—
Pneu 3 BS-5	—	—	—	Lys	Ala	—	—	—	Glu	—	—	—	—	—	—	—
Pneu 3 BS-1	—	—	—	Lys	Ala	—	—	—	—	—	—	—	Ser	—	—	—
Pneu 8 3315	—	—	—	—	Ala	—	—	—	—	—	—	—	Ser	—	—	—
Strep C 4135	—	—	—	—	Ala	—	—	—	—	—	—	—	—	—	—	—
AZBGG 2717	—	—	—	Thr	Ala	—	Ser	—	—	—	—	—	—	—	—	—
M. Lyso. 120	—	—	—	—	Ala	—	—	—	—	—	—	—	Ser	—	—	—

Fig. 6. Sequence of the segment of rabbit antibody light chain identified as the second hypervariable region in human κ chains (42). Data are from (15,31,33,34,36). Numbering and symbols are as in Fig. 5.

	88	89	90	91	92	93	94	95	96	97	A	B	C	D	98	99	100	101
Pneu 3 3374	Cys	Gln	Ser	Tyr	Tyr	Ser	Ile	Ser	Ser	Ala	---	---	---	---	Phe	Gly	Gly	Gly
Pneu 3 3368	—	—	Gln	Asp	Trp	Asn	Ser	Asn	Asn	Val	Val	Asn	Asn	---	—	—	—	—
Pneu 3 BS-5	—	x	Gly	Ser	Asx	Tyr	Thr	Gly	Thr	Val	---	---	---	---	—	—	—	—
Pneu 3 BS-1	—	x	Gly	Ser	Thr	Tyr	Gly	Gly	Gly	Tyr	---	---	---	---	—	—	—	—
Pneu 3 K7						Ile	Thr	Ala	Thr	Thr	---	---	---	---	—	—	—	—
Pneu 8 3315	—	Leu	Gly	Asn	—	Asp	Cys	—	—	Gly	(Asp)	(Ser)	Phe	Thr	—	—	—	—
Strep C 4135	—	—	—	Thr	—	Gly	Val	Gly	---	---	---	---	---	---	—	—	—	—
AZBGG 2717	—	Gly	Gly	Ala	Asp	Tyr	Thr	Gly	Tyr	Ser	---	---	---	---	—	—	—	—

Fig. 7. Sequences around the third hypervariable region of rabbit antibody light chains. Data are taken (from 15,31-34,36). Numbering and symbols are as in Fig. 5.

98 to end it, then its total length varies from five residues in 4135 to 11 residues in 3315. It is of considerable interest that cysteine is one of the residues which appears within the hypervariable region of 3315 (31).

Many of the same observations can be made with respect to the third hypervariable region as have been made previously with respect to the hypervariable region from 30 to 32. There appears to be no relationship between the length of the hypervariable region in this segment of the molecule and specificity. Of the four pneumococcal Type III specific antibodies in which an assessment of length can be made, hypervariable regions may be either seven or 10 residues in length. The azobenzoate-specific antibody sequence 2717 is seven residues in length, although the single pneumococcal Type VIII specific antibody and the single streptococcus C-specific antibody sequence appear to be either longer or shorter. The four Type III antibodies all exhibit a very different amino acid sequence and show no greater homology within the group than between the different antibody specificities examined. Only two sequences, BS-1 and BS-5, both with pneumococcus Type III specificity, appear to be somewhat similar (34).

Conserved Segments of the Variable Region and the Constant Region

In all rabbit κB chains sequenced thus far, cysteine has been found at position 80. We also previously demonstrated an extra cysteine in the constant region at position 171 (32) not found in human or mouse κ chains. The three constant region sequences available for comparison, 3315 (45), antiazobenzoate 2717 (15) and antistreptococcal type C 4135 (36), also show a half-cystine at position 171. We had previously postulated the existence of an interdomain disulfide bridge because rabbit κB light chains subjected to selective acid cleavage at aspartic acid 109 did not decrease in molecular weight until cystines were cleaved (46). On pepsin digestion of antibody 3315, a disulfide bond-containing peptide was isolated (47), the sequence of which proves that position 80 is joined to position 171. This unequivocally locates the position of the interdomain bond.

There is complete identity between the amino acid sequence of 3315 and 4135 in the constant region except for an amide. It should be noted, however, that position 174 appears to be variable in other incomplete light chain sequences (32). 3315 and 4135 have asparagine in this position; 2377 and 2388, valine; and nonimmune immunoglobulin light chains, leucine (32). All these sequences were obtained from rabbits light chains of b_4 allotype. All other positions examined were identical within the constant region.

Wu and Kabat pointed out that there were 11 invariant residues in human and mouse light chain variable regions. These include glutamine 6, cysteine 23 and 88, tryptophan 35, proline 59, arginine 61, aspartic acid 82, tyrosine 86, phenylalanine 98, and glycines 99 and 101. All of these residues are also invariant in rabbit antibody light chains sequenced thus far except proline 59. In seven chains on which data is available, proline occurs four times and serine three times.

Heavy Chain

Considerably less data is available as yet on hypervariable regions of rabbit antibody heavy chains. Fig. 8 shows available rabbit heavy chain sequence information in the region identified by Capra as the first hypervariable region in human heavy chains (48). There seems to be relatively little variability. Position 30 is a constant serine. Position 31 has two alternatives. Position 32 is tyrosine in all the sequences; 33 has three alternatives; 34 two; and 35 three. Positions 36 through 42 are invariant. The data is insufficient to identify a hypervariable region with certainty. It should be noted, however, that all the sequences are of the same length in this region, and there is no evidence of either insertion or deletion.

Fig. 9 shows the second hypervariable region. In this region of the sequence a cluster of five positions is identified in which three alternatives are seen among four sequences (positions 50, 52, 53, 54, and 57). Positions 47, 56, 61, and 62 have two alternatives. The remainder of the residues are invariant. The two pneumococcal Type III antibodies differ from each other in six positions in this region.

Fig. 10 shows a sequence segment homologous to the fourth hypervariable region defined by Kehoe and Capra (55). In the three sequences available in this region, residues 92 to 94 are invariant. Variability begins at

Antigen	Allo-type	ID	22	23	24	25	26	27	28	29	30	31	32	33	34	35	36	37	38	39	40	41	42
			Position																				
Pneu 3	A_1	BS-5	Cys	Thr	Val	Ser	Gly	Phe	Ser	Leu	Ser	Ser	Tyr	Asp	Met	Gly	Trp	Val	Arg	Gln	Ala	Pro	Gly
	A_1	3381-2	—	—	—	—	Glu	—	—	—	—	—	—	Ser	—	Ala	—	—	(—)	(—)	—	—	—
	A_2	K-25	—	—	—	—	—	—	—	—	—	Gly	—	—	—	Ser	—	—	—	—	—	—	—
Strep C	A_2	2690	—	—	—	—	—	Ile	Asp	—	—	—	—	Gly	Val	Ser	—	—	—	—	—	—	—

Fig. 8. Sequence of a segment of rabbit antibody heavy chain corresponding to the first hypervariable region of human heavy chain myeloma proteins (48). The cysteine nearest the amino-terminal is assigned position 22. Sequences are from (49-52).

Antigen	Allo-type	ID	46	47	48	49	50	51	52	53	54	55	56	57	58	59	60	61	62	63
Pneu 3	A_1	BS-5	Glu	Trp	Ile	Gly	Ile	Ile	Tyr	Ala	Ser	Gly	Ser	Thr	Tyr	Tyr	Ala	Ser	Trp	Ala
	A_1	3381-2	—	Tyr	—	—	Val	—	(Ser)	Ser	Gly	—	—	Ala	—	—	—	—	—	—
Pneu 8	A_1	325	—	—	—	—	—	—	—	—	—	(?)	—	Pro	—	—	—	Gln	Ser	—
Strep C	A_2	2690	—	—	—	—	Ala	—	Asp	Gly	Tyr	—	Thr	—	—	—	—	—	—	—

Fig. 9. Sequence of a segment of rabbit antibody heavy chain homologous to the second hypervariable region of human heavy chains (53). Sequences are from (49,50,52,54).

Antigen	Allo-type	ID	92	93	94	95	96	97	98	99	100	101	102	103	104	105	106	107	108	109	110	111	112
										Position													
Pneu 3	A_1	BS-5	Cys	Ala	Arg	Gln	Gly	Thr	Gly	Leu	Val	His	Leu	Ala	Phe	Val	---	---	---	Asp	Val	Trp	Gly
	A_2	K17	—	—	—	Ser	Ile	(?)	Thr	(?)	Ile	Asp	Ser	Ser	(?)	(?)	(?)	Phe	Leu	—	—	—	—
Pneu 8	A_1	3322-A	(—)	—	( )	Asp	Asn	Tyr	—	Asn	Ala	Gly	Tyr	Ile	(?)	Leu	---	---	---	---	---	—	—

Fig. 10. Sequence of a segment of rabbit antibody heavy chain including a hypervariable region. This segment is homologous to the fourth hypervariable region of Kehoe and Capra (55). Sequences are from (28,49,54).

residue 95. In each of the positions subsequent to residue 108 no homology is seen, each chain having a unique sequence except at position 98 where two chains share a glycine (BS-5 and 3322A). At position 109 and 110, BS-5 and K17 share the Asp-Val sequence, whereas there is a deletion in 3322A. Positions 111 and 112 appear identical in all three sequences with very little additional variation through position 121. All three antibodies have different hypervariable region lengths. The longest sequence is antibody K17, which appears to have a hypervariable region of 14 residues. BS-5 has a deletion of three residues while 3322A has a deletion of five residues. As in the first and second hypervariable regions of the heavy chain, there appears to be no sequence homology between the two antipneumococcal Type III antibodies.

DISCUSSION

The observation that immunization of rabbits with bacterial vaccines frequently results in the production of antibodies in very high concentration which may be either homogeneous or readily fractionated into homogeneous components has facilitated the application of sequence analysis to elicited antibodies. Improvements in sequencing techniques (24,31) allowing complete sequence analysis of a variable region to be performed on as little as 2 micromoles of polypeptide chain will yield a great deal of information concerning antibodies which arise through conventional immunization. This allows a critical comparison between such antibodies and myeloma proteins with specific antigen binding properties. As indicated in the introduction, certain questions concerning the evolution of the immune response and the generation of diversity are more readily answered utilizing elicited antibodies than myeloma proteins.

The Significance of a Hypervariable Region

Wu and Kabat on the basis of a critical examination of available human and murine light chain sequences concluded that there were three areas of hypervariability which could be distinguished from relatively constant sections within the variable region of these chains (42). They also demonstrated that deletions were to be found in relation to two of these hypervariable segments. Capra and Kehoe analyzed variability within the heavy chain and postulated four areas of hypervariability (48,53,55). Early studies with affinity labeling reagents indicated that at least some of these hypervariable regions were especially close to the antigen binding site (56). Most recently, elegant crystallographic analyses of two Fab fragments (1,2) clearly indicate that two of the three light chain hypervariable regions and three of the four heavy chain hypervariable regions actually form the antigen combining site. It appears then that hypervariability alone is not a sufficient criterion for identifying an antigen binding region. Examination of the rabbit antibody light chain shows three regions of hypervariability, one comprising the three amino terminal residues, the second corresponding to positions 30 to 32 analogous to the first hypervariable region described by Wu and Kabat, and the third comprising positions 91 to 97 corresponding to the third hypervariable region identified by these investigators. Examination of the two crystallographic analyses of Fab indicate that the amino-terminal three residues of the light chain do not play a major structural role in the integration of the molecule and are quite distant from the antibody combining site. On the other hand, positions homologous with the first and third hypervariable regions of the light chain participate in antigen binding. Corresponding regions in rabbit light chains also show hypervariability. The segment homologous to the second hypervariable region identified in human and murine light chains does not participate in formation of the antigen combining cavity; the corresponding segment of the rabbit antibody light chains shows very little variability. Comparison of the two crystallographic analyses indicate that variations in the length of the hypervariable region are the principal determinants of the size and shape of the combining site cavity (2). It is of interest that in rabbit light chains, variation in hypervariable segment length is found only in areas homologous to the first and third hypervariable regions.

Heavy chain data is more sparse. A first hypervariable region cannot be identified with certainty. However, the two other regions which appear clearly hypervariable correspond to two of the four hypervariable segments identified by Capra and Kehoe. In one of these regions variations in chain length also occurs; they are homologous to two of the three variable region segments which have been shown to participate in forming the antigen combining cavity. The third hypervariable region of Capra and Kehoe (55) does not appear to be significantly hypervariable in the limited rabbit heavy chain data available nor does it participate in forming the antigen combining cavity. In both the heavy and the light chains of rabbit antibodies, the carboxyl-terminal hypervariable segments (91 to 97 in the light chain and 95 to 109 in the heavy chain) are of greatest length and also of greatest variability in length.

Kindt et al (21) have suggested that the amino-terminal sequences of light chains of rabbit antibodies might be useful genetic markers for the variable region of the light chain. Indeed, a number of investigators have attempted to classify rabbit light chain sequences into subgroups on the basis of homology with prototypes of human sequences (35, 38). The high degree of homology seen in all the rabbit chains reported here (~ 75% identity) tends to make division into subgroups difficult. In any event, Fig. 2 demonstrates that identical amino terminal sequences may be associated with different specificities and the same specificity may be associated with substantial differences in amino-terminal sequence. If amino-terminal sequence differences are indeed to be markers for germ line genes, these findings suggest that the same antibody specificity may be associated with very different sets of germ line genes. Conversely, if amino-terminal sequence identity defines a single germ line gene, then one germ line gene may code for disparate specificities. Moreover, chain length does not appear to be correlated with antigen specificity. The distribution of chain length among pneumococcal antibodies does not differ significantly from that in the nonimmune pool. Antistreptococcus polysaccharide antibodies show a bias toward shorter light chain length. This may be related to inbreeding of the immunized population. Perhaps the phenotype of chain length is hereditable.

When two or three antibodies of the same specificity appear at one time during immunization, they often have different amino-terminal sequences, indicating that at least among the set of antibodies studied here, there does not seem to be a close relationship between "framework" sequence and specificity. Selective evolution of hypervariable regions with maintenance of a constant framework is not noted in these examples. A comparison of the amino-terminal sequences of antibodies 3322A and B allows a more critical examination of this question. Both of these pneumococcus Type VIII specific antibodies were isolated from the same antiserum which also contained several other Type VIII specific antibodies; both can be specifically eluted from Type VIII polysaccharide immunoadsorbant with cellobiose, indicating that this disaccharide segment of Type VIII polysaccharide is the immunodominant group (28). Nevertheless, they exhibit markedly different amino-terminal sequences.

The general lack of correlation between hypervariable region sequences of both light and heavy chains and antibody specificity indicates the very high degree of variability among antibodies specific for the same simple antigen. The greatest amount of data is available for antibodies specific for pneumococcal Type III polysaccharide, an unbranched repeating disaccharide polymer. While it is possible to conceive of several different ways of binding this antigen, it is already apparent that the number of unique hypervariable sequences in Type III specific antibodies is large. In contrast to these observations, studies of the first and second hypervariable region sequences of heavy chains of elicited antihapten antibodies from inbred guinea pigs show considerably more uniformity (57). Since other hypervariable regions which may participate in antigen binding have not yet been reported from these antibodies, an assessment of the uniformity of their combining sites cannot be made.

We previously reported unique changes in circular dichroism pattern in each of three pneumococcal Type III specific antibodies isolated from the same antiserum (58). On close analysis, the difference spectra indicated changes in the microenvironments of either tyrosine or tryptophan. An examination of the hypervariable regions of five pneumococcal Type III specific antibodies shows that 3374 has a tryptophan at position 32, and tyrosines at positions 91 and 92; 3368 tryptophan at 92; 3381 tryptophan at 32; BS-5 tyrosines at 30 and 93; and BS-1 tyrosines at 30, 93, and 97. Each of these antibodies thus have either tyrosine or tryptophan in one or both light chain hypervariable regions which appear to be associated with the antigen combining site. The varying interactions between these aromatic residues and the antigen may account for the changes in circular dichroism spectral observed. These aromatic residues are frequently found in antibody combining sites.

Protein 3315 appears to have a unique half-cystine within the third hypervariable region of the light chain (31). While no prior antibodies or myeloma proteins with antibody binding activity have been shown to have a cysteine within a hypervariable region, the human lambda chains X (59) and Bau (60) were demonstrated to have a half-cystine within the first hypervariable region.

The Interdomain Bridge

The presence of additional cysteines within the variable region at position 80 and within the constant region at position 171 is now well confirmed in a number of sequences, as is the location of the interdomain bridge by direct sequence analysis of a peptic peptide containing the disulfide bond. In examining the crystallographic models of the light chain dimer Mcg (61) and Fab' λ New (62), it is apparent that the homologous positions to 80 and 171 approach one another sufficiently closely within the three-dimensional structure to permit the presence of a disulfide bridge. This indicates that the domain structure of the rabbit light chain need not differ from that of other species (43). Since rabbit antibody light chains either contain five or seven half-cystines and never six, there presumably exist two constant region kappa isotypes as well as two sets of variable regions uniquely associated with each.

Invariant Regions

Invariant amino acids within the set of rabbit antibody light chains correspond very closely to invariant residues found in human and murine light chains with but one exception. Examination of crystallographic structure indicates that many of these residues are necessary for maintaining the overall conformation of the polypeptide chains. For example, the invariant glycines are all associated with either hairpin turns in the chain or with positions in which the presence of a side chain would not fit with a necessary structural feature (62). These observations indicate an evolutionary conservation of structural features necessary for the conformation and consequently the function of these molecules.

CONCLUSION

The study of the structure of elicited antibodies is still in its early stages. While only a few variable region sequences are available, it is already apparent that the simplicity and relative uniformity of the immune response suggested by studies of myeloma proteins with antigen binding properties may not reflect the complexity, diversity, and degeneracy of the normal elicited immune response. If the total number of germ line variable genes is to be estimated from the number of different immunoglobulin sequences outside of the hypervariable region and somatic mutation assessed from an examination of changes within hypervariable regions, it may well be necessary to wait until a great deal more sequence information on elicited antibodies becomes available.

Supported in part by a grant from the National Institutes of Health AI04967 and a Grant-In-Aid from the American Heart Association.

Michael N. Margolies is an established investigator of the American Heart Association.

REFERENCES

(1) L.M. Amzel, B.L. Chen, R.P. Phizackerley, R.J. Poljak, F. Saul, in Progress in Immunology II, vol. 1, Immunochemical Aspects, eds., L. Brent, J. Holborow (North-Holland Publishing Co. Amsterdam, 1974) pp. 85-92.

(2) D.M. Segal, E.A. Padlan, G.H. Cohen, E.W. Silverton, D.R. Davies, S. Rudikoff, M. Potter, in Progress in Immunology II, vol. 1, Immunochemical Aspects, eds., L. Brent, J. Holborow (North-Holland Publishing Co., Amsterdam, 1974) pp. 93-102.

(3) H.G. Kunkel, V. Agnello, F.G. Joslin, R.J. Winchester, J.D. Capra. J. Exp. Med. 137 (1973) 331.

(4) J.D. Capra, J.M. Kehoe. Advan. Immunol. (in press).

(5) M. Potter, R. Lieberman. J. Exp. Med. 132 (1970) 737.

(6) M. Potter. Physiol. Reviews 52 (1972) 631.

(7) L. Hood, J. Prahl. Advan. Immunol. 14 (1971) 291.

(8) F.F. Richards, L.M. Amzel, W.H. Konigsberg, B.N. Manjula, R.J. Poljak, R.W. Rosenstein, F. Saul, J.M. Varga, in The Immune System--Genes, Receptors, Signals. eds., E.E. Sercarz, A.R. Williamson, C.F. Fox (Academic Press, New York, 1974) pp. 53-67.

(9) D.W. Talmage. Science 129 (1959) 1643.

(10) P. Barstad, V. Farnsworth, M. Weigert, M. Cohn, L. Hood. Proc. Nat. Acad. Sci. 71 (1974) 4096.

(11) M. Cohn, B. Blomberg, W. Geckeler, W. Raschke, R. Riblet, M. Weigert, in The Immune System--Genes, Receptors, Signals. eds., E.E. Sercarz, A.R. Williamson, C.F. Fox (Academic Press, New York, 1974) pp. 89-117.

(12) R.M. Krause. Advan. Immunol. 12 (1970) 1.

(13) E. Haber. Fed. Proc. 29 (1970) 66.

(14) B.K. Seon, O.A. Roholt, D. Pressman. J. Immunol. 108 (1972) 86.

(15) E. Appella, O.A. Roholt, A. Chersi, G. Radzimski, D. Pressman. Biochem. Biophys. Res. Com 53 (1973) 1122.

(16) R.H. Painter, M.H. Freedman. J. Biol. Chem. 246 (1971) 6692.

(17) M.H. Freedman, R.B. Guyer, W.D. Terry. J. Biol. Chem. 247 (1972) 7051.

(18) J.-C. Jaton, M.D. Waterfield, M.N. Margolies, K. J. Bloch, E. Haber. Biochemistry 10 (1971) 1583.

(19) F.W. Chen, A.D. Strosberg, E. Haber. J. Immunol. 110 (1973) 98.

(20) T.J. Kindt, R.K. Seide, V.A. Bokisch, R.M. Krause. J. Exp. Med. 138 (1973) 522.

(21) T.J. Kindt, A.L. Thunberg, M. Mudgett, D.G. Klapper, in The Immune System--Genes, Receptors, Signals. eds., E.E. Sercarz, A.R. Williamson, C.F. Fox (Academic Press, New York, 1974) pp.69-88.

(22) E. Haber, A.D. Strosberg, in Specific Receptors of Antibodies, Antigens and Cells. eds., D. Pressman, T.B. Tomasi, A.L. Grossberg, N.R. Rose (S. Karger, Buffalo, 1972) pp. 236-258.

(23) I. Gibbons, R.N. Perham. Biochem. J. 116 (1970) 843.

(24) A.W. Brauer, M.N. Margolies, E. Haber. Manuscript in preparation.

(25) G. Braunitzer, B. Schrank, A. Ruhfus. Hoppe-Seyler's Z. Physiol. Chem. 351 (1970) 1589.

(26) K.J. Fraser, K. Poulsen, E. Haber. Biochemistry 11 (1972) 4974.

(27) M.N. Margolies, A.D. Strosberg, K.J. Fraser, D.J. Perry, A. Brauer, E. Haber. Fed. Proc. 33 (1974) 809.

(28) F.W. Chen, E. Haber. Unpublished results.

(29) W.C. Cheng, K.J. Fraser, E. Haber. J. Immunol. 111 (1973) 1677.

(30) J.-C. Jaton, M.D. Waterfield, M.N. Margolies, E. Haber. Proc. Nat. Acad. Sci. 66 (1970) 959.

(31) M.N. Margolies, L.E. Cannon, A.D. Strosberg, E. Haber. Manuscript in preparation, 1975.

(32) A.D. Strosberg, K.J. Fraser, M.N. Margolies, E. Haber. Biochemistry 11 (1972) 4978.

(33) J.-C. Jaton. Biochem. J. 141 (1974) 1.

(34) J.-C. Jaton. Biochem. J. 141 (1974) 15.

(35) D.G. Braun, J.-C. Jaton. Immunochemistry 10 (1973) 387.

(36) K.C.S. Chen, T.J. Kindt, R.M. Krause. Proc. Nat. Acad. Sci. (1974) 1995.

(37) L. Hood, M.D. Waterfield, J. Morris, C.W. Todd. Ann. N.Y. Acad. Sci. 190 (1971) 26.

(38) L. Hood, K. Eichmann, H. Lackland, R.M. Krause, J.J. Ohms. Nature (London) 228 (1970) 1040.

(39) T.J. Kindt, R.K. Seide, H. Lackland, A.L. Thunberg. J. Immunol. 109 (1972) 735.

(40) A.L. Thunberg, H. Lackland, T.J. Kindt. J. Immunol. 111 (1973) 1755.

(41) M.D. Waterfield, J.W. Prahl, L.E. Hood, T.J. Kindt, R.M. Krause. Nature, New Biol. 240 (1972) 215.

(42) T.T. Wu, E.A. Kabat. J. Exp. Med. 132 (1972) 211.

(43) J.A. Gally, G.M. Edelman. Annual Review of Genetics 6 (1972) 1.

(44) L.E. Cannon, M.N. Margolies, A.D. Strosberg, E. Haber. Manuscript in preparation.

(45) M.N. Margolies, A.D. Strosberg, K.J. Fraser, E. Haber. Manuscript in preparation.

(46) Poulsen, K., K.J. Fraser, E. Haber. Proc. Nat. Acad. Sci. 69 (1972) 2495.

(47) A.D. Strosberg, M.N. Margolies, E. Haber. Fed. Proc. 33 (1974) 726.

(48) J.D. Capra. Nature New Biol. 230 (1971) 61.

(49) J.-C. Jaton. Biochem. J. 143 (1974) 723.

(50) M.S. Rosemblatt, D.W. Andrews, L.E. Cannon, E. Haber. Fed. Proc. (in press) 1975.

(51) J.-C. Jaton, J. Haimovich, Biochem. J. 139 (1974) 281.

(52) J.B. Fleischman. Immunochemistry 10 (1973) 401.

(53) J.D. Capra, J.M. Kehoe. Proc. Nat. Acad. Sci. 71 (1974) 845.

(54) A.D. Strosberg, J.-C. Jaton, J.D. Capra, E. Haber. Fed. Proc. 31 (1972) 771.

(55) M. Kehoe, J.D. Capra. Proc. Nat. Acad. Sci. 68 (1971) 2019.

(56) D. Givol, in Contemporary Topics in Molecular Immunology, vol. 2, eds. R.A. Reisfeld, W.J. Mandy (Plenum Press, New York, 1973) pp. 27-50.

(57) J.J. Cebra, P.H. Koo, A. Ray. Science 186 (1974) 263.

(58) D.A. Holowka, A.D. Strosberg, J.W. Kimball, E. Haber, R.E. Cathou. Proc. Nat. Acad. Sci. 69 (1972) 3399.

(59) C. Milstein, J.B. Clegg, J.M. Jarvis. Biochem. J. 110 (1968) 631.

(60) K. Baczko, D.G. Braun, M. Hess, N. Hilschmann. Hoppe-Seyler's Z. Physiol. Chem. 351 (1970) 763.

(61) M. Schiffer, R.L. Girling, K.R. Ely, A.B. Edmundson. Biochemistry 12 (1973) 4620.

(62) R.J. Poljak, L.M. Amzel, B.L. Chen, R.P. Phizackerley, F. Saul. Proc. Nat. Acad. Sci. 71 (1974) 3440.

DISCUSSION

M. TEODORESCU: A short comment on your speculation that the antibody producing cell was transformed in continuous line. First of all, the kind of cultures that you described could be easily obtained from any normal spleen without any virus. It is probable that what you obtained is evidence for a communication between tumor cells *in vitro* by breach or by passenger cell fusion and that the immunoglobulin gene was transferred to a fibroblast, so that you actually did not transform an antibody producing cell into a continous cell line. We have failed to obtain established cell lines from rabbit so far, probably because rabbits do not have tumors of the lymphoid system.

E. HABER: The first part of your comment is rather easy to answer. This is a transformed cell line, as evidenced by the presence of the viral antigen (T-antigen) on its surface and by the fact that the virus can be rescued as infectious virus from the culture itself by fusion with indicator cells. The second part I cannot really address. There has been no rigorous test of the identity of this cell line as a lymphoid cell line. It is clear, however, that this is a population of cells capable of producing antibodies.

M. TEODORESCU: Is it an antibody producing or containing cell?

E. HABER: Well, it is an antibody containing cell, which has the capacity to synthesize the antibody which it contains.

G. KRAMER: Using your technique did you obtain from the same spleen, different clones making different antibodies?

E. HABER: No, this investigation is presently underway. The information I presented was on the only clone which we have successfully cultured from that spleen.

E.A. KABAT: The hypervariability shown in positions 1, 2 and 3 might just be a consequence of pieces of precursor molecule that are not split uniformly and the chain length differences found from the hybridisation data might not be really relevant to the main structure of the antibody.

E. HABER: I certainly do not wish to pretend that either hypervariability or variation in chain length have important structural connotations with respect to the structural integration of the molecule or the combining site. This is not, however, the result of variable deletion of the amino-terminal segment of the precursor molecule. When we subject the sequence data to objective computer analysis in order to line them up according to maximal homology the deletions do not fall at the end. They fall at either positions 1, 2 or 3. This suggests that the amino-terminal deletions do not simply represent ragged ends.

R.C. LEIF: Since you have a limited number of specific immunoglobulins, have you tested if they are inherited? This would be a test of the somatic mutation theory, even with the use of outbred animals, because even if only one of the hypervariable regions were inherited it would be strong evidence against somatic mutation.

E. HABER: We have not studied inheritance of structure phenotypes in the rabbit. The data available from Krause's lab on streptococcal antibodies suggests inheritance of partial idiotypic cross-reactivities. Until these are defined in structural terms we cannot be sure that they represent combining site information or even what the structural meaning of such cross reactivities are.

C. MILSTEIN: I was struck by the difference in the pattern of variability of the kappa chain in the rabbit compared to that of the human kappa chain. This brings in rather dramatically, especially because of the deletions and additions, the gap region after the second cysteine. In human kappa chain, there is only one example of deletions in that region. In contrast the rabbit seems to have found it very convenient to introduce deletions and additions quite often there. It strikes me that this may well illustrate how each species may find their own solution to the problem.

E. HABER: We started to work in the rabbit not simply to gather more data in another species, but because of the conviction that antibody molecules might be subjected to different kinds of selection pressures than those to which human and mouse myelomas are subject. If you looked at elicited antibodies in the mouse or the human you might find the same kinds of differences. Are you not jumping too far when you say this is the rabbit's solution to this problem, whereas the human or mouse solution might be different? Might we not be comparing apples and oranges?

C. MILSTEIN: I think the myeloma is representative of the population and that in the human the solution is as we see it from the myeloma protein.

E. HABER: If what you say is really true, that is if the three species are comparable, then the rabbits must find it advantageous to change the shape and the size of the combining site cavity by adding to or deleting from the third light chain hypervariable region.

C. MILSTEIN: Right, but there must be some underlying mechanism, a genetic mechanism that is either in the germ line or in the somatic mutation process.

F. HAUROWITZ: Does the amino acid composition of the antibodies change after injection of the virus and does it remain constant after infection? I am asking the second question because the cell might differentiate.

E. HABER: The evidence to answer the first question is limited only to information on the isoelectric point of the antibody protein. If there are substitutions balanced according to charge or neutral substitutions we would not detect them. To answer the second part of your question we have subcultured this line for many many generations and it appears to be constant in respect to all the properties we have examined.

M.M. SIGEL: I would like to ask a couple of related questions. In your fusion experiments on monkey kidney cells, were you able to demonstrate antibody synthesis in the fused cell?

E. HABER: It wasn't looked for.

M.M. SIGEL: And, secondly, have you tried fusion with lymphocytes?

E. HABER: Not yet.

M.M. SIGEL: It is known that many of these viruses cause fragmentation of chromosomes, deletions and translocations. Might not their use be an approach to some of Dr. Williamson's questions this morning? The origin of diversity or relation to translocation of the V and C regions.

E. HABER: Karotyping of this cell line indicates that it is heteroploid-the number of chromosomes are not quite twice the normal diploid number.

E. BRILES: You have shown us that rabbits are able to make many different antibodies to the pneumococcal carbodrates; the same is true for inbred mice immunized with streptococcal group A carbohydrate. Why are only one or a few antibodies made in each individual animal?

E. HABER: I wish I knew the answer to that - Mel Cohn told me that I was going to be asked that question and I have been thinking about it for considerably longer than the last hour. In general a pattern of evolution is seen - in each rabbit the first antibodies are of relatively low affinity; there is a recruitment of affinity with time as in many other systems. The appearance of the products of a new clone always seems to occur at a time when antibody concentration has first fallen and then is rising very rapidly. Because of the very high concentration of plasma antibody in these animals it may well be that there is intense competition for antigen between circulating antibody and cell receptors. As the concentration of antibody rises there is not enough antigen present to continue stimulation of the clone. A new clone then arises, which has receptors of higher affinity for the antigen. This explanation tells you something about why new clones are continually appearing. However, the reason why only a small number of clones arise at any one time is unclear. I doubt very much that we are dealing with a T-independent antigen here because the rabbit does not at all respond to soluble polysaccharide. The immunizing antigen must be a vaccine; presumably the organism itself or some cellular proteins act as carrier. This must be a relatively complex antigenic stimulus. The reasons for the magnitude and simplicity of the response are not at all clear.

C. BELL: I would like to ask a question and to make a comment. Do you detect host rabbit immunoglobulin at the secreted level, that is in the culture supernatant or on the membrane, or at the total cellular level?

E. HABER: The antibody can be found in both the supernatant and within the cell sap, the concentration of antibody is low in both places.

C. BELL: I have experienced a similar low incidence of secretion of immunoglobulin by rabbit spleen and lymph node cells following treatment with exogenous RNA. These lymphocytes secreted little immunoglobulin and retained almost equal amounts of immunoglobulin at the cellular and membranal level. Although when the exogenous RNA was obtained from cells expressing an allelic allotype for the kappa light chain and for the variable V_H (a locus) chain, allelic immunoglobulin markers were selected at the membranal and cellular level essentially in a similar fashion to the expression of SV_{40} antigens by your rabbit transformed cells. would not call the RNA treated lymphocytes transformed cells. I do know, however, that they are lymphocytes, perhaps nucleated cells or precursor B-cells which have translated the exogenous RNA but either have not yet fully differentiated to plasma secreting cells, or have remained arrested at some level leading to the retention of the cellular immunoglobulin. Did you determine the total amount of secreted immunoglobulin antibody with reference to the allotypic specificity and did you look for surface immunoglobulin expression in the transformed cells?

E. HABER: We looked for immunoglobulin on the surface with fluorescent staining and there must not have been enough to see. More sensitive methods need to be applied. Immunoglobulin concentration was measured in two ways, by affinity chromatography with antigen or by precipitation with anti-IgG; both methods gave approximately the same result.

C. BELL: Were your reagents directed to the V regions of the immunoglobulin?

E. HABER: Antibodies were not specifically directed to the variable part of the synthesized immunoglobulin.

REPETITIVE HINGE REGION SEQUENCES IN A γ3 HEAVY CHAIN DISEASE PROTEIN-ISOLATION OF AN 11,000 DALTON FRAGMENT

B.F. Frangione, J.B. Adlersberg and E.C. Franklin, Dept. of Medicine, Irvington House Institute, New York University Medical Center, New York, N.Y.

The heavy chain of IgG3 subclass of human immunoglobulins (γ3) has a molecular weight of 60,000 daltons, instead of the 50,000 dalton value reported for γ1, γ2, and γ4 heavy chains. Using protein OMM, a γ3 Heavy Chain Disease protein, it was possible to isolate and analyze the extra fragment. Protein OMM had a molecular weight of 39,000 daltons, Gly as its NH_2-terminal, and contained only the hinge region, C_H2 and C_H3 domains. CNBr cleavage at Met 252 (γ1 numbering, protein Eu[1]) yielded the hinge fraction (Fh fragment). On the basis of molecular weight of Fh fragment (10,800 daltons), its amino acid composition, its partial sequence, and its unexpectedly low number of tryptic peptides, it is postulated that i) the extra fragment in γ3 Heavy Chain Disease protein OMM represents a series of similar or identical duplication of sections of the previously reported γ3 hinge region[2,3]; ii) this unusual structure is not a product of gene aberration but is a normal feature of intact γ3 heavy chains. Although the biological significance of these findings is not known, the relationship of the primary structure of the hinge region among different immunoglobulins supports the concept that this region is coded by a unique piece of DNA which has evolved by partial duplications and/or crossing over.

REFERENCES

(1) G.M. Edelman, A. Cunningham, W.E. Gall, B.D. Gottlieb, V. Rutishauser and M.J. Wardal, Proc. Nat.Acad.Sci.(USA), 63 (1969) 78.
(2) B. Frangione and C. Milstein, Nature, 224 (1969) 597.
(3) B. Frangione and C. Wolfenstein-Todel, Proc.Nat.Acad. Sci. (USA), 69 (1972) 3673.

STRUCTURAL CHARACTERIZATION OF A MUTANT HUMAN LAMBDA TYPE L-CHAIN IMMUNOGLOBULIN

Fred A. Garver, Lebe Chang, Takashi Isobe and Elliott F. Osserman, Medical College of Georgia, Augusta, Georgia and College of Physicians and Surgeons, Columbia University, New York, N. Y.

Recently, Isobe and Osserman described the first case (Sm) of a plasma cell dyscrasia associated with the production of a defective IgG molecule containing lambda (λ) type L-chains (1). In addition, the λ chains possessed a substantial quantity of carbohydrate. The molecular weights of both the γ and λ chains were considerably smaller than those of normal subunits. In order to define the molecular nature of the deletion, we have determined the partial amino acid sequence of the urinary Sm λ chain. The protein had a blocked N-terminus presumably pyrrolidone carboxylic acid (PCA). After chymotryptic digestion, the amino-terminal peptide was selectively isolated from a column of Dowex 50x2 equilibrated with water. A ninhydrin negative peptide was detected with the chlorine-starch iodide reagent after paper chromatography; it had an amino acid composition of (GLU,SER,ALA,LEU). Treatment of the peptide with carboxypeptidase A released leucine (96%) and alanine (24%), and hydrazinolysis removed serine establishing the N-terminal sequence as PCA-SER-ALA-LEU. After hydrolysis of the protein with trypsin, the peptides were separated on a Dowex 50x2 column, followed by chromatography on Dowex 1x2 columns. All of the expected eleven tryptic peptides of the constant (C) region were recovered. The C-region of protein Sm contains an arginyl residue at position 191, which is correlated with the Oz^- factor, and a glycyl residue at position 154, associated with the $Kern^+$ isotype. In addition, a large glycopeptide consisting of 32 residues was isolated, which corresponded to the N-terminal region. This peptide was further split with thermolysin, and eight peptides, covering the entire region, were purified and sequenced with the Edman-dansyl technique. The C-terminal portion of this peptide terminates with GLN-PRO-LYS, which is the initiation of the C-region corresponding to positions 110-112. The Sm V-region of 29 residues is very homologous to protein NE1 (2). Thus, protein Sm has an internal deletion of 82 amino acid residues, which is entirely restricted to the variable (V) region.

REFERENCES

1. T. Isobe and E. F. Osserman. Blood 43 (1974) 505.
2. F. Garver and N. Hilschmann. Eur. J. Biochem. 26 (1972)10.

HETEROGENEITY OF THE C-REGION OF AN IgG1 IMMUNOGLOBULIN: THE STRUCTURE OF γ-HEAVY CHAIN DISEASE PROTEIN BAZ

Fred A. Garver, Lebe Chang and Byron McGuire, Medical College of Georgia, Augusta, Georgia.

Heterogeneity of the constant (C) region of immunoglobulins results from two types of sequence variability, isotypic and allotypic variants. Allotypic variants are allelic markers which segregate in the population and are inherited in simple Mendelian fashion,such as the Gm factors of IgG proteins. The Gm markers were first detected serologically and subsequent sequence studies showed that they were usually associated with single amino acid exchanges. In the process of delineating the structural defect of a γ-heavy chain disease protein (BAZ), we have found an amino acid substitution in the C-region which has not been described before. Protein BAZ contains two methionyl residues, and cyanogen bromide cleavage yields three fragments which were separated on Sephadex G-100 in 30% formic acid. The last peak (CB III) represents the C-terminal octadecapeptide of the polypeptide chain. The amino acid composition of this peptide revealed an absence of alanine and an additional mole of glycine. Using the Edman-dansyl technique, the sequence of the C-terminal region of protein BAZ was shown to be: 431 HIS-GLU-GLY-LEU-HIS-ASN-HIS-TYR-THR-GLN-LYS-SER-LEU-SER-LEU-SER-PRO-GLY. (440)
Therefore, protein BAZ has an exchange of ALA→GLY at position 433, using the numbering system of protein NIE (1). Fragment CB I contained 176 amino acid residues and had an N-terminal isoleucyl residue and a C-terminal homoseryl residue. Therefore, CB I represents the interior of the polypeptide chain from position 255 to 430. The second Sephadex peak, CB II, was a glycopeptide with a blocked α-amino group and a C-terminal homoseryl residue. This peptide corresponded to the N-terminal portion of the chain. According to the amino acid composition, CB II contained 38 residues. This fragment also lacked cysteine, further supporting the dissociating studies in 6 M guanidine HCl which indicated an absence of disulfide bonds joining the γ chain dimer (2). Therefore, protein BAZ has a deletion of 212 amino acid residues and the deletion encompasses the hinge region of the molecule.

REFERENCES

1. N. Hilschmann, and H. Ponstingl. Hoppe-Seyler's Z. Physiol. Chem. 353 (1972) 1369.
2. L. L. Smith, B. P. Barton, F. A. Garver, C. L. Lutcher and G. B. Faguet. Fed. Proc. 32 (1973) 3507.

GROWTH FACTOR FOR A VIRAL TRANSFORMED CELL FROM RAT LIVER AND HEMICORPUS PERFUSIONS

A. Lipton, C.J. Roehm, J.W. Robertson, J.M. Dietz and L.S. Jefferson, The Milton S. Hershey Medical Center, Hershey, Pennsylvania, 17033.

Serum has been shown to contain several macromolecules necessary for the growth and survival of cultured 3T3 mouse fibroblasts (3T3) and SV40 virus-transformed 3T3 cells (SV-3T3). The 3T3 growth factor specifically promotes the growth of 3T3 cells, while the SV-3T3 growth factor promotes that of SV-3T3 cells.[1,2]

Perfusion of either rat liver or rat hemicorpus results in the production of a factor that promotes the growth of SV-3T3 cells. This material does not promote the growth of sparse 3T3 cells or the initiation of DNA synthesis in confluent 3T3 cells.

Gel infiltration of the liver perfusate thru Sephadex G-100, pH 7.4, 0.01 M NaCl, Tris buffer reveals the SV-3T3 growth-promoting activity to be a large molecule (35,000 daltons). This activity is not dialyzable. The activity is completely destroyed by treatment with pepsin and 50 per cent of the activity is removed by trypsin treatment. It is not destroyed by treatment with bovine pancreatic DNAse I or RNAse-A. It has the same heat and pH stability as does the serum SV-3T3 growth factor.

REFERENCES

(1) Holley, R.W. and Kiernan, J.A., Proc. Natl. Acad. Sci., U.S.A., 60 (1968) 300.

(2) Paul, D., Lipton, A. and Klinger, I. Proc. Natl. Acad. Sci., U.S.A., 68 (1971) 645.

LYMPHOCYTE RESPONSES TO MITOGENS AND ANTIGENS IN AGAROSE-GEL CULTURES.

E. Kondracki and F. Milgrom, Department of Microbiology, State University of New York at Buffalo, Buffalo, New York.

It has been suggested that cell-to-cell contact is a necessary early step for lymphocyte proliferation in response to antigens or mitogens (1).

In order to study further this possibility, we have developed a technique to examine the lymphocyte response to stimulating agents in agarose-gel cultures. The lymphocytes were separated by Ficoll-Hypaque density gradient centrifugation from peripheral blood of healthy human donors, and $4x10^5$ cells were mixed at 40°C with 100 µl of melted 0.5% agarose in RPMI 1640 medium. After solidification of the agarose, the vast majority of cells remained separated from each other. The gel was overlaid with 400 µl of RPMI 1640 containing 10% autologous serum and a suitable dose of mitogen or antigen. After incubation at 37°C in 5% CO_2 atmosphere for 2-4 days, 0.2 µCi of ^{3}H-thymidine were added to each tube and 3 hours later, the cultures were terminated by freezing at -20°C. Afterward, the tubes were heated at 100°C and centrifuged at 56°C. The pellet was washed twice with 5% TCA, solubilized with NCS solubilizer, and mixed in scintillation vials with a toluene-based "scintillation cocktail". The samples were counted in a liquid scintillation spectrometer.

The response to PHA-P in agarose gel cultures was at most 10% of that in liquid cultures. This response could be increased 3-5 fold by incorporating into agarose (a) autologous erythrocytes, (b) untreated erythrocyte stromata, (c) sonicated stromata or the (d) supernatant fluid from sonicated and centrifuged stromata. The efficiency of these preparations in increasing the lymphocyte response was a>b>c >d. It was also shown that lymphocytes in agarose gel responded hardly, if at all, to Con-A, PWM, Zn^{++} and $NaIO_4$. For studies on antigen stimulation, the effect of PPD on lymphocytes from tuberculin-sensitive subjects was examined. No response in agarose cultures was noted and incorporation of erythrocytes had no effect.

Our results are consistent with the suggestions that cell-to-cell contact is very important for lymphocyte stimulation. Furthermore, we have shown that erythrocytes or even their membrane fragments are capable of providing necessary conditions for proliferation of separated lymphocytes.

(1) J.H. Peters, Exptl. Cell Res. 74 (1972) 179.

STEROL SYNTHESIS IN NORMAL, PHYTOHEMAGGLUTININ-STIMULATED, AND LEUKEMIC MOUSE LYMPHOCYTES

H.W. Chen, H.J. Heiniger, and A.A. Kandutsch, The Jackson Laboratory, Bar Harbor, Maine

Normal peripheral blood lymphocytes synthesize cholesterol at a very low rate. Incubation of these mouse lymphocytes with phytohemagglutinin stimulated the incorporation of thymidine into DNA of lymphocytes as they transformed into large lymphoblasts. DNA synthesis began after about 24 hours of incubation and reached a peak at 48 hours. The *de-novo* synthesis of sterols from acetate was stimulated much earlier beginning at 4 hours of incubation and reaching a maximum at 24 hours, approximately at the time DNA synthesis began. The rates of ^{14}C incorporation from ^{14}C--acetate into fatty acids and into CO_2 by phytohemagglutinin treated blood cells were not significantly different from control values. Phytohemagglutinin stimulation of sterol synthesis could be abolished by the addition of certain oxygenated derivatives of cholesterol (e.g., 25-hydroxycholesterol and 20 -hydroxycholesterol) which specifically depress the activity of the regulatory enzyme in the sterol synthesis pathway, 3-hydroxy-3-methylglutaryl CoA reductase[2]. This treatment also abolished DNA synthesis and blastogenesis which otherwise followed the peak of sterol synthesis. Furthermore, DNA synthesis was repressed only if the inhibitor was added early enough to prevent sterol synthesis from reaching its usual maximum.

Peripheral lymphocytes from leukemic AKR/J mice synthesize sterols from acetate at a vastly greater rate, 20- to 100-fold, than the respective cells from normal AKR/J mice[1]. This great rate of sterol synthesis in leukemic lymphoblasts is only partly reduced upon addition of the oxygenated derivatives of cholesterol in concentrations which abolish the synthesis in PHA-stimulated lymphocytes.

REFERENCES

(1) H.W. Chen and H.J. Heiniger, Cancer Res. 34 (1974) 1304.
(2) A.A. Kandutsch and H.W. Chen, J. Biol. Chem. 248 (1973) 8408.

Supported by Research Contract N01 CP 33255 of the National Cancer Institute and Research Grant CA 02758 of the same Institute.

CAN PROTEIN SYNTHESIS IN CULTURED CELLS BE REGULATED BY MEMBRANE-MEDIATED EVENTS ?

G. Koch, P. Bilello, R. Mittelstaedt, A. Hoffman and L. Fisher, Roche Institute of Molecular Biology, Nutley, New Jersey

Membranes are thought to play a key role in the regulation of basic functions of the cell such as DNA replication, gene expression and transport of nutrients. They carry specific receptors for hormones and for cell-cell interactions[1]. Infection by viruses, especially by oncogenic viruses, causes alterations in membrane structures[2]. Cells are released from contact inhibition by exposure to trypsin or pronase[3]. Addition of pronase-released membrane glycoproteins to suspended cells results in a rapid inhibition of protein synthesis[4]. Exposure of several tissue culture cell lines to medium hypertonicity[5] (exerted by addition of either sucrose or salts), to DMSO[6] and to L-1-Tosylamido-2-Phenylethyl Chloromethyl Ketone (TPCK)[7] triggers an immediate blockage in the initiation of protein synthesis. However, protein synthesis in cell-free extracts prepared from these cells continues in the presence of either sucrose, glycerol, DMSO or TPCK. These observations suggest that membrane-mediated events are involved in the regulation of protein synthesis in cultured cells.

REFERENCES

(1) O. Mechter and I.D.K. Halkerston, In "The Hormones" 5 (1964) 697.
(2) L. Warren, J.P. Fuhrer and C.A.Buck, Proc. Nat. Acad. Sci. USA 69 (1972) 1838.
(3) M.M. Burger, Nature 227 (1970) 170.
(4) G.Koch, H. Kubinski and F. Koch, Hoppe Seyler's Z. (1974) in press.
(5) J.L. Saborio, S.S. Pong and G. Koch, J. Mol. Biol. 85 (1974) 195.
(6) J.L. Saborio and G. Koch, J. Biol. Chem. 248 (1973) 8343.
(7) S.S. Pong, D.L. Nuss and G. Koch, J. Biol. Chem. (1974) in press.

ALTERATION OF MEMBRANE ANTIGENS BY TRYPSIN

J.A. Molinari, S. Sinka and D. Platt, Univ. of Pittsburgh, Pittsburgh, Pennsylvania

Transformed cells are capable of being agglutinated by plant lectins, such as wheat germ agglutinin[1] and concanavalin A,[2] while normal cells remain unaffected. When normal fibroblasts are treated with trypsin they likewise are agglutinated in the presence of these lectins.[3] Since the immunologic implications of these phenomena remain to be clarified, the present study examined alterations in antigenicity of normal (3T3) and polyoma virus-transformed (PY-3T3) mouse fibroblasts following mild treatment with trypsin.

The cell lines were grown in Dulbecco's modified Eagle's medium and harvested 5 days after subculturing. Cell layers were obtained for immunization employing either mechanical scraping or treatment with 10 μg/ml twice crystallized trypsin for 3 min. Washed cell preparations were resuspended in physiological saline to a concentration of 3×10^5 cells/ml and diluted 1:2 with complete Freund's adjuvant to form stable emulsions. ICR/CD-1 mice were immunized with 0.2 ml subcutaneously and foot pad tested 7 days later to detect delayed hypersensitive reactions. The extent of pad swelling following challenge with 0.05 ml of an appropriate test suspension was compared to that measured for a control hind pad injected with 0.05 ml sterile physiological saline. Measurements were taken 4 and 24 hr after challenge.

Mice immunized with untreated PY-3T3 cells gave positive delayed hypersensitive responses (24 hr) when challenged with homologous antigen, but mild treatment with trypsin prior to sensitization abrogated the ability of the viral-transformed cells to induce a 24 hr reaction. None of the animals given untreated 3T3 fibroblasts responded to foot pad challenge with a similar cell preparation. However, mice immunized with trypsin-treated 3T3 cells showed positive 24 hr reactions after challenge with either homologous antigen or untreated PY-3T3 cells.

REFERENCES

(1) J.C. Aub, B.H. Sanford, and M.N. Cote, Proc. Nat. Acad. Sci., U.S.A. 54 (1965) 396.
(2) M. Inbar and L. Sachs, Nature 223 (1969) 710.
(3) M. Burger, Fed. Proc. 32 (1973) 91.

IgM Complex Receptors on T and B Lymphocytes

H. Whitten[1], E.W. Lamon[1] and B. Anderson[2]
1-Department of Surgery and Microbiology, University of Alabama in Birmingham School of Medicine, Birmingham, Alabama and , 2-Department of Tumor Biology, Karolinska Institute, Stockholm, Sweden

CBA mouse antiserum was harvested five days following a primary injection of sheep red blood cells (SRBC). Using this antiserum (heat inactivated) coated on SRBC the extent of rosette formation with non-immune spleen, lymph node and thymus lymphocytes was determined. The macroglobulin nature of the antiserum was evidenced by a hemolytic titer of 1:1024 and an extreme 2-mercaptoethanol sensitivity of hemagglutination activity. A zenith of rosettes was observed with a 1:32 dilution of antiserum with all three types of lymphocytes. 25% of spleen cells, 10% of lymph node cells and 7% of thymus cells exhibited SRBC rosettes at this dilution of antiserum. No rosettes were observed when the lymphocytes were incubated with SRBC alone. Subsequent fractionation experiments employing rabbit anti-Ig serum, rabbit anti-T serum and macrophage removal by iron powder and magnetism showed that sub-populations of both normal T and B CBA splenic lymphocytes possessed receptors for the IgM-SRBC complexes. The receptor was insensitive to trypsin. The functional significance of a receptor for IgM complexes on a thymocyte subpopulation may be correlated with the recently demonstrated destruction of Murine Sarcoma Virus (MSV) induced tumor cells _in vitro_ by normal thymocytes in conjunction with MSV tumor specific IgM (Lamon, Whitten, Skurzak, Andersson and Klein, unpublished data).

B AND T LYMPHOCYTES IN DYSGAMMAGLOBULINEMIA

B. Q. Lanier, A. S. Goldman, and N. S. Harris, Shriners Burns Institute, and The University of Texas Medical Branch, Galveston, Texas

The immunological surface characteristics of T and B lymphocytes was investigated in patients with primary immunodeficiencies. T lymphocytes were enumerated by the E-rosette assay. In addition, the E-rosettes were also examined after *in vitro* treatment of lymphocytes with thymosin[1]. B lymphocytes were determined by fluorescent staining using heavy chain specific antibodies to IgA, IgG, and IgM, as well as a specific antisera to plasma cells which was prepared by using an *in vitro* culture of human plasmacytoma cells as the antigen. This antisera recognizes a population (11.5%) of human blood lymphocytes with a surface plasma cell antigenic marker[2].

Twenty patients were studied. They ranged in age from six months to 45 years and had one of the following immunodeficiencies: severe combined immunodeficiency, Bruton's x-linked agammaglobulinemia, x-linked dysgammaglobulinemia, variable hypogammaglobulinemia, or isolated IgA deficiency. The most significant aspect of this study was the relationship of the number of lymphocytes with the plasma cell antigen (PC) and the type of immunodeficiency. Blood lymphocytes bearing PC were deficient in x-linked agammaglobulinemias and certain other diseases. The levels of PC bearing lymphocytes correlated with the number of Ig bearing cells in some of these disorders, but not in others. These studies suggest that the measurement of the plasma cell antigen on lymphocytes is an additional tool for the investigations of primary immunodeficiency diseases, and may aid in further understanding and categorizing them. (This study was supported in part by NCI R01 CA 15278 01.)

REFERENCES

(1) A. L. Goldstein, A. Guha, M. A. Hardy, and A. White, Proc. Nat'l. Acad. Sci. 69 (1972) 1800.

(2) N. S. Harris, Nature 250 (1974) 507.

THE ROLE OF THYMIC EXTRACT IN TRANSFER OF DELAYED HYPERSENSITIVITY (D.H.S.) AND IMMUNOSTIMULATION

Elias G. Elias, M.D., M.S., F.A.C.S. and Robert M. Cohen, B.S.
Roswell Park Memorial Institute, Buffalo, New York

The first objective was to transfer cell-mediated immunity to guinea pigs (G.P.) and man, utilizing a non-cellular thymus extract (TE) from previously sensitized G.P. Twenty-two G.P. less than 3 months of age were the donors of TE. Three of them were not sensitized and these donated TE^{o}. Another 9 animals were sensitized with dinitrochlorobenzene (DNCB) and donated TE^{DNCB}. The remaining 10 G.P. were sensitized with BCG and were the donors of TE^{PPD}. Forty-four adult G.P. received different thymic extracts: 12 received TE^{o} by different routes and none of these developed D.H.S. to DNCB or PPD. Sixteen adult animals received TE^{DNCB} and were divided into 2 groups that were tested 12 hours and 6 days later and both groups developed D.H.S. to DNCB. The last 16 adult G.P. received TE^{PPD} at different dose levels (.1, .3, .5 of thymus) and were tested for PPD skin reactions at 24 h, 1 and 2 weeks, and at 3 months. D.H.S. to PPD reached maximum at 2 w period post-transfer as 13/16 turned positive to PPD.

Eight patients - with metastatic carcinoma that showed no DNCB response on 2 or more occasions for over 2 months - received TE^{DNCB} intradermally (I.D.) and 6 of them developed D.H.S. to DNCB. Another 9 patients that were PPD negative received TE^{PPD} I.D. and 7 of them developed D.H.S. to PPD between the 4th and 6th day.

The second objective was non-specific immunostimulation in man. Eight patients received TE^{o},which resulted in a rise in peripheral lymphocyte count, PHA stimulation or T cell rosette formation.

It seems that D.H.S. to DNCB and PPD could be transferred cross-species with small doses of acellular thymic extract, even in the immunosuppressed subjects. An intact bone marrow may be essential to establish such transfer. Furthermore, non-specific thymic extract can re-institute immunocompetence in cancer patients.

GROWTH PROPERTIES AND ALLOANTIGENIC EXPRESSION OF MURINE LYMPHOBLASTIC CELL LINES GROWN IN SUSPENSION CULTURE

R.K. Zwerner and R.T. Acton, University of Alabama in Birmingham, Bimingham, Alabama 35294

In an endeavor to culture cells expressing Thy-1 and TL cell surface "differentiation alloantigens" in mass volume, preliminary investigations on growth properties and alloantigenic expression have been carried out on murine lymphoblastic cell lines. Growth curves initiated with various cell concentrations, per cent of new medium, and cells from various phases of a growth curve, have permitted a better understanding of the growth properties of lymphoblasts when cultured in 8-L spinner flask, 3-L vibrofermentor or 14-L fermentor. Cells cultured in these three types of suspension culture vessels attained a density of 2-6 x 10^6 viable cell/ml. In addition to the growth studies, the expression of TL and Thy-1 has been quantified. While all but one cell line investigated was demonstrated to have Thy-1, the precise amount expressed varied by as much as 50-fold. Cells examined at different phases of the growth curve showed a variation in the amount of Thy-1 expressed while TL expression was more constant. These studies indicate that murine lymphoblastic cell lines can be grown to a high density providing certain culture conditions are achieved which continue to express Thy-1 and TL cell surface antigens.

REGULATION OF Ab ACTIVITY OF RABBIT (Rab) Ig^+ LYMPHOCYTES (LC) BY PRODUCTS OF Rab Ig^-LC.

Clara Bell, U. of Illinois, Chicago, Illinois.

Synthesis by mouse (Mu) B-LC of Ab against some Ag depends on a helper function by T-LC or T-LC products[1]. Rab show LC with Ig receptors and expressing PFC (Ig^+LC), like Mu or human (Hu) B-LC, and LC undergoing blast transformation with anti-Ig (Ig^-LC), like Mu or Hu T-LC[2]. This indicates that Rab may have analogous, functionally distinct LC types tho it is unclear if they possess T-LC.
LC of Rab homozygous for the K-L-chain (b4 or b5) and for the V_H-chain (a1, a2 or a3) allotypes, have been separated into Ig^+LC and Ig^-LC[3] by rosetting with complementary Ig-SRBC target indicator cells[4]. The Ig^+LC showed Ig-receptors, bound ^{125}I labeled or fluorescein-conjugated anti-K-L-or V_H-Ig, formed RFC or PFC of K-L- or V_H-specificity and responded to SO, PLS or dextran polyclonal stimulation. The Ig^-LC lacked Ig-receptors, bound labeled or fluoresced anti-brain Ig and responded to PHA stimulation[3].
In this study, Ig^-LC from unimmunized (NI) or immunized (I) Rab were cultured with SRBC or with mitogens and the cell-free supernatants (S) analyzed for effect on the response of Ig^+LC to SRBC, BSA-SRBC or mitogens. S from NI or primary I Ig^-LC had a facilitating effect on Ig^+LC. S from secondary I had a suppressive effect. Pre-treatment of the Ig^-LC with anti-brain Ab and complement abrogated abt 70% of responsiveness to PHA and rendered the S ineffective. Pre-treatment of Ig^+LC with anti-brain Ab did not abrogate their responsiveness to mitogens or to S of Ig^-LC.

REFERENCES

1. Feldman M. and A. Basten, Nature New Biol. 237 (1972)13.
2. Sell S. and H.W. Shepperd, Science (1973) 586.
3. Bell C., N.Y. Acad. Sci. "Conference on Thymus Factrs in Immunity", April 3, 1974. Discussion Paper. In press.
4. Coombs R.R.A., B.W. Gurner, C.A. Janeway, A.B. Wilson, P.G.H. Gell and A.S. Kellus. Immunology 18 (1970) 417. Molinaro G. and S. Dray, Nature 248 (Apr.5 1974) 515.

Supported by PHS-Al-10138. Recipient of Career Development Award PHS-Al-70235.

EVIDENCE FOR THE GENETIC CONTROL OF ANTIGENIC MODULATION

W. Liang and E.P. Cohen, La Rabida-University of Chicago Institute, Chicago, Illinois 60649

Thymus cells of several strains of mice and murine leukemias form thymus-leukemia (TL) antigens; in the presence of TL antisera, the TL antigens reversibly disappear from the cells (antigenic modulation). Studies of the metabolism of TL antigens of leukemic cells reveals that modulation results because in the presence of TL antiserum the rate of antigen degradation exceeds its rate of synthesis (1,2). Further growth in the absence of specific antiserum leads to re-expression of TL antigens. The capacity for modulation exceeds the host's immune capacity and permits neoplastic TL(+) cells to grow without inhibition in specifically preimmunized recipients.

A somatic hybrid of TL(+) and TL(-) cells was formed which continued to express TL antigens; however, it lost the capacity to undergo antigenic modulation. ASL-1 leukemia cells ($H\text{-}2^a$, theta-C3H, TL 1,2,3, modulation (+)) were fused, with the aid of inactivated Sendai virus, with $LM(TK)^-$ cells ($H\text{-}2^k$, TL(-), theta (-)). The hybrid cells were selected _in vitro_ in HAT medium. They formed both $H\text{-}2^a$ and $H\text{-}2^k$ antigens and possessed a hybrid karyotype. They were theta (-). The hybrid cells as their ASL-1 parents formed TL 1,2,3 antigens. The concentration of TL antigens in the hybrid paralleled that of F_1 hybrids of TL(+) and TL(-) strains and was less than that of ASL-1 cells. Hybrid cells failed to undergo antigenic modulation in the presence of high titers of TL 1,3, TL 2, or TL 1,2,3 antisera. Exposure to TL antisera for up to five times as long as that required to modulate parental ASL-1 cells was used in the attempt. Both direct and indirect immunologic means were applied. Persistance of TL antigens after prolonged exposure to TL antisera was found by immune cytotoxicity, immunofluorescence, mixed hemagglutination and TL antibody absorption by hybrids as well as by the direct isolation of TL antigens from the cells.

REFERENCES

(1) A. Yu and E.P. Cohen, J. Immunol. 112 (1974) 1285.
(2) A. Yu and E.P. Cohen, ibid, 112 (1974) 1296.

THE RESPONSE OF CONGENITALLY ATHYMIC (NUDE) MICE TO INFECTION WITH *MYCOBACTERIUM BOVIS* (STRAIN BCG)

N.A. Sher, S.D. Chaparas, L.E. Greenberg, E.B. Merchant, J. Vickers Bureau of Biologics, FDA, USPHS, Bldg 29, Rm 406, NIH, Bethesda, Maryland 20014

The host response to *M. bovis*, strain BCG, in immunosuppressed subjects is of importance with the widespread use of BCG in cancer patients. Mice homozygous for the mutation *nude* (nu/nu) are athymic and lack T-dependent lymphocytes. They are hairless, have retarded growth and die of a "wasting" syndrome. Nude mice and heterozygote (+/nu) controls which are phenotypically and immunologically normal were infected with 1.0×10^6 colony forming units of Phipps strain BCG, i.v. There was a significant decrease in morbidity (wt. loss) and mortality of the nude mice infected with BCG versus the saline treated nudes. In the +/nu spleens, there was progressive growth of BCG up to the second week followed by a gradual decline. In the nude mice, BCG growth was progressive after the second week until death at 5-6 weeks. In the lung, significant differences were not noted until after the second week, at which time there was a rapid growth in the nude mice, with an increase of more than two $\log_{10}$. No significant growth occurred in the livers of either group.

Changes in the normal histology of the lung were striking and included a massive influx of monocytes during the first two weeks, which peaked at day 21. In the +/nu, there was considerable granuloma formation by day 28, consisting of monocytes and small lymphocytes. In the nu/nu lung, the granulomas were made up primarily of monocytes with a lack of small lymphocytes. Acid fast stains confirmed the presence of large numbers of organisms in the nu/nu macrophages which gradually destroyed the cells. It is hypothesized that in the nude mouse, the lack of T cells resulted in a decreased ability to produce lymphokines to the mycobacterial antigens. Subsequently the nude macrophages, although present in adequate numbers, are not sufficiently activated and are unable to suppress the proliferation of organisms.

NONSPECIFIC STIMULATORS OF THE IMMUNE SYSTEM

Benjamin Becker and Julian R. Kaufman, Purdue University, Fort Wayne, Indiana

BCG (Bacille Calmette Guérin) is thought to be a strong nonspecific stimulator of the immune system and has found use in cancer therapy. BCG is an attenuated strain of *Mycobacterium bovis*, a cause of tuberculosis in animals. However, the side effects of BCG therapy can be unpleasant and dangerous. Thus a search is being made for other microorganisms or macromolecules which are nonspecific immunostimulators with less toxic side effects.[1]

Mycobacterium is a genus of the bacterial order *Actinomycetales*. All mycobacteria have polysaccharides consisting of major amounts of arabinose and galactose. Chemical analyses of the hydrolysates of the cell walls of members of the order *Actinomycetales* reveal the presence of arabinose and galactose in the following genera: *Nocardia*, *Thermomonospora* and *Micropolyspora*.[2] The sugar combination was not found in *Streptomyces*, *Micromonospora*, *Actinomadura*, *Thermoactinomyces*, *Actinoplanes*, *Streptosporangium*, and *Dermatophilus*. Thus members of the genera *Mycobacterium*, *Nocardia*, *Thermomonospora* and *Micropolyspora* have a cell wall polysaccharide content similar to that of BCG and are valuable candidates for the role of nonspecific immunostimulators.

REFERENCES

(1) J. L. Marx, SCIENCE 184 (1974) 652.
(2) B. Becker, M. P. Lechevalier, and H. A. Lechevalier, Appl. Microbiol., 13 (1965) 236.